"You're the First One I've Told"

[

"You're the First One I've Told"

New Faces of HIV in the South

KATHRYN WHETTEN-GOLDSTEIN

TRANG QUYEN NGUYEN

RUTGERS UNIVERSITY PRESS
New Brunswick, New Jersey, and London

Library of Congress Cataloging-in-Publication Data

Whetten-Goldstein, Kathryn, 1963–
    You're the first one I've told : new faces of HIV in the South / Kathryn
    Whetten-Goldstein, Trang Quyen Nguyen.
        p.   cm.
    Includes bibliographical references and index.
    ISBN 0-8135-3114-4 (cloth : alk. paper)—ISBN 0-8135-3115-2 (pbk. :
    alk. paper)
    1. AIDS (Disease)—Southern States.   I. Nguyen, Trang Quyen, 1976–
    II. Title.

RA643.84.S68 W48 2002
362.1'969792'00975—dc21

                                                          2001058668

British Cataloging-in-Publication data for this book is available from the British Library

Manufactured in the United States of America

This work is dedicated to the people who shared their lives and hearts with us during the summer of 1998. Their honesty, laughter, and tears have influenced the lives of all who have been involved in this project. Additionally, the case managers and HIV providers of North Carolina taught us so much in the first few years of our HIV work. You have responded to our frequent questions, requests, and surveys. Your willingness to share with us made this work possible. Thank you.

Contents

Part V   Theory and Policy

Acknowledgments

Many people have contributed to the ideas presented in this book through their research assistance and by working with us in the field. First we would like to thank the primary interviewers for this work, Alyson Roberts and Steve Heasley. You were wonderful to work with and your voices will ring in our heads always. Traci Dreher, Anahita Homayoun, Josh Reaves, D'Anna Saul, Melinda Steele, and Julia Wang were each research assistants who contributed to the interview process and data entry for the book. The contributions of Melissa Moore, Rachel Stevens, Jeremy Sugarman, Leslie King, Stephanie Harrell, Clark Smith, and Gini Whetten were invaluable. Thanks to Phil Cook, Fritz Meyer, and Robert Sember for our informational discussions. We thank Jeremy Sugarman for helping us learn how to use the quantitative data software. The vision of Mirtha Beadle, Barnie Singer, and Sandy Gamliel were greatly appreciated and, we believe, made this a better book.

We thank the North Carolina Services Integration Project (NC SIP) team for their dedication and support: Frank Lombard, Priscilla Miller, Kimberly Scott, Mat Despard, Liyun Yu, Jenny Flythe, Margaret Farrell, Mike Belden, Susan Reif, Robin Swift. Y'all are great. We thank the lead physicians from each site: John Bartlett (and thank you for your cabin!), Joe Eron, Jeff Engel, Alison Heald, and Nathan Thielman. Thank you to the staff in the North Carolina AIDS Care Unit, including Stacy Smith, and the HIV/STD Prevention and Care Section chief Evelyn Foust for being so willing to work with us. We hope to continue this work in the future.

Finally we would like to thank our families for their support of this work.

Kathryn Whetten-Goldstein and Trang Nguyen

This work was supported in part by the HIV/AIDS Bureau's Special Projects of National Significance Project from the Health Resources and Services Administration, of the Department of Health and Human Services [Domestic Assistance number 93-928]. We thank them for their support of NC SIP. The content is solely the responsibility of the authors and does not necessarily represent the official view of the funding agency.

Part I   Background

Chapter 1   Setting the Stage

Sometimes I feel as though I care more
about the lives of my patients than they do
[for] themselves
> —North Carolina physician, 1996

Fʀᴏᴍ ᴛʜᴇ ᴘᴇʀsᴘᴇᴄᴛɪᴠᴇ of a health care provider, policymaker, or citizen with knowledge of the consequences of human immunodeficiency virus (HIV), it may seem incomprehensible, and possibly unforgivable, when patients do not make HIV the top priority in their lives. HIV kills people at a young age. HIV will kill the people to whom a patient transmits the disease. Most HIV-infected persons will cost society vast sums of money in medical expenses before dying (Holtgrave, Pinkerton 1997). From either a humanistic or an economic perspective, the consequences of HIV are serious.

Considering the effects of an HIV infection, how could it not be *the* most important circumstance in an HIV-infected person's life? Physicians who have worked in infectious diseases clinics for more than a decade say that, earlier in the HIV/AIDS (acquired immunodeficiency syndrome) epidemic, it was not unusual to have patients come to their appointments with long lists of questions and sometimes more information about the most recent therapies than the physicians themselves had. Partners and friends often came with patients to help ask the right questions, understand the answers, and provide emotional and physical support. This group of people infected with and affected by HIV were their own health policy advocates. They pushed the Food and Drug Administration to allow patients to take new drugs earlier in clinical trial phases and influenced policymakers to provide greater levels of financial support (Crimp, Rolston 1990). Today, infectious diseases physicians are increasingly concerned and frustrated that their

3

HIV-positive patients frequently miss appointments. Physicians are concerned that the new powerful medications, requiring multiple pills throughout the day, are difficult to adhere to. Patients, usually taking at least three medications from among the various available classes of drugs, must follow the prescribed regimen in their own home on a daily basis for an indefinite period of time (Bartlett, Gallant 2000). Taking this "three drug cocktail" can involve ingesting more than twenty pills each day, some of which need to be taken with meals and others on an empty stomach, which often make the patient feel very ill at first. In urban areas, keeping medical appointments is a strong measure of medication adherence (Lucas et al. 1999). Physicians report having insufficient information concerning the lives of their rural-living patients to decide whether the patients will be able to adhere to such complicated medication regimens.

The responsibility being placed on infectious diseases physicians today is intense and rare in the field of medicine. Generally, physicians are trained to focus on the individual patient when patients present in clinic. Physicians are not well trained either to adequately assess the environment in which patients live or to determine factors that promote or deter patients from taking medications. Often, in specialty training, physicians are trained to focus even more narrowly on specific body system(s). In contrast to this training, treatment of infectious diseases necessitates holistic understanding of physical functioning, treatments and patients' potential for adherence to medications. With HIV, a treatment not adhered to may introduce an even more dangerous agent to the public, a drug-resistant virus (Wainberg, Friedland 1998), in which case the physician would be culpable in creating more harm to human health than good.

In the early 1990s, at the same time that treatments for HIV were becoming more powerful and complex, the characteristics of the typical patient entering infectious diseases clinics were also changing (Centers for Disease Control and Prevention (CDC) 1997; Song 1999; Deeks et al. 1997; Freedberg et al. 1998; Stephenson 1998; Palella et al. 1998; Marwick 1998; Voelker 1998). The well-educated, gay white men who engaged fully in HIV treatment and often brought family and friends to the clinic became less prevalent. By 2000 more typical are patients who either appear complacent about their care or even show aggression. Patients have multiple life needs that are at the very base of Maslow's hierarchy of needs (Maslow 1987): housing, electricity, food, clothing, and a telephone (Whetten-Goldstein et al. 2001b). For individuals with such needs, maintaining good health through nonurgent medical care ranks lower in priority than obtaining food and shelter.

Background

As we begin the twenty-first century, the HIV epidemic is represented by a relatively large proportion of poor and disenfranchised people. The epidemic continues to spread in resource-poor rural areas (Voelker 1998), which already experience higher age-specific mortality (Nickens 1995) and morbidity rates from chronic diseases other than HIV (General Accounting Office 1991). In the late 1980s and early 1990s, the southern region of the United States experienced the largest proportionate increase in persons with HIV and AIDS. The proportion of persons with HIV and AIDS rose most dramatically in the African American community and among women (CDC 1998a).

In the Southeast, nearly 80 percent of new cases are among African Americans (NC DHHS 1999). Even the race and ethnicity of HIV-infected individuals who identify themselves as men who have sex with men are now more likely to be nonwhite than white (CDC 2000a). Nationally, women account for 32 percent of new HIV cases (CDC 1999a); moreover, trends indicate that women in the Southeast will eventually represent half of those newly infected with HIV (NC DHHS 1999). Of those women with HIV, 69 percent have children under the age of eighteen living with them (Whetten-Goldstein et al. 2001b). CDC data indicates that as of June 1999, those newly infected with the disease are as likely to acquire the disease through heterosexual sex and injection drug use as through homosexual sex (1999a). The mean education level of groups newly infected with HIV was low as the complexity of the therapeutic regimens was increasing (Von Bargen 1998; Stephenson 1998; Lishner et al. 1996). Exacerbating these changes in the HIV epidemic are data indicating that residents of rural areas have been found to receive less aggressive care (Ford, Cooper 1995) while simultaneously costing the care system even more (Ricketts et al. 1994).

In rural areas, the barriers to care are already great for all persons with chronic diseases (Schur, Franco 1999). HIV carries with it the added stigma of a deadly disease transmitted through behaviors that are taboo for discussion, particularly in rural areas where the stigma of AIDS is overwhelming (Heckman et al. 1998a, b; McKinney 1998), even among health care professionals. Furthermore, the majority of people infected in these areas is sufficiently poor in order to meet Medicaid eligibility criteria (Levi, Kates 2000).

Clients have difficulty accessing medical care in their communities. When the number of possible HIV-related therapies was few and the medication-related complications minimal, infectious diseases clinicians were trying to identify ways to convince local rural physicians to treat clients. However, as therapies became more complex and resources ever more restricted, it became apparent that the primary HIV providers for rural areas would be, at least for the interim, academic medical centers and large hospitals that care for high numbers of HIV-positive persons.

Therefore, the stereotype, never truly accurate, of the HIV-positive person being a well-educated, urban-living, white gay male has been shattered. Since the first known HIV cases in the United States, the disease has attacked a disproportionately large share of socially marginalized persons, first in the gay community and then among poor and disenfranchised persons. Although social marginalization continues to go hand-in-hand with HIV, those with the disease in 2001 are poorer and live further outside the primary structures of our society than ever before, making clinic visits and medication adherence difficult.

Yet for the patient and for the public's health, the peril of nonadherence is great because the virus may become resistant not only to the medication(s) being taken but also to other drugs similar to the original medications. Physicians have no reliable way of knowing the level of drug resistance a patient has achieved without genotyping or, through trial and error, prescribing many different costly therapies (Chaix et al. 2000; Matsushita 2000). In addition, should the patient with a drug-resistant virus infect another person, the virus in the new person will also be drug resistant (Boden et al. 1999). Therefore, the same drug therapies will be ineffective in the newly infected individual in just the same way that they are ineffective in the original patient.

HIV is extremely costly to both the infected individual and society. Medications can cost close to $1,000 per month. Lifetime costs per person with HIV are estimated to be between $55,000 and $155,000 (Holtgrave, Pinkerton 1997). Society pays for inappropriate medication use that leads to drug-resistant HIV strains in two ways. First, society must pay for new drug therapies to be developed, tested, and marketed, at an estimated cost of $65 million (Office of Technology Assessment 1993). Moreover, there is no guarantee that such monies will actually discover a new useful medication. Second, the health of the infected individual is directly affected by the more dangerous and deadly mutant virus, and the cost to treat the person will be even higher than if the person had a virus that was not drug-resistant; thus, society pays higher costs through taxes or insurance premiums.

From an altruistic perspective, society should be interested in having people seek best care, which includes not only adherence to medications and care appointments but also risk-reduction counseling and treatment of comorbidities such as substance abuse and mental health needs. Such care can improve the patient's quality of life and health outcomes. A self-interested perspective may also drive society's desire to improve HIV prevention activities and medication adherence because the risk of HIV transmission is lower when the amount of HIV in the body (viral load) is lower. Reducing viral load can be achieved through medication adherence, thereby reducing the overall risk of further infection throughout society.

In summary, HIV is a costly infectious disease that requires a complicated set of service visits and medication adherence rules that must be followed both to slow health declines in the individual and to spare the public from drug-resistant forms of the deadly virus. The care-seeking and adherence behavior of individuals with HIV greatly affects costs for their own care and care of anyone whom they subsequently infect. Additionally, any propensity of infected individuals to engage in high-risk behaviors (i.e., unprotected sex) also has a great impact on society in terms of lives lost and future costs for newly infected persons. Out of consideration for society's interest both in keeping people healthy, as demonstrated by our nation's desire to meet health goals such as those outlined in "Healthy People 2000" (Public Health Service 1990) and "Healthy People 2010" (Office of Disease Prevention and Health Promotion 2000), and in reducing or preventing increases in health care costs, it is critical to assist people in using health services and drug therapies appropriately.

Action

In 1996, clinicians from North Carolina Infectious Diseases clinics at East Carolina University School of Medicine, Duke University Medical Center, and the University of North Carolina at Chapel Hill Hospital decided that, to provide adequate care, the model of care for the state where 75 percent of clients seen in these infectious diseases clinics came from rural areas (Whetten-Goldstein et al. 2001b) had to change. The isolation of the clinics from the patients' communities meant that the physicians needed a better link to their patients' lives that could come through contact and coordination with local health care and social service providers (Berry et al. 1997). Thus HIV researchers, practitioners, and administrators in North Carolina wrote a grant proposal to connect case managers in the community with the infectious diseases clinicians (Nguyen, Whetten-Goldstein 2001). Physecally

Case managers are key providers because these professionals help poor people manage and negotiate their lives and needs. Case managers help patients find housing, apply for Medicaid, pay utilities, and search for income supports and other life necessities, all within existing systems of health care and human services. In rural areas, case managers meet with clients most often in their homes and work primarily on the road by negotiating the crises in their clients' lives immediately. The case managers know their clients well, and physicians need that knowledge to create the best possible care plans. Similarly, case managers need information from the physicians, such as written verification of an HIV diagnosis, in order to access Medicaid benefits. Managers also need to know the medications their clients were prescribed to assist in securing medications. As well, information about basic lab results aids case managers in helping their clients negotiate systems such as Medicaid and Social Security.

From 1996 through 2001, dedication to integrating care services brought together this newly formed group of HIV physicians, social workers, case managers, regional administrators of Ryan White Comprehensive AIDS Resources Emergency (CARE) Act funds (federal government funding is designed to provide care for HIV infected individuals who do not have alternative sources of care payment), and administrators from the North Carolina Department of Health and Human Services to form the North Carolina Services Integration Program (NC SIP) (Whetten-Goldstein et al. 2000a). The groups worked separately and together to understand and outline what we as providers, policymakers, and researchers considered to be the best care and practice for people living with HIV.

Discussion during one meeting of physicians exemplified the continuing frustration they faced when treating HIV-positive patients. The goal of the meeting was to outline the best care practices for patients in different stages of HIV. Recently distributed federal guidelines stated that all persons with HIV should be placed on aggressive medication therapy. One physician in particular wanted to simply comply with the federal recommendations. Others argued that not all patients were ready to make the life changes and commitment necessary to facilitate adherence to aggressive complex therapies; furthermore, prescribing aggressive therapy for someone who is not ready to adhere endangers that individual patient as well as others who might become infected by that patient. The lone physician retorted that his job was to be a physician and not a public health practitioner; therefore, when he prescribes therapy he thinks only of the health of the individual patient. When asked if he actually prescribed aggressive therapy to all of his patients, he replied negatively. Embarrassed, frustrated, and angry, he then retracted his previous statements by stating that he had tried, during national meetings, to argue against aggressive therapy for all patients but had "tomatoes thrown in [his] face." His national colleagues thought that he was being neither fair to his patients nor faithful to his oath by withholding aggressive therapy. In truth, this physician believed that the doctors and researchers making national recommendations regarding aggressive therapy wore "golden gloves" and had no understanding of what it was like to treat his patient population. The national guidelines have since been changed and concur with North Carolina guidelines, but this incident exemplifies the unique and intense concerns that clinicians struggle with when treating their infectious diseases patients. In no other area of medicine must clinicians daily balance individual with public health concerns.

The dialogue and process of creating an integrated network of care, which continue today in North Carolina, allow providers, researchers, and policymakers to gain a deeper understanding of the difficulties. For example, case managers in several southern states are not allowed to explicitly bill Medicaid or Ryan White CARE Act funds for providing counseling related to medication adherence, yet some would argue that adherence counseling is exactly what clinicians and patients need most from case managers. Adherence is often the performance objective by which other HIV providers and administrators judge case managers as well as a means by which case managers often judge their own client care. This policy has also meant that case managers are not officially trained on helping clients with adherence. As a second example of difficulties in patient care, providers have reported anecdotally that they assist patients in meeting their Medicaid deductible (also known as a "spend-down") to become Medicaid-eligible: a process by which people must periodically requalify for Medicaid in part by incurring medical expenses for which the patients (or the hospitals) pay. (See chapter 2 for more details about Medicaid.) Providers may help their patients incur expenses in order for patients to maintain access to medications; often un- or underinsured patients will not be able to get their medications consistently if they are not receiving Medicaid. Further, in North Carolina persons with HIV have limited access to mental health and substance abuse services (Whetten-Goldstein et al. 2001a). Because of financial difficulties and systematic barriers, mental health professionals have referred HIV patients back to their HIV case managers for treatment, but case managers are neither trained to provide such treatment nor can they be reimbursed for this time even if they were trained to do so.

Monetary and transportation barriers are not the only obstacles to care. For example, one of our grants provides free health care services along with child care and transportation, but often patients still do not make their appointments. The project arranges for taxis to pick up patients at their homes (and confirms the appointment with the patient the previous day), only to find that the patients are not home when the taxi arrives.

These difficulties and limitations make us realize that HIV is presenting health care and social service providers and policymakers with a complicated situation. If we want people to have the opportunity to use services appropriately and to make informed decisions about their treatment plans, then we need to better understand the lives of those who represent the new face of the disease: the woman who comes to the clinic and appears to agree to everything; the woman who laughs and for whom the provider feels sympathy and a connection, but who then does not return for services; the woman who yells or walks out of clinic without receiving treatment; and the men who do the same. What does HIV mean to patients representing the new face of HIV? Where and how does HIV enter into their lives? What *is* important to the patients? What would an arrangement of optimal care for patients look like? What health policies need to change to create such care, and what would be their impact?

The Hidden Face of HIV

Structured survey instruments do not allow for the exploration of human behaviors beyond the realms of previously determined and constructed domains. Such instruments allow us to test hypotheses about a person's life but do not facilitate open-ended inquiry into new aspects unknown to researchers, such as what their life priorities are and what dilemmas they face. The authors explored this uncharted territory of patients' lives by conducting twenty-five oral life histories with patients across the eastern half of North Carolina, the area in the state with the highest rates of HIV and some of the highest rates of sexually transmitted diseases in the country (HIV/STD Prevention and Care Branch, Epidemiology and Special Studies Unit 1999a,b). Mid-year 2000 HIV disease prevalence rates indicate that in several North Carolina counties nearly 3 percent of the African American male population and more than 2 percent of the female population are infected with HIV. We supplement the life histories with data from surveys linked with chart abstraction data of HIV-positive persons living in North Carolina, South Carolina, and Alabama—the largest survey of its kind. The surveys were initiated in 1997, prior to and separate from the case studies. We also include results from: qualitative data from three focus groups held to receive client input about confidentiality in rural areas; a survey of 101 randomly selected North Carolina health care and social service providers offering HIV-related services; and in-patient and out-patient data from HIV-infected individuals who received Medicaid reimbursement at some point in time between 1996 and 2000 and who were cared for at one of three academic medical centers. (See appendix A for details regarding each data collection activity.)

The development of grounded theory from qualitative data collection dictates that, when investigating a new area of study, researchers should allow what is relevant to emerge from the data rather than begin with a theory that the researchers attempt to prove or disprove (Strauss, Corbin 1998). We used grounded theory and strict rules of qualitative data collection and coding. Open-ended interview scripts were altered as themes emerged.

It is difficult to imagine another group of people in the United States who would present a stronger study of those who face the greatest obstacles to care. If we can understand and reduce barriers to care faced by individuals who represent this HIV-positive population, then the results should be applicable to other poor, disenfranchised, and rural-living persons in need of health care.

Book Outline

The objective of this book is to grasp the basic foundation of the lives of HIV-infected persons who represent the new wave of the epidemic and whom we serve as current or future clinicians, practitioners, policymakers, and researchers. The book concludes with health policy recommendations drawn from the data and information presented. This book is also for people infected with HIV who can be supported by learning about the lives of others infected and affected by this virus. Chapters 3 through 10 are unprecedented in the amount of space provided to the voices of case study participants and our refusal to overanalyze their stories. It is our conviction that people can speak for themselves, thereby helping us hear and understand their voices when we take time to listen and listen carefully. We feel that we have sufficiently manipulated the information presented simply through categorization and summarization.

The remainder of part I presents a brief history of the course of the HIV epidemic in the United States, rural areas, and the South with general information on the geographic distribution of other chronic diseases (chapter 2). The structure of health care and social services for poor, HIV-infected persons is described. The life histories are presented thematically throughout parts II through IV. Exploration of the case study participants' lives prior to their HIV infection is the focus of part II (chapters 3 and 4). Chapter 3 introduces the reader to each of the twenty-five participants through narrative excerpts. Participants were asked, for example, to describe their parents, care takers, siblings and their best and worst memories. They spoke of interactions with school systems, people they learned the most from, and the dreams that they once held for their futures. Chapter 4 presents current thought on the importance of childhood and past adult experiences to understanding current behavior. The chapter focuses on themes presented by the case study participants and the relevance of these themes to understanding the new face of the HIV epidemic.

Part III consists of four chapters exploring the participants' discovery of their HIV-positive serostatus and their subsequent lives. The chapters move from HIV diagnosis (chapter 5) to support systems including desires and attempts to form long-term relationships (chapter 6) to the role of children in the lives of participants (chapter 7) and finally to current hopes for the future (chapter 8). Some data from the Southeast HIV Patient Survey (SHIPS) are presented in discussing support systems and children.

Part IV explores the participants' trust of those in power positions and the participants' interactions with their HIV providers and attitudes toward medications. Chapter 9 explores the participants' belief that the government created HIV and participants' fear of breaches in confidentiality. Results from a series of focus groups conducted by the authors around confidentiality issues are presented in addition to the life experiences of case study participants. Chapter 10 examines relationships with infectious diseases clinicians and case managers as well as adherence to medication and clinic appointments. Data analyses from the SHIPS and the North Carolina HIV Provider Survey are presented in this chapter.

Part V (chapter 11) places the information presented throughout the book into a theoretical framework that describes determinants of health-related behaviors, including attending clinic appointments, adhering to medications, and engaging in activities that are high risk for HIV transmission. The book concludes with recommended areas of policy investigation and changes.

If future studies find the lessons from these life histories to be generalizable to a broader population of HIV-positive persons living in southern or rural areas and/or poor, risk-taking populations living in urban areas, then decisions can be made regarding the extent to which services can be made more accessible. If future studies find that the hypotheses do not hold up, then the results still indicate the need for sensitivity to the lives of patients. By better understanding the context of patients lives, we can better understand how desired behavior changes might occur. More boldly, some trends presented herein are so striking in their prevalence, such as trauma, that we argue a need for immediate rethinking of care systems to cope with the presenting lives of patients while epidemiologic data is being collected.

THE FABRIC OF OUR society becomes visible and magnified through examining the lives of people infected with HIV. Listening to the lives of those representing the new wave of the HIV epidemic in the United States tells not just of HIV but also about the experience of living marginalized lives from childhood to adulthood. Being able to successfully care for persons who have lived marginalized lives involves more than knowledge of the most recent drug treatment regimens. Appropriate care involves knowledge and understanding of people whose life experiences are profoundly different from those of most health care providers, researchers, and policymakers in the United States. Life experiences teach us how to best survive and navigate systems. As children, we learn whether authority figures can be trusted with our innermost thoughts and doubts. We learn whether those in authority are there to assist us or to be avoided unless avoidance becomes impossible. No doubt, few individuals have not had negative experiences with parents, teachers, or other organizations that were intended to be helpful. However, the individuals represented in this work, at an extreme point on a life experiences spectrum, may therefore perceive structures intended to be helpful to them, such as health care, as systems to be manipulated and better avoided. If this is true, then providing such individuals with care will require a much greater emphasis on engagement and retention activity, as well as meeting what may seem like ancillary needs of patients.

HIV, the South, and Benefits

Chapter 2

HIV offers a lens through which the under-
lying problems of the U.S. health care
system can be examined.
                    —LEVI, KATES 2000

THE STATES OF Alabama, Georgia, Louisiana, Mississippi, North Carolina, and South Carolina form a band along the Southeast in which we find a con-centration of the highest age-adjusted mortality rates in the United States. The upper end of the band is concentrated in the eastern half of North Car-olina. Low birth-weight rates, often used as a sensitive predictor of the health of a population, are also among the highest in this region as are syphilis rates and age-adjusted HIV/AIDS mortality rates. These high mortality rates include such chronic conditions as heart disease, stroke, diabetes, and even asthma. Lack of medical care professionals is often blamed for these poor health statistics, yet the South is no more rural than the Midwest, where health indicators are better, and the South does not have fewer providers per population than other rural areas according to defined primary care health professional shortage areas. (Data compiled by the North Carolina Rural Health Research and Policy Analysis Center at the University of North Car-olina at Chapel Hill.) The South is a region of high morbidity and mortality for diseases considered to be caused by genetic predisposition, environmental factors, and behavioral factors. HIV is a lens to understanding the faults in the care system. As we discuss throughout this book, persons who represent the new face of HIV present complex challenges to health and social service providers. However, these very care structures also present their own unique challenges to persons infected with HIV.

The United States Census Bureau and Centers for Disease Control and

Prevention define the southern region of the United States as comprising sixteen states that extend from Delaware to Florida and from the eastern seaboard through to Texas. However, six of these states (Alabama, Georgia, Louisiana, Mississippi, North Carolina, and South Carolina) are uniquely similar in that they have: (1) population densities under 200 per square mile (U.S. Bureau of the Census 1997); (2) populations that are more than 20 percent African American (U.S. Bureau of the Census 1998), representing more than 70 percent incident HIV or AIDS cases; and (3) women comprising approximately 40 percent of incident HIV and AIDS cases. These six southern states are most similar to the eastern half of North Carolina, from where we draw the life histories, focus groups, and provider survey. In addition, three of these six states are included in the Southeast HIV Patient Survey (SHIPS) discussed in later chapters.

The Changing Face of HIV/AIDS in the United States and the South

When the CDC began collecting data on AIDS cases in the United States, the South accounted for barely 17 percent of all U.S. AIDS cases between 1979 and 1983 (see graph 2.1a). By 1990 that percentage had increased to almost 35 percent. The continuing disproportionate increase in the AIDS rate of this region highlights the seriousness of the epidemic in the South (see graph 2.1b). Graph 2.2 illustrates the proportionate changes in AIDS rates experienced from 1989 to 1999. More than twenty-three thousand new AIDS cases in rural areas were reported by the CDC between March 1994 and February 1995, with the highest increases in the rural South (Sowell, Christensen 1996). From 1989 to 1993, the South experienced higher proportionate increases of AIDS cases than did the rest of the United States. Then, in 1994, when the United States began to experience decreases in AIDS incidence (Palella et al. 1998) with the successes of combination drug therapy, the decreases in the South were generally less than the decreases in the rest of the United States. Limiting the scope to the previously indicated six states further exaggerates the differences in disease trends with the rest of the country (see graph 2.2).

Beginning in the mid-1990s, AIDS case reporting indicated rising proportions of infections among African Americans, Hispanics, and women. HIV transmission among women was via intravenous drug use and heterosexual relations (CDC 1999b). The demographic changes in the epidemic led to the debilitation of already disenfranchised populations. Minority populations, particularly those living in the rural South, have historically experienced barriers to medical and social services care, which has created a dangerous situation for the care and spread of HIV.

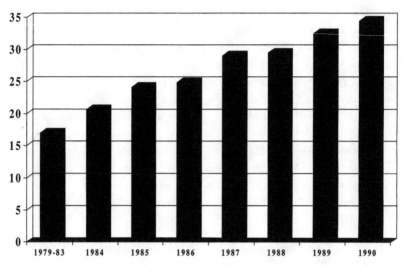

Graph 2.1a. Percent of U.S. AIDS Cases in the South. Source: *CDC. Summary of Notifiable Diseases, United States, [1989–1999].* Morbidity and Mortality Weekly Report *1990(38(53)); 1991(39(53)); 1992(40(53)); 1993(41(53)); 1994(42(53)); 1995(43(53)); 1996(44(53)); 1997(45(53)); 1998(46(54)); 1999(47(53)); 2000(48(53)).*

Studies including HIV-infected people in the South find that a substantial proportion of individuals migrated to these states after being diagnosed with HIV in other states (Cohn et al. 1994; Lansky et al. 2000). Injecting drug users were more likely than those of other modes of transmission to have been diagnosed out of state. Studies from other rural areas have found similar patterns of inward migration and spread (Davis, Stapleton 1991; Graham et al. 1995; Lam, Liu 1994). HIV-related funding allocations are based on the number of identified HIV/AIDS cases in a state. When cases are consistently identified in states and counties other than where the person lives, resources are misdirected; monies flow to the state and county of diagnosis rather than the place of residence, which further limits care options.

Rural Living

The U.S. Census Bureau defined "urban" as all territories, populations, and housing units in urbanized areas and in places outside urbanized areas of more than twenty-five hundred persons (or at least one thousand persons per square mile). Approximately 43 percent of persons living in the South live in rural areas. This percentage represents a higher proportion of rural-living residents than in other clusters of states as defined by the U.S. Census Bureau (1995). SHIPS indicated that 76 percent of the HIV-positive, poor patients receiving

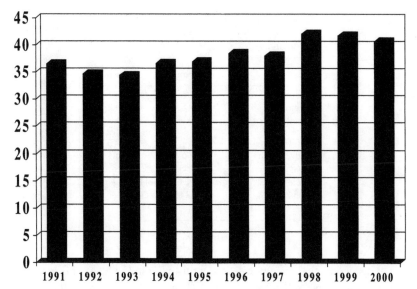

Graph 2.1b. Percent of U.S. AIDS Cases in the South. Source: CDC. *Summary of Notifiable Diseases, United States, [1989–1999]*. Morbidity and Mortality Weekly Report *1990(38(53)); 1991(39(53)); 1992(40(53)); 1993(41(53)); 1994(42(53)); 1995(43(53)); 1996(44(53)); 1997(45(53)); 1998(46(54)); 1999(47(53)); 2000(48(53)).*

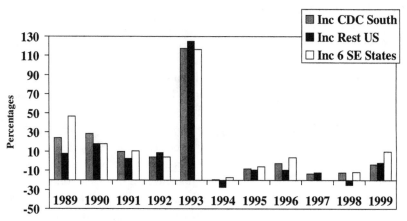

Graph 2.2. Proportional Change in AIDS Rates. Source: CDC. *Summary of Notifiable Diseases, United States, [1989–1999]*. Morbidity and Mortality Weekly Report *1990(38(53)); 1991(39(53)); 1992(40(53)); 1993(41(53)); 1994(42(53)); 1995(43(53)); 1996(44(53)); 1997(45(53)); 1998(46(54)); 1999(47(53)); 2000(48(53)).*
NOTE: Inc = Increase

Table 2.1
Urban and Rural Residents, 1990 (in
percentages)

State	Urban	Rural
Alabama	60.4	39.6
Georgia	63.2	36.8
Louisiana	68.1	31.9
Mississippi	47.1	52.9
North Carolina	50.4	49.6
South Carolina	54.6	45.4

Source: U.S. Census Bureau, 1990 Census of Population and Housing, "Population and Housing Unit
Counts," CPH-2-1.

care at academic medical centers were rural-living individuals who travel an
average of forty-five miles to reach care (Whetten-Goldstein et al. 2001b).
Care for most HIV-infected persons in the six southern states is primarily
located in large hospitals in the urban centers of the states (see table 2.1).

Poverty in the South

Federal guidelines dictate whether an individual or family is considered to live
in poverty; the degree of poverty serves as a basis for qualifying for specific
financial and health care assistance. The Federal Poverty Measure can be
explained in two ways: poverty thresholds and poverty guidelines. Poverty
thresholds are defined yearly by the United States Census Bureau for statistical
purposes, such as in estimating the number of people in the United States in
poverty each year. A person or household can be above the poverty threshold
and still be eligible for benefits as defined by program and state guidelines.
Louisiana, Mississippi, and eastern North Carolina have particularly high rates
of poverty, with approximately 18 percent of the population living in poverty
compared to about 13 percent nationally from 1996 to 1998 (table 2.2). The
six southern states had a higher rate of poverty than the Northeast or Midwest.
Furthermore, during this time period the United States saw increases in
income and declines in the poverty rate, and, even though the South experienced an all-time low poverty rate in 1998, the South still had higher poverty
rates than other regions and urban states (Dalaker, US Census Bureau 1999).

As we discuss in chapter 11, those demographically representing the new
HIV epidemic in the South—people who are rural living, female, African

Table 2.2
Three-year Average (1996–1998) of Residents Living in Poverty

	Living in Poverty (%)	Standard Error
Alabama	14.7	1.29
Georgia	14.3	1.12
Louisiana	18.6	1.36
Mississippi	18.3	1.38
North Carolina	12.5	0.88
South Carolina	13.3	1.30
Average of six SE states	15.3	1.22
South[a]	14.9	1.19
Northeast[a]	10.9	1.00
Midwest[a]	10.6	1.02
West[a]	13.1	1.14
United States	13.2	0.15

[a]Geographic regions are used as defined by the Centers for Disease Control and Prevention.

American, and poor—represent people who face extensive barriers to care. In fact, they face barriers regardless of the condition for which they seek care, be it diabetes, cancer, or HIV. However, HIV creates unique challenges of specialized care, such as serious stigma and confidentiality concerns and treatment protocols that are difficult to adhere to.

Benefits

Individual states, with federal financial backing, provide monetary and medical assistance to HIV-infected persons, through programs for people who are financially needy and/or disabled by AIDS. There are resources available to HIV-infected individuals, but the system of access is complex and fragmented.

Social Security programs pay a minimum level of income to people who are disabled and needy. Medicaid and Medicare provide health care to poor and disabled individuals, respectively, whereas Ryan White CARE Act funds, designated solely to persons living with HIV, seek to fill service and treatment gaps. We discuss these federal and state financial and medical resources in detail later in the chapter, but only to the level needed to understand the basic eligibility requirements and coverage of each program for people living with HIV. Additional information can be obtained from local and federal agencies.

The Federal Register of the Department of Health and Human Services sets income levels each year that are used nationally to define poverty. These thresholds are used for administrative purposes to determine eligibility for

Table 2.3
2000 Health and Human Services Poverty Guidelines (in dollars)

Size of Family Unit	48 Contiguous States and D.C. ($)	Alaska ($)	Hawaii ($)
1	8,350	10,430	9,590
2	11,250	14,060	12,930
3	14,150	17,690	16,270
4	17,050	21,320	19,610
5	19,950	24,950	22,950
6	22,850	28,580	26,290
7	25,750	32,210	29,630
8	28,650	35,840	32,970
For each additional person, add:	2,900	3,630	3,340

SOURCE: *Federal Register*, 65, no. 31, February 15, 2000, pp. 7555–7557.

federal and state programs, such as Social Security and Medicaid. Table 2.3 provides the poverty guidelines for the year 2000. Income limits can vary depending on the organization. For example, one state may limit program eligibility to 150 percent of the Federal Poverty Level (FPL) for one person, thereby allowing program access to people whose income and resources are at or below $12,525 per year. Another state may define eligibility for the same program as 350 percent of the FPL, which makes eligible those individuals with an annual income of $29,225. This state variability augments the already disproportionate access to services and treatment for people living with HIV (Levi, Kates 2000).

SOCIAL SECURITY PROGRAMS

The Social Security Administration offers a number of programs with the goal of providing needy individuals with financial assistance to live in health and security. Some of its programs are retirement insurance, disability insurance, unemployment insurance, and public assistance (Social Security Administration 1997a). Two programs utilized extensively by people living with HIV/AIDS are SSDI (Social Security Disability Insurance) and SSI (Supplemental Security Income). SSDI is available to people who paid Social Security taxes while working and have become disabled. To qualify for SSDI, a person must have earned approximately twenty work credits in the ten years prior to the year of disability onset, but the number of work credits needed depends on the age when an individual becomes disabled; that is, younger workers can qualify with fewer credits. A work credit depends on the amount of earnings and increases as nationwide wage levels increase. Only four work credits can be earned per year. For Social Security purposes, a person who cannot work as she previously did for at least one year is considered disabled. For those who do not have consistent work histories, such as many of those representing the new HIV epidemic, these requirements may be difficult to meet.

Consistent with all federal and state assistance programs, proving disability, illness, and work history is a tedious process. The Social Security Administration reviews information to ensure that an individual meets the basic requirements and then forwards the application to the state's Disability Determination Services office. This office conducts a full review of the medical information provided and talks with an applicant's medical caregivers to determine whether the person's impairment does in fact make working impossible. Therefore, unless a patient is symptomatic (and has probably already progressed to AIDS) and has worked previously, an HIV-infected person will not likely qualify for SSDI. If a patient does qualify, then Social Security payments are not paid until the sixth month after disability status is determined, and the amount paid is determined by the average pay a person earned while covered by Social Security. The average SSDI monthly benefit is $790. SSDI recipients are also eligible for Medicare after receiving SSDI benefits for twenty-four months (Social Security Administration 1999).

SSI is guaranteed as a minimum level of income for needy, aged, blind, or disabled persons in order to supplement incomes to enable living at a certain financial level. Disability is defined by SSDI standards, so usually only symptomatic HIV-positive persons are eligible. A supplemental income cannot exceed the current federal benefit rate, which is used in computing the allowable SSI benefits for individuals and couples. As of January 2000, the monthly rate was $512 per person and $769 per couple; that is, if either an individual's or a couple's income was higher than the monthly federal benefit rate, then the paid SSI benefit is reduced by the difference. Less than half the states pay higher SSI payments than the average $512 per month, but states do have the option of supplementing the monthly payment (Social Security Administration 1997b; Office of the Chief Actuary 2000).

Therefore, a person who worked under Social Security–covered employment, became disabled due to HIV, and met income level requirements could receive both SSDI and SSI. Those disabled by HIV who did not work to earn sufficient work credits will most likely receive only SSI payments ($512 per month) as their primary income.

MEDICAID

The federal government provides at least half of every state's Medicaid costs through the Health Care Financing Administration (HCFA), but, unlike Medicare, these programs are state operated. Medicaid provides medical assistance to individuals with limited income and assets, but Medicaid is not automatically guaranteed for all poor persons. Although income level is a primary eligibility measure, to qualify applicants must also fit into one of many possible categories, such as being a pregnant woman or a child. In most, but not all, states, SSI recipients are automatically eligible for Medicaid. Medicaid programs for each state must include hospital care (inpatient or outpatient), doctor visits, laboratory tests, X rays, nursing home, and home health services. The states then have the option of providing other services, such as prescription drug benefits, clinic services, and case management services (Hoffman et al. 2000).

Medicaid is the venue through which the largest portion of federal money is spent on health care for people living with HIV. With more than half the people living with AIDS estimated to be receiving Medicaid, federal/state spending on Medicaid for people with AIDS in 1999 was approximately $3.8 billion (Levi et al. 2000). A person living with HIV must be poor to qualify for Medicaid, but the degree to which the person must live in poverty and be disabled to qualify is determined by each state (Center for Medicaid and State Operations 2000). Most often, poor people living with HIV cannot receive Medicaid until they have progressed to AIDS, which allows them to qualify under the disabled category. They are therefore limited in their access to medical treatments that could actively prevent progression of their illness. Maine is the first state to have received approval from HCFA to include poor individuals with HIV in its Medicaid program, but, for the program to remain cost-neutral, the state limits the number of people who can enroll and requires medication discounts from pharmaceutical companies (Levi, Kates 2000).

Some states allow people who would not qualify for Medicaid because of their higher-than-permitted income or resources to become eligible by incurring medical expenses out-of-pocket to meet a deductible. The deductible is calculated by subtracting the income level designated by the state for eligibility from the total net income of the family for one month and then multiplying that answer by six (because Medicaid eligibility has to be reestablished every six months). The difficulty of applying for and meeting eligibility requirements for Medicaid in North Carolina can be seen by this example. A person under the age of sixty-five who is, disabled due to AIDS:

- must not be able to work for at least twelve months;
- have a monthly income of no more than $716 (income includes Social Security, veteran benefits, pensions, or other retirement programs and wages);
- have resources of no more than $2000 (resources include cash, bank accounts, a second car, retirement accounts, stocks and bonds, and real estate that is not the primary residence).

The application must include documentation to validate all income, resources, and disability statuses. If the sum of income is, for example, $800 per month, then the applicant must incur $504 (calculated as: ($800 − 716) × 6 = $504) in out-of-pocket medical expenses before qualifying for Medicaid. Therefore, the applicant must incur medical costs equal to 70 percent of a month's income as soon as possible to then receive Medicaid, which will cover the person for only six months before the process must start again (North Carolina Division of Medical Assistance 2000). Meeting this deductible is sometimes referred to as spending down.

The patient's disability status is determined, in part, by interviews with doctors or other hospital or clinic providers and by directly answering questions about how HIV/AIDS has affected activities of daily living, such as cleaning, shopping, cooking, and taking the bus, and employment over the past fifteen years. Even with this information, though, processing a Medicaid application can take a long time, so it is helpful if the applicant can produce supporting documents including a calendar or short notes about possible daily activities, a log of daily health, and the kinds of things that require help—all of which is meant to provide specific information about physical or psychological problems since becoming sick with AIDS. Other supporting information can also include notes from a doctor or case manager who has tracked health problems over the course of the illness (Social Security Administration 1995). Then, repeated every six months, all eligibility requirements (income, resources, disability) must be verified.

MEDICARE

Medicare, administered solely by the federal government through HCFA, is a national insurance program that provides health care security to (1) seniors, (2) people under age sixty-five who have become disabled, and (3) patients with end-stage renal failure. Most people are eligible for Medicare if they are sixty-five and older and have had Medicare-covered employment for at least ten years. Younger people with a disability, such as AIDS, can also qualify if they have been receiving Social Security payments for two years. Medicare is the second largest federal payor of HIV care.

Medicare insurance is offered in two parts: hospital (Part A) and medical (Part B). Hospital insurance includes coverage for inpatient hospital, nursing facility, hospice, and some home health care. Medical insurance covers doctor visits, outpatient hospital care, some health services, and other medical services not covered by Part A, including physical and occupational therapists. Prescription drugs are usually not covered by medical insurance, nor are dental care, eye examinations, or hearing aids. Most people can choose from three plans to cover these two insurance parts: (1) The Original Medicare Program in which any provider who accepts Medicare can be seen and the patient makes copayments; (2) Medicare Managed Care Plans where there is limited choice of providers but copayments may be lower, and (3) Private Fee-For-Service Plans, which are available only in some regions but accept any provider.

Because most people living with AIDS who qualify for Medicare are under age sixty-five and receive Medicare owing to their disability, we discuss Medicare from that perspective. Consider the example of the woman previously mentioned: if she has been receiving Social Security benefits, then she is automatically enrolled into Medicare in the twenty-fifth month of receiving Social Security. She does not have to pay for hospital insurance but needs to pay, in the year 2000, $45.50 per month to receive medical coverage. If she is not receiving Social Security, then she needs to contact her local Social Security Administration office to apply for Medicare hospital insurance. If her income level does not enable her to pay the premiums to receive medical insurance, her state may have a program that can cover those payments (Federal Medicare Agency 2000). Although she no longer needs to meet Medicaid deductibles (paid for by Medicare), Medicare does not cover prescription drugs, so she is suddenly faced with paying approximately $1,000 per month ($200 more than her income) for HIV-related medications.

THE RYAN WHITE CARE ACT

The Ryan White CARE (Comprehensive AIDS Resources Emergency) Act is a federal funding program enacted in 1990 and reauthorized by Congress in 1996 and 2000. It is the second largest provider of federal health care and supportive services funding for people living with HIV. The Ryan White CARE Act primarily serves people who are either not eligible for Medicaid or do not have private insurance. The program requests that the federal government form partnerships with state and local governments, community-based organizations, and AIDS service organizations to provide care and services to HIV-infected persons, but ultimately the states are responsible for their CARE Act funding. There are five Titles under the CARE Act:

- *Title I* provides emergency assistance for heavily affected cities and metropolitan areas. In fiscal year 1999, fifty-one metropolitan areas received Title I funding.
- *Title II* authorizes funds to every state, Washington, D.C., Puerto Rico, and other territories to provide HIV-related services. Title II covers prescription drugs, primary AIDS care services, health care insurance continuation, and home health care. Funds cover urban, suburban, and rural communities. Funding for AIDS Drug Assistance Programs (ADAPs) comes from Title II funding. ADAP funding is limited for each state and often has to cover medication costs for people who are disabled with HIV whose Social Security Disability Insurance or other income exceeds Medicaid limits for medications.

ADAP is funded primarily from three sources: Title II Base funds, Title II ADAP Earmarked funds, and state support. A portion of the funds that states receive in Title II Base funds from the federal government can be used for ADAP; the amount is determined by each state. With the increased demand for financial treatment support, in 1996, Congress began to earmark additional Title II funds to be used specifically for ADAP. Furthermore, by the year 2000, thirty-seven states had decided to designate state funds toward ADAP, including five of the six southern states of interest, all of which varied in the portion of their ADAP budget drawn from state funds: Alabama (3 percent); Georgia (17 percent); Mississippi (14 percent); North Carolina (51 percent); and South Carolina (6 percent). The total use of these federal and state funds and the formularies designated to determine how the funds are spent are state regulated (HIV/AIDS Bureau 2000a).

ADAP eligibility is also state regulated in both medical and financial components. All states ask for medical proof of HIV status, while ten states require laboratory documentation of HIV progression (i.e., CD4 tests). Financially, each state uses the federal poverty level as the guideline to determine eligibility. Of states and ADAP grantees 30 percent require ADAP recipients to live at 101 to 200 percent of the Federal Poverty Level (FPL), which equates to income ranging from $8,434 to $16,700 per year; 41 percent establish the income eligibility at 201 to 300 percent FPL, 28 percent allow income levels of more than 300 percent FPL, and one state uses a sliding fee scale for incomes of 201 to 500 percent of the FPL (HIV/AIDS Bureau 2000b). Table 2.4 provides the state-determined eligibility guidelines for the six southern states of focus in this volume.

Table 2.4
AIDS Drug Assistance Programs (ADAP) Eligibility for Fiscal Year 2000

	HIV + Diagnosis	CD4 Count <500	Specific Criteria for Protease Inhibitors	Financial Eligibility (% FPL)
Alabama	Yes	No	No	250
Georgia	Yes	Yes	No	300
Louisiana	Yes	Yes	Yes	300
Mississippi	Yes	No	No	400
North Carolina	Yes	No	No	125
South Carolina	Yes	Yes	No	300

SOURCE: Health Resources and Services Administration, HIV/AIDS Bureau AIDS Drug Assistance Programs (ADAPs) Fact Sheet.

- *Title III* funds community-based clinics and public health providers to develop and deliver early and ongoing comprehensive health services on an outpatient basis as a form of capacity building. Title III can fund rural and underserved urban areas, particularly among women, adolescents, and people of color.
- *Title IV* funds HIV services and clinical research programs targeting children, youth, women, and families to provide direct primary medical care.
- *Title V* covers AIDS Education Training Centers (AETC), HIV/AIDS dental reimbursement programs, and SPNS (Special Projects of National Significance). AETCs educate health care providers on advances in HIV disease, while the dental program trains dentists and reimburses dental schools that address oral and dental needs of indigent HIV-infected patients (HIV/AIDS Bureau 2000c). SPNS supports grants to develop and evaluate unique models of care delivery to improve HIV care provision for vulnerable populations (i.e., incarcerated persons, migrant farm workers, rural-living individuals, people with AIDS in need of palliative care).

OTHER ASSISTANCE PROGRAMS

Additional assistance with medication procurement comes directly from some pharmaceutical companies that have developed Prescription Drug Patient Assistance Programs (although each company has a different name for its program) to assist patients who cannot financially afford drug treatments. Each pharmaceutical company defines differently the eligibility criteria, medications, and time frame for the assistance program. This assistance is not limited to HIV-related medications. For example, Agouron Pharmaceuticals, Inc. offers the VIRACEPT (an HIV medication) Assistance Program, which provides a month's supply of the drug to a patient via her physician for four-month periods. Each case is handled individually and through the physician. Glaxo Wellcome, Inc., through its Glaxo Wellcome Patient Assistance Program, has another approach: the company makes available any of its marketed prescription drugs for patients being seen in outpatient settings. Patient eligibility for this program is analyzed on a case-by-case basis using the federal poverty guidelines. For up to ninety days, the program will provide treatment assistance with minimal copayments until financially disadvantaged persons can find other alternatives (PhRMA 1999). Because these programs are meant to be viewed as payors of last resort and are provided as a philanthropic endeavor of the company, meeting eligibility can be time- consuming and difficult. Although this additional support is needed because of the high demand for medication assistance for resource-poor individuals, case managers and social workers have yet another maze of programs and eligibility rules to learn about and through which to maneuver their clients.

The U.S. Department of Agriculture sponsors the Food Stamp Program to help low-income families buy food. The potential recipient cannot have a large accessible savings, and each unemployed adult must make an effort to find work. Food stamps are used like cash, but sales tax is not charged on food stamp items. However, food stamps cannot buy everything that cash can; alcohol or tobacco products, restaurant foods, household supplies (such as soap or paper products), vitamins or medicines, foods that are ready to eat (prepared deli or hot foods), or pet foods are excluded. Food stamps can be used to purchase seeds or plants and to pay for programs such as Meals on Wheels or other elderly and handicapped communal dining facilities. Eligibility is based on resources (not to exceed $2,000 in countable resources), income (as limited by an income chart of allowable gross and net income amounts), deductions, and work (Food and Nutrition Service 2000).

Housing Opportunities for People Living with AIDS (HOPWA) provides housing assistance and related supportive services for low-income persons with HIV/AIDS and their families. States and metropolitan areas with the largest numbers of cases and incidence of AIDS receive grants based on formula calculations. Additionally, state and local governments and nonprofit organizations provide local housing funds through grant competitions (US Department of Housing and Urban Development 2000).

Low-income persons with HIV appear to have available to them several major sources of federal and state support. However, it should be clear that accessing these support mechanisms is often difficult. The complexity of the multiple systems makes them inaccessible to many; one must be fairly savvy and have time to negotiate the system. Moreover, one must be ready to reapply to agencies when first turned down and willing to argue with "the system."

Given this basic understanding of HIV in the South and the consideration of issues of poverty, ruralness, and resources, the reader is better prepared to hear and understand what the case study participants' stories teach us. The new face of the HIV epidemic is poor in personal finances, community and provider education, state resources, and support. But their HIV status is not the only difficulty persons recently infected face in finding care and following treatment regimens. As their stories tell us, people in the new wave of the HIV epidemic have always lived in poverty in the South. Their barriers are exacerbated by their HIV status, which joins the multitude of problems that they have continually faced in life.

Part II

Life before Diagnosis

Chapter 3   Voices of the Past

*I know my mama loved me, but I really had
a hard life. I mean a really rough life.*

*I can remember some good times, but my
basic memories: [mama] was always working, I was always cold and raggedy, and my
lazy-ass sisters wouldn't comb my hair.
Dirty little raggedy thing running around the
neighborhood, you know.*

FOR CLINICIANS AND PROVIDERS, a person's disease usually defines the patient;
we take people where they are and move forward. But diseases do not enter
people's lives in isolation from their own histories; the disease is simply one more
characteristic of their lives. Good clinicians assess their new patients' health history, while social workers and case managers evaluate a new client's current life
necessities (e.g., food, housing, electricity), home life, and even social support
systems. Although health and human service providers do not generally conduct
extensive life histories of their clients, individuals have unique histories of childhood, adolescence, familial and school experiences, childhood community experience, and environmental influences, all of which affect a patient's condition or
treatment. A patient's disease enters into this individual's complex past experiences and present existence. One's history, influencing the perceived importance
of services and medications, can facilitate or create barriers to care, thereby influencing the ability and willingness to adhere to appointment schedules and medication regimens. This information—patients' lives before they entered the
health care system with HIV—is usually missing from what we know about the
people for whom we are trying to arrange health care and social services.

To assess the influence of a biased sample on the impressions given, read-
ers should remember how the individuals were chosen for inclusion in this
study. We asked HIV case managers in the eastern half of North Carolina,
where the state's highest rates of infection are concentrated, if they had
clients who would be willing to speak to an interviewer about their lives. The
case managers selected several clients who would be amenable to such a study
and provided their demographic information. Project staff then selected a
sample of persons who demographically reflected the HIV epidemic in North
Carolina.

In total, thirteen women and twelve men were interviewed; 72 percent of
the clients were African American (table 3.1). Nineteen participants were
rural-living, and six lived in mid-sized cities. Fifteen of the twenty-five interviewees were born and spent most of their childhood years in rural North Carolina; the other ten moved to North Carolina when they were either very
young or in their early teens. By their own account, ten clients contracted the
virus from heterosexual relations, and six reported IV drug use as their mode
of transmission. Five men said that they contracted HIV through homosexual
relations, while four clients were not sure if they became HIV-positive from
heterosexual contact or IV drug use.

The reader should expect the selection method to lead to two biases.
First, to meet eligibility requirements for having a case manager, the respondents were most likely uninsured or receiving Medicaid; they were poor. More
than 50 percent of HIV-positive persons in North Carolina are either uninsured or receiving Medicaid. Second, the respondents were willing to speak
with a stranger about their lives, which means that they were probably more
accepting of "the system" than others who refused such an interview. With
these caveats in mind, we introduce the pre-HIV lives of our sample of
twenty-five participants living in eastern North Carolina.

Table 3.1
Demographic Characteristics of Case Study Participants

	Race		Mode of Transmission			
	BLACK	WHITE	MSM	HETEROSEXUAL CONTACT	IV DRUG USE	HETERO OR IVDU
Female	9	4	NA	7	5	1
Male	9	3	5	3	1	3

NOTES: MSM = men who have sex with men. IVDU = intravenous drug use.

By moving from the life history of one person to the next with no commentary, we allow the reader to get a sense of each person as an individual with a story to tell. After approximately eight hours of interviews per person, we could present a chapter on each person, but we prefer to summarize, through the participants' voices, major life events and feelings. The presentations are not equal in length because participants differed in how much they shared. The women are presented alphabetically, followed by the men. All names have been changed to protect the identities of the respondents.

The Women

AMY

Amy, who was adopted and raised by her aunt and uncle, stated that her biological mother did not want her because she was too black. Amy's biological sister was able to stay with their mother because she had light skin like their mother. Amy never met her biological father, although she is still looking for him.

Amy's biological mother did not want her sister (Amy's aunt) to adopt Amy and instead had left Amy with another woman; however, the aunt fought for, and was awarded custody of, Amy in court. Amy became the oldest sister in a family with three other girls where she was treated as "a servant." Her adoptive parents did not work outside the home; her father was "a drunk" who picked tobacco "at times." Amy described her childhood home as a "shack" that the owners would not fix. A wood heater supplied warmth, but there was no running hot water, and the house was cold when it rained. Amy states that her mother always made sure that they had enough warm clothes and other necessities that were provided for by relatives who lived in the North. Amy's other aunt and uncle from the North showed their love "by buying me gifts on Christmas and bringing me gifts to show their love." Before school each day, Amy had to work in either the garden or the house. While at school, Amy was regularly teased because her clothes were old and she smelled. She felt like an outcast from both her family and the schoolchildren.

At home, her father regularly beat her mother. The four girls would hide when the beatings and arguments took place.

> I can remember when I was a little girl I played in the mud and made pancakes and stuff, you know right by my little self. You know when you are a little child and growing up you be thinking, and I was thinking. I see how mama and them were doing fighting and fussing, carrying on and fussing and stuff and I would be by myself and they would be fussing and I would be like this [imitating being scared]. I

must be in the way or something; you know I couldn't stand it. Then
I would run under the house.

The girls feared for the life of their mother and worried about what would
happen to them if the mother were killed. On more than one occasion, Amy
used a neighbor's telephone to call the police on her father.

When asked to recall a happy childhood memory, Amy reported: "The
only happy memory I can think of is I played with other kids, just playing,
shooting marbles. . . . I don't think I ever had a birthday party because mama
couldn't afford those things when I was coming up as a kid."

Amy quit high school because she was too embarrassed about always
arriving late and the way she looked, both of which she felt powerless to
change.

> I had stopped [in the tenth grade] because my mama always had me
> going somewhere. And I got kind of scared walking in the [class]
> room because I was late all the time. And the teachers are always,
> they'd say, "Amy, you're late again." And then my mama would have
> me doing something before I could get to school, and I was shy then,
> and I'd say "Yeah," you know, she'd have me going to places. And I'd
> say, "Mama, I've got to be in school." "You go where I tell you." You
> know. "Do this and do that." And I would go to school. . . . Every
> time I would walk in the classroom, and they'd look at me. You know,
> I'd try not to look at them but I know they was looking at me. . . . I
> quit school because . . . I didn't dress like. . . . [cries] I didn't have the
> clothes like, you know, the other children that went. They all would
> tease me. They was always teasing me about, you know, the way I
> looked. That's another reason why I had quit.

When asked about her ambitions as a child, Amy reported that she
simply wanted to help other people: "You know, be treated not like I had been
treated like my mama and daddy treated me. I want to treat somebody nice
and, you know, respectful."

Amy remembered between interviews that she had been gang-raped
when she was between fourteen and sixteen years of age:

> I have never told nobody this, I never have told my family. I never
> . . . I remember I went into the woods and I thought I had a
> boyfriend and he was taking his brothers to work and he said, "Do
> you want to ride with me?" He said, "I'm gonna take my brothers to
> work." I said, "Okay, all right then." And I can remember he didn't
> take them to work. I was in front with him [in the car] and there was
> three in the back. He took me in the woods, I can't tell you, I don't

know how to tell you. Well it just seems like I was raped by all four of them. I never told nobody that. All four of them . . . I never told nobody but you, . . . I was young, it was a dirt road down low and all four of them. . . .

Following this incident Amy was often sick:

My head would hurt all the time. I said, "Mama I have a headache," like that, and I remember that they took me in the woods and stuff and I always stayed sick. Then mama took me to the doctor but the doctor said; "Give her these for her headaches," and "she has a little bit of heart trouble," so the doctor checked. He said, "Ma'am, I can't see what else is wrong with her right now." I remember that. But I ain't told nobody all them guys took me into the woods. I just remember that. I saw one of the brothers, I think it was last week, and he said, "Amy, do you remember me, do you remember me?" I said, "Yeah." He said, "Don't you remember you were going with my brother." I said, "Oh yeah." He said, "You act like you don't know nobody," you know, try to sweet talk me then. I said, "Okay, yeah, I remember," and that's what made me remember.

Another time, Amy was badly scared when a fire started on the other side of the duplex in which her family lived. The neighbors were drinking "just like my mama and father." That night the neighbors had a bad fight:

"Mama," I says, "this [neighbor], he beating her up. He beating her up." . . . He always would beat on his wife. I can remember, I can just imagine something going to happen. Mama said, "Shut up, it's nothing. Just go ahead and sit down and stop being so nosy. . . ." "But Mama," I says, "they just over there fighting. He beating her. He's hitting her." . . . Mama said, "Y'all get back and take your bath and go to bed." . . . Yes. I did never go to sleep. My eyes were open all that night. That oil heater, it was burning; it lit up the floor. All of the sudden, I smelled smoke. I jumped up, and I went and I said, "Mama! Mama! Mama! Smoke! The house is on fire! The house is on fire!" Mama said, "The house isn't—" [sniffing sounds]. All of the sudden she says, "I do smell smoke. Get up children! Get up!"

Like many of our participants, Amy also experienced hurricanes and floods, and she remembered being taken from her house by boat on one occasion.

For Amy, though, one of her most difficult memories was when she found out in the health department that she was four months pregnant and HIV-positive. The news of her serostatus was made more difficult because the health department staff convinced her that she had to have an abortion, telling her that the baby would probably have HIV, live a terrible life, and die. Amy could not stop crying when they told her that she had to get an abortion: "I was bringing out the tears. Lady had to go get another lady to calm me down. And I was four months [pregnant], and I was HIV-positive. And she talked to me. She said, 'Now, Amy, you know, you don't want your baby to come out like that.' I was crying because I didn't want to go through [an] abortion, and that's what happened." Amy did have the abortion. The baby's father, serving life in prison for raping two girls, had been very physically abusive to Amy.

ANGEL

Angel grew up with one older sister in a mid-sized North Carolina city. Angel never stayed at the same school for very long because her family moved often within the city. Her father was in the military and her mother, who was disabled from childhood polio, had use of only one arm and received disability payments. Regarding her mother, Angel said:

> We knew that [our mom] loved us from just the way that she was taking care of us. Even when I was growing up as a young child up into my teenage years, my mom would even spank me. I realized, I knew that she was doing it for my own good because I had done wrong. . . . Because she had one hand [to use due to polio], we had to put our hands up under our belly and lay down on the bed so that our hands would not get in the way of the belt or whatever she was using to spank us with. So we had a lot of respect for her.

Both of Angel's parents consumed a lot of alcohol. Her father would drink six to twelve beers a night, but he was not an "angry or sloppy drunk." Angel's parents divorced when she was between the ages of six and nine. After the separation, Angel's mother moved in with a boyfriend, while Angel stayed with her sister, her father, and his girlfriend so that she would not have to change schools. When Angel was a teenager, her father would touch her in places "where he should not" when he was drunk. Angel told a social worker, who proceeded to tell the family; Angel felt strongly that the social worker had violated her confidentiality and made the situation worse within the family, especially between her father's girlfriend, on whom Angel was dependent, and her.

When Angel was about fifteen, her mother's boyfriend tried to get her into bed with him when her mother was out of town. Angel escaped by running on foot to her own boyfriend's house, but her mother's boyfriend drove there and was waiting when she arrived. When Angel saw her mother's boyfriend, she started running back to her mother's house, but that was also where her mother's boyfriend was staying:

> Here I was running to his house, through the woods and by the pond, and running from this man because he had a gun. He always carried a gun because he always carried a lot of cash on him. So here I was hiding from him, at their house, and here he was following me in the car.

When she finally reached safety and called her mother to explain what had happened, her mother told Angel that she was lying. As Angel recounted the story, she said that what hurt her most deeply was that her mother had not believed her. When Angel's mother returned home and confronted her boyfriend, he admitted to the incident. A short time after this incident, Angel slit her wrists and began seeing a counselor.

Later that year, Angel quit school and married her father's girlfriend's son; her father said that, because they were having sex, they should get married. As a teenager, Angel very much wanted to have a baby to love and care for. She reported that she felt no attachment or need to go to school.

Angel continued to experience difficulties with men into adulthood. Before turning eighteen Angel left her first husband after he threw her across the room. She married a second husband who had a teenage son on probation because of violent threats made at school. Angel feared for her life when she was alone with him:

> I slept with a knife under my bed because his father would go outta town, ummm, like on weekends, he was doin' truck driver trainin' and, uhh, this child was getting very big. . . . His son was getting bigger than me. . . . It was really a rough road, and finally I had just had enough. After two and a half years.

Angel started working in construction when she was sixteen. She worked in construction for most of her life, but, at the time of the interview, had become a secretary.

BETTY

Betty was the oldest of ten children whom she helped raise. She grew up in a very small North Carolina town in a four-room house on her mother's farm with cold indoor running water but no electricity or indoor bathrooms. The boys had one bedroom, and the girls slept in another, with five to six children per room. Betty's father drank and "used to fight when he get drunk." Betty describes both parents as very strict, but loving and good. All the children were so well-behaved that people in the grocery stores and doctors' offices would comment on her mother's ability to keep so many children quiet and orderly. In reference to helping to raise the other children, Betty reports, "It wasn't hard. I had to do it, so I might as well say it wasn't hard. Diaper changes: we didn't have no washing machine; we had a scrub board."

Betty grew up in the 1950s in a segregated community. She remembered that there was separate seating for blacks at the movies and she "had to go to the back door to go to the restaurant." She reported that "black people stayed in their place and the white people stayed in their place." Each morning Betty took two buses to get to an all-black school far from her home. When asked if going to a segregated school affected her in any way, she replied, "No. It didn't bother me. There wasn't anything that bothered me when I was growing up; I did my work. I did what I was supposed to do. I was happy just baby-sitting." Betty's younger brother and sister went to a "black-and-white" school when the schools were being integrated. She recalled that her brother "stayed out of school more than he went because he was tired of them calling him 'nigger.' They sent him home every day for beating up a white boy." Betty felt lucky that she did not have to experience school integration.

Betty enjoyed school as an escape from home: "I used to love to go to school. I rather go to school than stay home because mama would put you to work." Betty also wreaked havoc in school: "I used to fight all the time. Taking up for my sisters and brothers because they would fight. . . . I used to have to take up for my brother that passed [from HIV]. He was supposed to take up for me."

Betty's dream had been to join the Army.

CHRISTINE

Christine grew up in "a little three-room house" in rural western North Carolina with four older sisters and two younger brothers. She could not remember her father, who had died when she was very young. Her mother had a number of boyfriends, including one fairly stable boyfriend who was the father of one of her younger brothers. This boyfriend, whom Christine considered a father figure, died from a heart attack when Christine was in her early teens.

Christine's family had a big garden, where they grew much of their food. Throughout Christine's childhood, the rest of their food came primarily from one of her mother's male friends who had a large farm. The children had "good department store clothes," "good food from the gardens," and received Social Security payments through the father figure. The community was "close-knit" where "everybody tended to each other's children."

Christine recalled that her mother and the stable boyfriend used to drink a lot. As well, Christine still has scars on her legs where she was beaten with notched switches and anything else that her mother could grab:

> I mean I got my share of whippin's, and I sort of think that
> sometimes my mama had a resentment because our father died and I
> was the last [daughter]. I mean, I can remember the time my mama
> whipped me with no clothes on with drop cords, with dogwood
> switches, and they don't break. . . . (pause) Yeah, I really do feel like
> my mama abused me when I was small because I got scars on my legs
> now from some of the whippin's with the switches that she used that
> had notches and things in it.

Christine reported also being verbally abused constantly while growing up. Her mother, convinced that Christine would end up a teenage mom, repeatedly told Christine that she was good only for having children: "I used to think we were living in hell. I said, 'It can't get no worse than here' because what I was going through with the resentment my mama had toward me, the beatings that I had, I just knew I was living in hell, and I used to say it. I say, 'This hell where I'm living.'"

Christine felt that she was constantly fighting against her mother's negative image of her and that this inner turmoil kept her from advancing in school:

> School was divided into poor, average, medium and high-class, and I
> used to hang with the medium . . .because I did not think that I was
> smart enough and I had a mother that she kept me down. . . . When
> I was in junior high, I remember my mama tellin' me that, "You are
> going to have a house full of younguns before you get in high school,
> you just gonna have a house full of younguns," and I used to run from
> guys, you know, and stay far away from them. . . . When she would
> threaten me with things like that when I got into high school, I took
> the easiest courses that I could take to make sure that I passed to
> show her. Instead of taking college prep courses or something another
> that I might still could have passed, I didn't. . . . That wasn't a good
> feeling.

Christine spoke of good times that she had with her grandparents, who would take her on the weekends. She reported that she "enjoyed the love that [her grandmother] used to share" with her. "On the weekends, me and my other sister, we used to go spend the weekend with my father's mother and father and go to church with them on Sunday, and then they would bring us back Sunday evening. I enjoyed that."

Christine attended three years of college, but she could not afford expenses of the fourth year; Christine deeply resented that her mother did not financially support her the way she did her sisters. Soon after leaving college, Christine gave birth to a daughter and moved in with a female friend who was "shooting up." When this friend sold the house for drug money, Christine then had no place to live. She moved in with a girlfriend's father, where life was a "nightmare":

> Me and my baby would be sleeping in the bed, and [the girlfriend's father] would come in there and try and get in the bed, and then if I wouldn't let him, he would get mad. And his two sons stayed with him, and he would get mad at them, and I mean, that was a nightmare too. So by that time, I had started getting my unemployment check and I was saving some, and my sister, she helped me get a three-room house, and I moved into that. . . . Sometimes I had to do it [sleep with the girlfriend's father], you know, because I didn't have nowhere else to go, and he just didn't have no kind of respect for my child being, you know, laying there.

Christine, later, pregnant by another man, gave birth to a son, but she could not support her family with the job that she had:

> But eventually I had to take welfare because I was, like, having to pay for a ride to work and back. I was having to pay my sister to keep my daughter after she got out of school. Having to buy groceries, having to pay rent, and I wasn't making that kind of money on minimum wage back then. And so my daughter got up one night, me and her were laying on the couch, and I had about three to four cigarette lighters laying around, and she got up messing with one and I woke up, and she had set this box, that I had in a corner, on fire, and we lost everything in that fire, and then they put us on HUD [Department of Housing and Urban Development] and put us in another house. . . . Then after a year, I think you had to stay in that house a year, then I moved to this other house where we had a gas stove and stuff like that. That is when the trouble started. That is when I had my little boy, and that's when he died, and then I started going to heavy drugs and stuff.

Christine's neighbors offered her drugs to ease her pain over her son's death; she had not tried illicit drugs previously. Soon after Christine went to New Jersey to take care of a sister who had been stabbed. By then, she was heavily using drugs and was stabbed herself:

> These three people, I knew two of them, but to this day I don't know who that third person was. I was at the house. See a lot of times when I

get high or drunk, I like to listen to Christian music, and this lady that sings a lot at her church, she had this building not too far from the house, and they would be up there practicing. I [had] just left up there from listening to her sing, and I was in there trying to help her sing too because I was drunk. So I came back to the house and I was laying there on the couch. These three people came to my house. This one girl . . . said, "We want to do some drugs." I say, "I don't want any more drugs in my house tonight, I don't want any more." Because I had been doing it all day long, dragging and going on. . . . When I walked around the coffee table and to the door, the girl stabbed me, and I went into the kitchen. This other girl . . . she was in the kitchen counting her money or something. I say, ". . . that bitch done stabbed me." Just like that, I used to curse. I say, "That bitch done stabbed me." [She] ran out and left me, everybody ran out and left me. It just so happens the lady next door to me is my sister's mother-in-law, and I went over there. I say, "[Neighbor's name]," I say, "That girl done stab me." She don't even let me come in the house; she said, "Stay on the porch." She called the police and rescue squad for me.

Christine was dismayed that her neighbor would not let her come in the house when she was scared and injured.

GINA

Gina, born in 1961, grew up outside Philadelphia in a three-bedroom, two-story house, with seven brothers and three sisters. They had "a big old back yard, plenty of grapes. We had a grapevine, it just spread out all over the place. I loved it." Their father would wake the children at five a.m. to work in the garden before school. Gina's mom worked as a custodian in an elementary school, and her father worked in a paper company. Gina reported having the best, but strict, parents:

Girl, they, um, they didn't take no mess. [laughs] They just had a whole lot of values. They didn't believe in disorderly children. Didn't believe in no violence and fightin' and tellin' lies, stealin'. So we had to walk strict, strict, strict, STRICT—Extra Strict Line! . . . From the day I was born until the day they died, I did pretty good, and then I just went wild after they died.

While the house and family were wonderful, the neighborhood was not: "It was rough. It was bad, terrible. Lots of gangs, fightin' going on. People gettin' killed on the step where you live at." Gina was also regularly chased home by the schoolchildren: "I had to have my brothers and them come walk me home from school."

Gina began school after racial integration, but her three older brothers experienced the onset and turmoil of integration: "They used to have to fight all the time and get called names and stuff." When Gina was in ninth grade, her father moved them to North Carolina into a triple-wide trailer in the country because "my father did not want his children up there in all that violence. There was too much violence and crime going on." However, the trailer had not been inspected, so the family had to sleep in a tent for three months. For Gina, the trailer was "just too far out in the country on a dirt road. I didn't like living on no dirt road."

Gina participated in lots of sports and had strong support from her father to finish high school:

> I ran track, I took sewing classes, cooking classes, I liked math, I did not like history, I didn't like biology either. . . . I was the only one that wanted to finish school [in my family] because everybody else was dropping out, and so my father told me, he said, "You finish high school and graduate, and I will give you a car." I got ready to go to the twelfth grade, and the day school got ready to start back, that is the day he died. So I ain't never get my car, so I ain't never thought about driving. I said, "Forget it, I ain't going to learn how to drive."

Gina dreamed of being a "computer whiz" or going into cosmetology, but instead she married a man with whom she frequently fought. On at least two occasions, her husband attempted to throw her out of a window and once tried to push her in front of a train. During their marriage Gina had three miscarriages, with at least one of them being directly caused by her husband's abuse: "Me and [my husband] got in a fight. He kicked me in the stomach. . . . Then I went to work the next day and, one day, I went to work—I was workin' in . . . [a] rest home . . . and, I went in that, the, the boss-man's office, and told him, I said, 'God, my stomach hurts so bad.' I passed out on the floor." Gina reports that she has not thought about having children since the miscarriages because they were the worst experiences of her life.

Gina's husband died of AIDS not long before the interviews were conducted. She went to the hospital every day while he was sick. Her brothers did not understand how she could care for the man who had infected her with HIV and abused her. She responded to them by saying, "It ain't about me today. It is about trying to help somebody else. . . . He suffered something fiercely."

JOANNA

Joanna was one of four children raised in a metropolitan city in North Carolina. Joanna's father was a truck driver who would at times go on drinking binges that kept him out of work for weeks at a time. Her mother would go without food and decent shoes to make sure that the children had food and shoes without holes in the bottom. Joanna reported that her mother "instilled a lot of things in me, you know, [about] what I would have to deal with through life as I was growing up." Joanna's fondest memories were of the holidays:

All of our Christmases were good. Thanksgiving was good. Any holiday that came and it pertained to children or family together: ours was good. And sometimes my daddy would dig a hole in the yard and cook us a hog. Fourth of July, okay, you all get in the car and we are going to get the hog and we would go all the way to [name of city] and get a hog and bring it back, and my daddy would cook us a hog. My mama would make the old fashion, old timey, old, old, timey lemonade. Squeeze the lemon.

To Joanna, her father demonstrated his love by confronting a boyfriend who had hit her; Joanna recalls: "When my daddy got there and I told my daddy, my daddy told him, 'I don't care what you do, but when you go to hitting on my daughters and you done messed around and hit my daughter, I will kill you.' My daddy like to have killed him too. So when it came to us girls, my daddy, he was a fool."

In high school, Joanna recalls getting into trouble with a group of girl friends:

We drank on the school yard. In back where we had our lunch at, we drank, and our favorite drink was Thunderbird and Kool-Aid, and we smoked weed, smoked cigarettes. We just had a ball at school. We were always in something. I was on the marching unit. We used to fight, good God. They barred me from going to the games, me and about six girls on the marching unit. . . . Shoot, we would get there and get to fighting. . . . They swore that I was the ringleader. All of us went and got all our hair cut off. . . . We called ourselves having our little gang. Boy, I thought my mama was going to beat me to death because my hair was down to here and I cut it all off. . . . We had Mohawks and had great big earrings, and when we got tired of Mohawks, we shaved our heads.

Joanna quit school after she was suspended for setting a disliked teacher's trash can on fire.

Joanna was a victim of abuse; she put her husband in jail for beating her, but she continued to fight as well:

My baby boy's daddy, I broke his nose with one of those cast-iron frying pans; I hit him with the butt of it. He was going to slap me from behind and tell me that I think more of that damn baby than I did him, and when I turned around and said, "I sure do," he slapped me from behind and I'm standing at the stove. When I hit him in the face, all of this right here [points to areas of the face] broke. . . . He stayed in the hospital for a long time. They put me in jail for that one [for] five months. I stayed in jail for about a month. . . . Then another guy I was going with, we were at the club and drinking and he done slapped me, and I tried my best to cut his head off. I cut him from here to here. I stayed in jail for that for about a month.

Joanna turned twenty-five years old in a women's correctional facility.

JONI

Joni grew up in a mid-sized North Carolina town in a "big old raggedy house" heated with a wood stove. The kids (four girls and two boys) slept four to a bed. Joni's only knowledge of her father is that he was a soldier from Puerto Rico. Joni reported:

I can remember some good times, but my basic memories: [mama] she was always working, I was always hungry, cold and raggedy, and my lazy-ass sisters wouldn't comb my hair. Dirty little raggedy thing running around the neighborhood, you know.

Okay, what I remember is that everybody was poor, you know pretty much so, but we are always the poorest, okay? I remember when if you talked back to an adult, they would whoop your ass and then take you home to your mama, and she would whoop your ass again.

Joni, who was in her late thirties at the time of the interviews, recalled the streets on which black people could live and those on which white people lived, a distinction that caused her to be wary of white people. She recalled some racist incidents from her childhood: "I can remember it so vividly: I saw this pretty white girl with blonde hair, she had such a pretty tan, and I was looking at her, you know how little kids do, and she said, 'What you looking at, nigger?'"

Joni remembered being raped on two occasions as a child:

The first time . . . I believe I was about seven. My brother-in-law, he didn't penetrate me or anything, 'cause my two brothers were young. They were curious, and they came in on me, and they told my sister, and you would have thought she would have put the bitch out, [but they] kept right on living together. And then, girl, if you knew the history of my life, you would shoot dope too. And then, when I was

eleven, Mama was working up in New York. And I was staying with
my sister. . . . And her boyfriend . . . used to babysit me. And this was
true rapes. He actually raped me when I was eleven years old. Sure
enough. Then what fucks me up, the big fat bitch that I hate, [my
sister] got the nerve to be a Jehovah Witness and come down here
and tell me she wanted to marry the mother-fucker when I told her
that he raped me when I was eleven. And then when I went berserk,
I went absolutely insane throwing and breaking [things], you know.
[I] turned into a fucking gorilla. He got the nerve to say [he] didn't
know it was going to haunt me for all my life. Well it haunts me,
mother-fucker, for all of my life, and you big dumb bitch. . . . What
. . . girl I got some shit in me, if it comes out, I be a dangerous critter.
I be real dangerous.

Joni witnessed her mother having a stroke from which she subsequently
died the year after they moved to New York City: "And I had wished her dead.
And then she actually died. It fucked me up, fucked me up good."

We was sitting at the table, having a cup of coffee, and she just went
slap [fell over on the table]. And she wouldn't say nothing else to me.
And our next door neighbor . . . I got her and she said, "Your
mother's had a stroke," and I went to the county hospital. They left
her laying out there [in the emergency room] seem like to me for
hours, probably wasn't, but it seemed like that for me. But nobody
was home but me.

Following her mother's death, Joni's sisters would beat her, deny her food, and
lock her out of the house when she was sick. She tried to kill herself when she
was fifteen with aspirin and again at sixteen with a knife.

But of all of these events, the following memory, drawn from Joni's childhood, was, in her opinion her worst memory:

Okay, I remember when my sister got married to [her] husband. And
they wouldn't let me go. They wouldn't let me go down to the
church. But I had a blue dress the lady down the street had given me,
she's dead. . . . She had given me a pretty blue dress, like royal blue,
and I went and got myself dressed with my little dirty feet and my
dirty hair, 'cause I had long hair and nobody had combed it. And I
went down to the church, and they were horrified. Okay?

Although she had experienced terrible and traumatic life events, Joni
maintained a strong sense of humor, and she laughed through much of the
interviews. While she laughed at her own trauma, she yelled about it at the
same time.

When asked to recall her happiest childhood memories, these events came to Joni's mind:

> One of the happiest memories, you're gonna think this is silly. Okay, I was back-talking [to] my mama, right. . . . I back-talked my mama . . . [My mama] was getting old by then, she was getting sickly. Mama threw a spoon and hit me dead in my fucking nose, yes she did. Well I guess I was smelling, what the old people say, you're smelling your musk, and I got to back-talking at the dinner table and I turned around on them steps because I knew I was free once I got to the steps, and I turned around and one of those big tablespoons hit me dead in the nose and, boy, I got to moving. I got to moving. Mama didn't play. I guess she said, "Well heck, no, you can't talk to me that a way."

She shared an additional "happy" memory representing how she enjoyed the feeling of deceiving others: "I'm ashamed to tell you this. Of course I went to church when I was growing up, and you know how the old people used to get the Holy Ghost and stuff like that. I was a little girl, and me and my girlfriend, we were little demons, and so we saw them dancing and getting the Holy Spirit and I got up, and I started having the Holy Spirit too. I ain't felt a damn thing. I was just doing what they were doing."

Joni was one of the few participants, even when asked directly, to mention a close childhood friend:

> [My friend was] much like me, she didn't have a whole lot, nothing like that, but you know she had like a solid family life, so she wasn't adrift. And so I kinda latched onto her, and we were best friends all the way through, 'til I went to the army. . . . She liked to read. We liked to talk about sex, but we never got none, you know what I mean. We wasn't getting any. We liked to talk about it; she was my best friend. A big influence on me.

The high school guidance counselor also played an important role in Joni's life. The counselor was the first person to tell Joni that she was smart and could go to college if she tried: "I didn't know I was smart. I didn't know I could go to college." Joni finished high school and made it through three years of college. She went to a private college in New York where she received a scholarship.

> Well, I always did like school, but I think I probably would have fared better if I hadn't gone to such a ritzy school. I always felt very self-conscious. You know, it's a drag to always be the poorest thing around, you know. It [was] always like that, you know, so I always had

kind of a complex about it. Not real high self-esteem. That's probably why I started getting high and I would always gravitate to trouble, I reckon. I was going into my senior year [of college] and I needed $900 and came down here to pick up $900, and the only one that was willing to give me the money was my brother-in-law. . . . So [he] said, "You know if we all contribute." He was willing to go borrow the money, and everybody else was telling me, "Well I got this to pay and I got that to pay" and this and that and other things. . . . I remember sitting on the porch crying, 'cause all of them had good credit. They could have borrowed that money, and it would have been money well-invested. Because who knows what I could have been today, and [I] might have given it back to them tenfold. . . . [Because I didn't finish college] it didn't do anything financially for me, so I just wasted the government's money, in my opinion. I'm living off the government now, you know what I mean.

Joni, who did not work at the time of the interviews, had wanted to go to Columbia School of Journalism and become a journalist.

While in New York City, Joni was raped again:

And the third [rape], I went to a party with my friend—dead now—she OD'd. We were doping. . . . We got up the street, way up here. And I thought we were [just] hanging out. Took me in a fucking—it looked like a house, I'm partying, thinkin' we going to shoot some dope. [The rapist] took my ass and kept me there all night long. I don't give a fuck about no man. A man is a dirty mother-fucker. I'm just sorry I ain't no mother-fucking lesbian.

Joni expressed her anger about the abuse that she had lived through in this way: "Did I deserve any of this shit? Am I innately—am I just bad? Fuck them mother-fuckers, I'll hurt one of them. I kill some mother-fuckers. Ain't nobody going to never touch me or hurt me again." Joni entered into several relationships as an adult that were very abusive, but she declined to describe these relationships in detail. She sought counseling at more than one agency for the rapes and tried to commit suicide on three different occasions. She claimed that the mental health system was a joke so she says she "don't talk about it, I don't deal with it, block it out."

JOY

Joy was raised in New York City. Joy said that her mom taught her "to be a woman. To cook. My mom taught me how to clean. So . . . she taught me that. Gotta give that to her!" Her grandmother in Mississippi was mostly of Native American descent and taught Joy about taking care of herself. Joy had one brother and one sister; each had different biological fathers. Her mom was a "sophisticated drinker," and her dad, an "expensive drinker," had extramarital affairs resulting in children with these other women. They lived in a nice house with three bedrooms, a living room, a kitchen, and a "loooong hallway," and always had plenty to eat.

Her parents argued frequently: "I never had a—I used to have a birthday party, but we never got to eat cake. . . . They used to fight—over my cake. That's the first thing my mom grabbed, was my cake! Boom! We never had cake!"

Joy hoped of graduating as a Licensed Practical Nurse (LPN). After attending vocational high school for nursing, she achieved her dream.

LISA

Lisa grew up in a small North Carolina town with one adopted brother and one biological brother. Lisa's father was killed when she was three, and her mom, who remarried the next year, supported the family by working in a cotton mill. Lisa's stepfather, who "fished locally, made nets, and hung out at home," "drank frequently and drank a lot"; he became violent when he drank, and once shot a gun at her mother "to scare her." Her parents fought at least once a week. Lisa remembered one fight that occurred when she was around the age of eight; she was so scared while watching her stepfather fight that she "peed" on herself. At other times, she watched her brothers be beaten so badly there would be "blood coming out their backs."

Lisa and her brothers would frequently be locked out of the house while their mother was locked inside with their stepfather. The children sometimes slept in the chicken coop:

> He [her stepfather] drinked, and my mama was a witch. So she would
> be thirty minutes late and he would swear up and down [that] she was
> screwin' around or whatever. So he would ahmm, what he would do
> was: she'd come in, she'd start naggin' so automatically, we knew
> where we was gon' sleep that night. And then he would start drinkin'
> and it would get worse, and then they'd throw dishes, food. We were
> doin' good if we eat supper that night, cause it would hit the floor,
> ahmm, up against the walls, but I mean we had good times. He was a
> good man. I mean, I don't fault him 'cause it's just as much my mom's
> fault as it was his.

Lisa's brothers were not as forgiving of their stepfather. Lisa's oldest brother tried to kill their stepfather but was stopped by their mother. Her stepfather died when Lisa was twelve, and her mother remarried again.

But with all of this violence around her, the event that Lisa said "changed her heart" was when her puppy died. Lisa had bonded closely with the puppy, even bottle-feeding it. The puppy was killed when, wrapped in a blanket in the hall, her mother stepped on it. Lisa reports never letting people close to her after that incident, but her relationship with her aunt was very important: "[My aunt] was just the ideal. She would sit out and talk to me and tell me, you know, what life's really about. 'If I could keep you, I'd keep you, but I can't. Your mama won't give you to me.' She'd a took me. Anytime. Anytime I'd a want to move in she'd a took me."

At school, Lisa was embarrassed by having to wear the same clothes each day: "My mother wasn't like everybody else's mother to go buy me clothes here and there and I could dress like other kids. I went [in]to my twelfth grade year. I went to school with three pair of pants."

Lisa's fantasy was to help other children not feel the pain that she felt: "To have a house full o' young uns. They didn't have to be mine. . . . Young uns that people didn't want. That they throw away, that they just didn't care about. . . . I wanted to build a great big house, two-, three-story house, and let these kids just stay here. How I'd a done that? I didn't have the money, but it was just a dream I always had."

When Lisa was seventeen, she started dating a close family friend (the family referred to him as a cousin). The boyfriend was very angry when they broke up:

He had a gun in my car one night and come to my house and said, "Look I got a gun in your car. You know me, if you don't go with me, then you know I'll shoot you." . . . At that point I didn't know he wouldn't [shoot me]. . . . So we went back to a camper trailer that he was living in. He was like, "This is one time you are going to do something I want to do." And he more or less forced me and . . . I try to block it out, just like push it right out of my head.

When Lisa was about eighteen, she married a man who also abused her. The first week that Lisa lived with her new husband, a male friend called her on the telephone. Her husband was furious that a man would call her so he beat her with the telephone. Lisa said, "Right then, I should've picked up and just walked out but I didn't. That was the ideal man I wanted: coal-black hair, he was slender, nice-lookin', that's what I wanted." Later, when Lisa got pregnant, her husband kicked her in the stomach, which caused a miscarriage, because he thought that she got pregnant by somebody else.

Lisa left this husband, who had also infected her with HIV. She entered another abusive relationship with a man who "ended up going to prison [because] he had hit somebody with a baseball bat and about killed them. So he went to prison, so when he got out of prison was when we got back together." Lisa later married another older man who she felt saved her from the abusive relationship. He was HIV-positive and gay, which Lisa discovered when she found him in bed with another man.

When asked if she had maintained any goals for the future as a child, Lisa said: "When I finished high school, the only thing I wanted to do was have me a baby [that] had black hair and coal-black eyes. . . . I had never really planned for a life. So I really didn't know what I wanted to do. I didn't want to work at fast food all my life, but that's what it looks like what I'm a have to do. . . . I guess I just thought I would get married and have a man to support me and, and have my children or whatever."

LORI

Lori spent her childhood in eleven different foster homes: "My mom would move me. She would find out that my dad would know where I was and she would have me moved to another foster home. . . . From what I could remember, I was in Virginia until [I was] eight years old. I was in foster homes then, but I moved to West Virginia into a foster home, and I was in there until I was seventeen." She was in the West Virginia foster home for the longest period of time with her brother and sister. The foster mother was a "Christian lady, and she had a front that everybody thought that she was all good." The house was in all-white "deep coal-mining country."

> One time, well when I first started my period I didn't know what it was, and I had a man teacher, and I told him I was bleeding, and when the teacher brought me home, [the foster mom] beat me for letting him know that I was bleeding. One time, the principal called home; I was sick throwing up and [the foster mother] slammed my head and leg in the door of the car because she didn't want me coming home sick. We weren't allowed to sit down and watch TV. We had to sit whenever she sit. She slept in the same room we slept in. The other bedroom that she had she wouldn't let nobody sleep in. If she would be gone, we would have to stay outside in the cold until whenever she came home, whenever she chose to come home. She would be out late and we would have to stay outside. We weren't allowed in the house when she wasn't there. There was one time that it was real cold and it was snowing out, and we went to our neighbors because we were cold, my brother and I. She beat us for that, telling us we weren't suppose to go to nobody's house. We were allowed to take a shower once a week. We sponged-bathed the rest of the time. She had an inside toilet, but we weren't allowed to use it; we had to

use the outside toilet. I wasn't allowed to have no friends. We wore the same clothes to school all week long, and we weren't allowed to change.

Lori and her siblings were not allowed to sit on the furniture that was "covered with plastic." The children were beaten and raped repeatedly in the foster home by the foster mother's daughter's father-in-law. Lori attempted to tell the social workers about their condition, but the social workers did not believe her; Lori would be beaten more after the social workers left. Finally, Lori went to the emergency room after a beating with a BB gun in her "private parts" and showed the doctors. Only then was she able to convince the social workers of the sexual abuse so that she and her brother and sister would be removed from the house.

When asked, Lori searched her memory for a positive childhood event. She remembered one home that seemed to be decent and recalled one small toy: "I remember one home I was in, it was a foster home. I wasn't in there long. I can barely remember, I had my own play-room and stuff, and I remember having a play snake. The main thing I can remember that you would hold him by the tail and it would wiggle. I don't know if you have seen them, but I had that as a toy, and I used to love that." Lori was frequently teased: "I was fat, which you can see I still am. My foster mother made me wear the same set of clothes all through the week. She wouldn't change clothes. I washed my hair once a week. I actually got in the shower once a week. I had low self-esteem. I didn't have many friends 'cause I wasn't allowed to have no friends."

Lori graduated from high school, went to college for a year, then got "into the drug scene," and quit college. She was raped again in 1987 at the age of twenty-one:

Yeah, my husband was out to sea. Me and my girlfriend, we were in a bowling league and we were going home one night, and I got a flat [tire] on the car. And in [name of city], the police officers have white vans and when that white van pulled up, I thought it was a policeman, but it wasn't. It was another man. He said he had to get a tire out or a tool or something to get the hubcap off our car. [My girlfriend] went around with him, and he had choked her, which I didn't know. Tied her up. I didn't know what was going on. He came to me from behind and done the same thing. Took us to a trailer, and then he asked us which one was first. She said, "What the hell. I'll go first. He ain't gonna hurt us." We didn't think he was going to hurt us. He shot her. He dumped her under an overpass. It was all on the news. Okay?

After five miscarriages, Lori finally gave birth to a son. In time, Lori divorced her husband when she caught him with another woman, Lori's best friend, who was staying with them. "He ended up having a child with her." This double loss of her two closest relationships led Lori to try to kill herself. She was admitted to a psychiatric ward, which in turn led to her losing custody of her son.

RHONDA

Rhonda was born and raised in New Jersey in the "projects." Her parents were married; her mom was a teacher, and her father worked for a moving company. She said that her parents provided her with the best of everything. Everybody in the projects knew her family. When her mom wanted her home, "she would just holler out the window." Rhonda reported of her childhood: "We had a ball. It was great growing up." Yet Rhonda had a difficult time remembering a happy time. Rhonda loved time that she spent with her grandparents:

> I just loved my grandmother to death. I just loved my grandmother. It was so bad, I used to be with my grandmother all the time. . . . [My grandparents shaped me by teaching me] morals and going to church. Being polite. I used to come down every summer and stay with [my grandfather] down here, right here. He said . . . something about a baby. I said, "Grandpa, you want me to have a baby?" He said, "Yeah, Rhonda, I want you to have lots of babies." That's what my grandpa told me, yep. Then I had a baby because, I guess, Grandpa said it would be alright, and that stuck with me.

Rhonda reported going to "a predominantly white school, you know, and grew up like regular children. I don't know, school was fun. Back then, we had gangs too now. Yeah, you know like the girls, this town against that town. We used to fight now. . . . I was a junior [in high school] and got introduced to heroin, and that was it. There was no more high school. Yeah, there wasn't no more high school, there wasn't no more nothing." Rhonda said that she "always wanted to be an undertaker or a doctor. . . . I was always fascinated by dead people." She was able to work in a funeral home in New Jersey for a time.

TERI

Teri was born in Virginia, the fourth of eight children. Her mom, a "lone parent," was an alcoholic, received welfare, and had "a little job on the side." Teri moved from apartment to apartment with her family, usually in "swamp areas," where there were lots of clubs, noise, and alcoholics. The biggest apartment they ever lived in had two bedrooms, so the children usually slept on the floor. It was not unusual for Teri and her siblings to watch her mother be beaten up by boyfriends or to wake up without their mother and have to find her beaten up in a park.

> Ah, I know my mama loved me. But I really had a hard life. I mean, a really rough life. You know, she—We didn't have much. Didn't get much, you know. We ate beans, weanies, grits, some—You know, we didn't, you know, we didn't eat good meals. But we really—lived hard. Yeah, I use—you know, fight. My brothers and sisters and me— we'd all fight, all the time. You know, we were never satisfied with what my mama would give us, we never were satisfied. I wasn't satisfied, you know. She tried her best. I know she did. 'Cause, you know, she, she—was on welfare.

Before the age of twelve, Teri was raped by one of her mother's boyfriends and lost her mother when one of her mother's boyfriends took her mom outside and "put a knife in her head and back," killing her. Teri and her siblings then moved in with relatives on the North Carolina coast. Teri was placed in a "crazy house" after her mother's murder: her anger over her mother's death was intense, and she confided that she would not travel to Virginia because she truly believed that, if she ever went back, she would try to find her mother's murderer and kill him.

Teri stopped going to school in tenth grade, a few years after moving to North Carolina: "I hate school! I got with the wrong crowd, start beatin' up white people in school. Got suspended for ten days. . . . And just said, 'Fuck it!' You know. I just can't cope. I just can't cope." She "got involved with drugs and stuff, you know. Started drinking first. I was an alcoholic. Then I had a baby." Teri, who reported that there were no positive adult role models in her life, never had any aspirations for her life other than to survive each day and make some money.

Like her mother, Teri wound up with men who abused her. She recounted: "And then, um, met up with this boy, met up with this drug dealer and that's when I started sellin'—I wasn't smokin' then. And he start beatin' me up and everything, you know. Broke my jaw and stuff. You know, like I caught hell most all my life, so—I depend on men all my life, you know, my family didn't come. We not close. We not close." Eventually Teri had two children. Her oldest daughter's father was her first love. He was an alcoholic and "user" who beat her regularly. Teri lived on the street then: "[My children] were very young, you know. They stay in the streets all night long and stuff. And my boyfriend beats my ass. You know, I'm goin' the same routine as my mother was. Choosing the wrong mens."

Teri's life on the streets was very rough. She was raped, regularly beaten, and experienced the deaths of close friends from overdoses. Her children were taken away from her. Given these experiences, Teri has great anger inside her. She was disturbed by her own reaction to a recent incident when another client in the substance abuse treatment center with her threatened her: "and for some reason I got too angry. . . . I had a butcher knife, and I just wanted to kill him."

Teri reported frequently thinking about suicide, which she attributed primarily to not having her children with her. At the time of the interviews, she was working to make herself better so that she could bring her children home.

WENDY

Wendy grew up in the woods of North Carolina. She, with three sisters and two brothers, lived in a trailer that was blue and white on the outside with wood paneling on the inside. Her parents both raised her, and her father worked very hard.

Wendy stopped going to school because she did not like the way that she was treated: "I just got tired of people's mess, mouth, picking and stuff. You know how people like to pick and stuff. It's hard." When asked about childhood role models, Wendy reported that she had none. "Myself. I made myself mean and hateful. Everybody says I'm mean like a rattlesnake, like I don't take no mess either."

She married into a two-year abusive relationship when she was nineteen and moved to upstate New York with her husband: "We'd fight. Girl, I'd throw plates at him. He throw something at me. He hit me one night, and downtown he went [to jail]. . . . That's what broke us up. Because I told him I wasn't living in a relationship like that. . . . He work all night, and then he come in and want to show his . . . m-hm. My daddy [taught] me if it's a man or not: if he hits you, you strike back."

Upon ending the relationship, Wendy was alone and far from home. It was winter when her husband moved out and stopped paying the bills: "He had the lights turned off in the apartment, freezing rain and snowing twenty-five inches, and I couldn't stay there with him. I just made up my mind I was coming home [to North Carolina]." Wendy told her husband that she was leaving with their child, but her husband and mother-in-law came and literally wrestled the baby from her arms in her driveway. Wendy went to the sheriff and asked if he would help her take her son so she could return home to North Carolina. The sheriff told Wendy that she could not take her son from the biological father without going to court and that if she tried to take him, they could arrest her for kidnapping. The sheriff told her that she would have to go to court to take her son out-of-state. Wendy, having nowhere to go and feeling cold and lonely, left New York without her son. She did try later to fight for her son, but her husband and mother-in-law hired a lawyer and eventually won custody because the court decided that the father was financially better able to care for the child.

The Men

ALBERT

After Albert was born, he lived with his parents in a shack on his grandparents' farm. The two-room shack was heated by a white kerosene stove and had running water, but there was no indoor bathroom—only an outhouse. When Albert was about eighteen months old, his mother gave birth to his brother. Six months later, both parents left him and his brother to be raised by their grandparents. Albert was regularly beaten by his grandfather with a razor strap, but to Albert, the emotional abuse from his grandfather was possibly worse than the physical abuse. Albert recalled: "I would never argue with [Grandfather] because he always telling me, he used to tell me that my mother was a tramp when I was younger and uh, I didn't have no right and [that] I would've wound up just like her. And that hurt me and hurt me and hurt me, and I listened to it every day at supper time."

When Albert was five or six, his brother died, which was incredibly upsetting to Albert. At age thirteen, Albert was placed in an orphanage. While in the orphanage, he started hallucinating and stopped speaking: "I was dreaming that I had seen a frog's legs as big as the danggone room was. Everything else when I was going to the hospital was upside down. If it wasn't upside down, it was straight up. I seen everything upside down. I didn't talk for three months." He was moved to a mental institution, where he stayed until age twenty-one.

Albert was able to recall positive memories, one of which was from fifth grade:

> The best teacher I had was in fifth grade, Miss [name of teacher]. I thought the world of her. She was real nice and she held me a lot and that's where I had a writing contest. They sent [my writing] upstairs. They said that everybody could read it plainer than they could read [the second-place winner's] because I really slant all my [letters] and everything was just perfect. I beat this other girl. I said, "I'm going to try to do the best I can." Then they put it in the county fair that year. That made me proud.

Albert reported that his happiest memory was the time that his father did not disappoint him:

> Last time I seen [my father] was back in the '70s. He was supposed to come down and see me, and what he done was he spent all his danggone money and asked me to give him money to get back with because he knew I didn't spend mine. I kept holding mine. So I told him I would [give him the money], and I gave him the money to go back with, and guess how much he sent me back? . . . Three times that amount!

Albert had two aspirations as a child: he wanted to be a Christian music singer, and he wanted to get his mom and dad back together so that they could be a family again.

In time, Albert married and became abusive toward his wife, even beating her when she was pregnant, which caused her to miscarry. Recalling this event, Albert said: "I really hate myself sometimes because that [child] would be the carrier of my name today." Albert lived on the street at the time of the interviews.

BILL

Bill was born in Virginia and, when he was three years old, moved to Long Island, where his mother got a job on a farm. He and six siblings were raised in a migrant labor camp with more than one family per house. The house had an outhouse, and Bill was bathed in the sink, even as a grown child. When Bill was nine and his brother was five or six, their uncle would get them drunk:

> [My parents] might have been raising me, but I was myself. But I blame myself, and [the migrant camp] is where I got started on alcohol and drugs. . . . I'd see the guys hanging out at lunchtime and some of them would be drinking, some of them would be smoking cigarettes, cussing goin' on. So to me, I thought that was a normal life. I didn't know any better; I was just a young child then. I don't think my parents were aware that I was picking up on the behavior of these other people. . . . I used to wait until they all went back to work and left their bottles there, and I'd go lay down somewhere where my parents wouldn't find me and they wouldn't know where I was goin' to, and I started feeling good. At least I thought I was feelin' good. My younger brother couldn't handle [getting drunk] . . . he was only like five. We used to go and see my uncle. . . . I guess he thought it was funny to be watching a child, to get high. Back in those days if you . . . for a kid five years old chewing tobacco, he was a man.

When asked specifically at the end of the final interview if he had ever been raped as a child, he said that his uncle had "done it" to him three or four times. Bill explained that his uncle was drunk when he committed the acts, but Bill still thought that the uncle knew what he was doing. The abuse ended when Bill got the courage to tell his father: "I hadn't told my father about it. I was scared to tell my father because he might have said, 'Boy, you always dreaming up some kind of crazy thing; go back to bed.' Finally, I went downstairs and told him. My brother went down there with me." Bill was very close to his younger brother who died when they were both young.

When the migrant farmers left in the fall of each year, Bill's family was the only black one in the area. Bill, who entered elementary school in the early 1960s, noted that going to an all-white school made him act "the fool" because he was afraid that he would "act different without realizing it." Bill reports consciously deciding to play the role of class clown: "They seemed to like [it]; they were all laughing at somebody acting like a fool. So I figured if, well, if you can make everybody laugh, everybody will like you. I picked that up. . . . I tried to be like a big brother image. I was probably a little bit older than everyone 'cause I stayed back a couple years of school because I was a slow learner."

One of Bill's happiest memories from childhood was when he made the final win for his high school team: "Anyway, I went into the long jump; that was the last event. In the whole track meet, we were behind by one point. The guy was good I was going against. He jumped. I jumped [further]. So we got first place. Everybody was cheering. Everybody was patting me on the butt. I felt like I was a hero."

Bill also reported a time when he was recognized in school for his work:

> I was kind of a slow learner at a certain age. I learned my mechanical skills by watching my father take things apart. I started doing that when I was real little. I would watch him take something apart and then when he wasn't looking, I would do it. I picked that up real quick. Back in 1978, I got a mechanical drawing board. I did some stuff on there most of the other students didn't realize what I was doing. My teacher took the blueprint. I don't know what he did with it. He gave me a good mark on it. He said, "I want to keep this." So I think I have qualities of learning to be better or better than my other classmates.

But as a teenager in New York City, Bill fought and was injured on several occasions.

BRAD

Brad was born in Connecticut and, in eighth grade, moved to rural North Carolina, which he did not like: "I was sad. I was depressed like any other child would be. Because I had my friends there [in Connecticut], then I had to move somewhere else. It took me a long time, I mean a very long time, to get adjusted to the school. Even to open up to some people at school—I mean it took me a long time." The middle of three children, Brad described his parents as very loving; however, he also reported that his only happy childhood memory was the day of his high school graduation. He wished that he could go back to that time and start over so that he would not be in the situation that he is in today.

CLARK

Clark was one of nineteen children, with nine brothers and nine sisters. He was born on the coast of North Carolina, and when he was four years old his family moved to New York; however, Clark continued to spend each summer and several of his school years on the North Carolina coast with his grandparents. Clark's father, a heavy drinker, was in the military and later became a truck driver. Clark's mother was a housewife and sometimes worked part-time cleaning the houses of others. One of Clark's happiest childhood memories was when a new television was given to his family by a brother in New York City. Although televisions were new for everyone at that time, the gift was particularly meaningful to Clark because it brought his family together and increased its prestige within his neighborhood:

> I can remember . . . our first television, we was down here when we got that. I was five then. I was about five 'cause I can remember, when we went to New York that was my first year in school, and I remember that. First time having a television. A little black-and-white television with an antenna on top. It was really nice. So people in the neighborhood they didn't have television, there was no television, and if you had a television you was doing good. You know? You was doing good.

Clark's father died when Clark was thirteen, and his grandparents died when he was in tenth grade. Clark's mother then moved the family back to the North Carolina coast and into the grandparents' home. "I wanted to come. My grandparents lived here, and this is where I guess I basically loved."

When Clark was about fourteen years old he witnessed the aftermath of a rape of a six-year-old girl. Clark and a friend were walking "in a wooded area that had a path where you could cut the walk in half across [to] the next block."

> [We were] just walking through there, and this little girl just shot
> right out in front of us. The guy came out with his thing in his hand.
> Bright bloody where he tried to penetrate this little girl. She was
> maybe half a block from home. Not even half a block; I would say
> that far. She ran home. I seen her daddy beat that boy half to death.

Clark and his friend were subpoenaed, but they did not have to testify in court because they were too young.

When Clark was in twelfth grade, his mother became ill with tuberculosis and was sent to a sanitarium for six months. Clark became the primary family caretaker for his siblings and worked very hard to stay in school while caring for the family:

> I don't know, I just got tired, I guess. I just got tired of school. You
> know, I guess it was like hard too because my mom had got sick, and
> she was in the . . . a sanitarium for tuberculosis. . . . And it was like
> me and my next younger sister was at home, and we, like, carried the
> load. For like six months or more, while I was in twelfth grade. . . . I
> went up and I done a lot of field work, cabbage and potatoes, and
> cucumber, I done a lot of hard work. I mean you wasn't making
> nothing, you know, 80 or 90 cents an hour, but it helped feed my
> younger brothers and sisters. We didn't have to borrow or beg nobody
> for nothing to eat.

The North Carolina community that Clark considered home was very nurturing: "We all lived neighborly. I was probably just as much as some of the neighbors' kid as I was my own parents' kid, because whatever they say do in the neighborhood, you did. You mind them and respected them, and that's how we lived, like a cluster community. Everybody looked after everybody's kids like that."

Clark was also proud of what he was able to accomplish under adverse conditions. He worked hard to finish high school while being a caregiver to his family:

> When I was in seventh grade, I lost [my father]. It took a long time
> to recover from that. A long time. I managed. I didn't quit school.
> There were many days I wanted to stop. I kept on pushing. After that
> I finished high school. That was a big highlight. Just to be able to
> graduate. Just to graduate is a basic thing because there's hundreds of
> things in the middle of these stories I'm telling you that I've been
> through. Graduation was really like a dream come true. I'm leaving

high school and going to college. Going into a world where either
you make it or you don't. I made it. Made it. Went to college.
Finished that.

Clark wanted to become a nurse and was able to do so, still practicing
nursing at the time of the interviews.

DAMON

From the age of two, Damon lived in rural North Carolina with his great-aunt
and -uncle on his dad's side of the family. The great-aunt and -uncle had a son
and a daughter who also lived with them. His mother and stepfather lived in
Virginia, and each had six children. His mother would send him clothes, and
his grandfather took special care of him.

Damon was raped by a family member when he was eleven. He was not
descriptive about events that had hurt him, but he did say, "Man done took
everything from me, so fuck it." When asked what he meant by "man" he
replied: "Well, whoever damaged my body. Whoever hurt me when I was
growing up. Whoever wasn't there for me when I needed it. . . . Physical and
mental. . . . Ain't nobody going to tell me everybody don't work through this
earth that ain't been physically hurt and mentally hurt."

Damon was openly gay in high school and associated with a group of
other gay boys. He finished high school and proceeded to take courses in different colleges for many years, wanting to become a nurse or an actor, but in
the end he did neither because he never stayed in one program long enough.

DEAN

Dean moved to North Carolina from Boston when he was six months old. He
had a biological father in Mississippi whom he did not know very well and was
raised by his mother and stepfather. By his own account his mother worked
hard in a vending company as a supervisor while his stepfather was a certified
public accountant. His stepfather used illicit drugs, and his mother drank.
Dean witnessed his stepfather beating his mother when the stepfather was
high:

> I was embarrassed, because he been drinking a lot, using drugs and
> stuff, and about my mom working, he would take out his frustration
> on her. And made my life like hell growing up as a child, because I
> couldn't focus on what I had to do. And constant fights, cursing each
> other every day all the time. . . . To escape from that, I would just go
> to school and focus myself a lot because I wanted to get out of the
> house.

Dean reported being raped when he was a child, but he declined to say anything more about the incident. Although Dean had two younger brothers, he remembered being very lonely as a child because he felt that his parents did not love him. While his brothers always got into trouble, Dean always tried to be the "good," kid, which endeared him to his great-grandmother. He felt that his great-grandmother was the most important person in his life, the person who really raised him. Dean noted that his mother and grandmother instilled in him a strong work ethic: "The main reason that I said I look up to those two women [mother and grandmother] is because they are very hard-working women. . . . Their hard work and determination made me realize what I had to do and put me in a place where I followed in their lead in what they did in the past as I was growing up, similar to what I have to do now." Dean's great-grandmother died when he was twelve: "It was the worst thing I thought could ever happen to me when I was a child is when my grandma passed, because she was always there for me, she was my great-grandmother, she was my grandmother's mom. And I was like more her child than my mom's child, and she kind of taught me some of the values that I have now. That was my girl."

Dean enjoyed the holidays, which he described simply as "Christmas was good. During Christmas, we had like big family dinners." Dean grew up in a small community where everybody knew each other and many were kin. Dean was ranked tenth in his class of 586 students and graduated with seventeen cousins. He reports:

> High school was good, I mean it was great, because I was in every club imaginable. I was president of FHA [Future Homemakers of America], I was vice-president of FBLA [Future Business Leaders of America], I was in track, in government. . . . I got a track scholarship at Appalachian. I didn't take it because I wanted to go to Boston [for college]. I got an academic scholarship, a partial scholarship. And then I was real popular, that [was] one thing that I loved, everybody knowing you, what you do. High school was good, but when I got to college, I had a lot of . . . once you leave high school, a bunch of things change. I never dealt with drugs. . . . The gay lifestyle and a lot of lifestyles that were being led, and a whole lot changed once you leave home. So I got myself into it, and that's what. . . . But I did finish school, though. I graduated [college] in Computer Science with a Bachelor of Science degree.

He felt positive about his accomplishments and the support that he received from home: "My mom said I was ambitious. 'Dean, you're very ambitious, you're going to make it. You're the only child to make it,' and I did. I was the first child in my family to graduate from high school with honors, and I went to college, first ever to graduate from college."

Dean, who worked with computers at the time of the interviews, explained his aspirations in this way: "I wanted to be a cook. My very first goal was to be a cook, I wanted to be a chef . . . but my typing teacher, she said, 'You [are] going to be a computer programmer,' and I said, 'That's what my father is,' and she said, 'Why don't you just follow,' . . . Then I wanted to be a lawyer. . . . Chef, lawyer and computer operator. [Those were] my career goals."

He then found himself in a scary relationship when he first started dating:

> When I started in this so-called lifestyle, I met this guy who was possessed, that's the only way I can put it. I was kidnapped. I couldn't prove it, but it was the worst thing that could happen, and he's very psychotic. He tried to make me into a servant/puppet, and I wouldn't let him do it. That's what I mean by a dramatic experience, it was like—have you ever seen the Tina Turner story? . . . [Turner's] life was more a reflection of my life. It was like that. Very abusive. He left marks on my arm, he stabbed me in my arm, cut me in my arm, he burnt my yearbook up, burned my pictures of my mother that I had up. He didn't want me to have any contact with my family. It was just him, nobody else. So I was, you know, held captive. He had a gun.

When asked about other traumatic events, Dean replied, "Yeah, I had a cousin that died of, that passed, she had AIDS and I didn't know about it until I went to her funeral. . . . She was a drug user. . . . But that was kind of traumatic back then, like five years [ago]."

GARY

Gary did not talk much about his home life as a child. He was born and raised with one brother in Plymouth Rock, Massachusetts. "My family came over on the Mayflower years, years, years and years ago, and we stuck around." His parents were married; his father worked hard at a gas station, at Burger King, and as a Bobcat driver, while his mother was a housewife. "Dad beat mom all the time. Dad used to go out drinking with his uncle after work, and he used to say, 'You have to go home and beat your wife.' Father said, 'You got to, got to go home and straighten her out.'" Gary reported that his mother beat him and his sibling regularly with "coat hangers, anything she could find," but Gary did not seem to think badly of this:

> [My mom] beat us. I mean not to the point we were in the hospital or anything like that, but if you didn't do your chores, your room wasn't

clean, or got a D, you just about had to drop your pants because you were going to get an ass-whooping. Coat hangers, anything she could find she would beat the hell out of you with. She realizes now that she was wrong, and she tries to make up for her mistakes.

Gary "always had food on the table . . . lousy food, but food." He added, "I always had bad self-esteem because I was missing teeth, you know. . . . I never smiled." Like Kevin, Gary decided to join the military before finishing school because he did not do well in school and did not feel supported: "My brother dropped out of high school on his junior year. My dad never graduated, my mom never graduated, so to me it was no big deal if I ain't got a diploma. So I joined the military."

Gary reported that most of his girlfriends were violent "psychopaths." He also said that he would hit his wives and girlfriends, arrested for two counts of assault and attempted murder of his first wife:

> I had just found out she had been sleeping with my best friend. Then one night, I was working night shifts at a trucking company, loading trucks, and I came home early at three o'clock in the morning one day and we were in bed, and I wanted to talk. I had to come home; that shit [her sleeping with his friend] been building up in my head. I wanted to get it off my mind, and she wouldn't talk to me, and the baby was crying. So I nudged her, nudged her, and nudged her, and she finally—she wouldn't get out of the bed, so I pushed her out of the bed. She got up to go to the baby, and the baby was crying. . . . She picked it up, and then she handed the baby to me and I turned around, she was gone. Well, [while] she [had been] screaming and punching me . . . I grabbed her by the throat, just holding her back. I wasn't intending to kill her or nothing like that. I was just fighting with her.

JAMES

James's parents "busted-up" when he was young. He and his two older brothers and three older sisters were raised by their mother, grandmother, and grandfather, but their mother was often away because she had a "sleep-in job" working in someone's house. When asked about his worst memory, James said it was that his mother had to stay away so much of the time, but overall he had experienced a good childhood. The family lived in rural North Carolina on a farm with cows, chickens, and hogs. James reported that his grandmother and grandfather taught him "right from wrong." He also enjoyed having his extended family from New York come home for the holidays—with lots of gifts. He had wanted to be a mechanic but eventually quit high school because he "started on other things, drinking and stuff."

JOEY

Joey had two older sisters and lived in the same small rural town until he was nineteen. His father, who worked in a fertilizer plant, died when Joey was about four years old but had fathered children with other women while married to Joey's mom. Joey's mother, who cleaned houses and motels, was strong and single minded, he recalls: "Mom—She said, 'You have to learn to do things for yourself.' She was a good teacher. The best teacher I have ever had. We didn't have to worry about getting whippings. She didn't beat you. She would talk to you, though. She would make it so bad by talking to you, I wish she would had went on and hit me." Joey identified not only his mother but also his grandfather as role models to him. "He said, 'Always think before you do anything.' He said, 'Always think before you talk. Figure out what you are going to say before you say it.'"

While growing up, Joey saw much violence. He recalled an incident when he was six:

> We were walking by there, me and some friends was walking by there at the time when the man knocked on the door. The man opened the door and shot him with a shotgun. . . . [I] seen all that blood come out. . . . That thing still, sometime, I don't care how bad things get, I always think about that. A six-year-old kid see a man get killed. Personally get killed, shot with a shotgun. All that blood coming out of there.

As a teenager, Joey got into "a lot of trouble" resulting in jail time:

> I remember one time, a friend of mine, we were at a service station and a woman had her pocketbook down here. . . . We didn't even see it. So this one guy, buddy of mine, he went in to her pocketbook and stole her purse out of it, full of money. So we getting on down the street, police come by, stop us, searched the other guy and found the money on that guy. We didn't even know he had took it. Now that was a bad memory. Yep, I got locked up at fifteen.

Also at the age of fifteen, Joey saw a man "pull a pistol" on his friend and shoot him:

> Fucked my head up for a long time. I couldn't think straight for a long time. I wanted to know why that man did that, you know, to him. He hadn't [done] nothing to him. Just shot him right there. I saw that man, you know when that bullet went in. I was looking right at it. When that bullet went in there. It was a long time before some blood came out. I mean that hole stayed there a long time. It

could have been a short time, being my mind might have been in
slow motion. I have seen a lot of death.

A few years later, he witnessed a girl's death from an overdose; the people he
was with hid her body in the basement.

When Joey was asked what growing up as a black person in North Carolina was like, he replied simply, "It was terrible." He went on to say that, if he
had had a bomb, he "would have dropped the bomb on [North Carolina] and
killed everybody there." He experienced some very frightening racist acts:

> Yeah, I've been through hell. I had one guy shoot at me with a gun.
> And we were out there just walking. He shot right out of the woods,
> man, people getting killed. Yeah, [my town] is a bad place. I love it,
> don't get me wrong now. I know a lot of white people around here
> that was friends, understand me? They were good friends. I know a
> lot of white guys, men that they all hang around black guys. . . . But
> then you got them kind, one of them belong to the KKK, whatever.
> They want to hang you, shoot you, run you all in the river.

However, when asked about what it was like growing up, Joey responded:
"Oh, man, I loved it. I wouldn't have no other place but this place. I loved it.
Everybody was nice around here." One of his happiest memories was being
surprised by the kindness of another person: "I was about seven years old. I'll
never forget this as long as I live. A friend of mine, his uncle come home. . . .
That man reached in his [pocket], gave, here is $5, and gave me $5 too. That
was a life's savings back then in the '50s, a lot of money. That thing always
stuck in my mind. . . . The $5, it won't the matter of money but the principle
of the thing. He gave me about the same. He gave everybody $5. That's what
I like about him, the man was straight up." Joey reported also loving school
and would have liked to have attended college but did not have adequate
finances.

KEVIN

Kevin grew up in the "projects" in a mid-sized North Carolina town. Kevin's
parents were not married, and he does not remember much about his biological father except that he "drank a lot" and "had a lot of women." His mother
held many different types of jobs at different times, such as being a school-
teacher, running a daycare center, and working in both a bus station and a
hospital. His mom got money from the Farmers Home Administration to buy
a house. Although Kevin's mom beat him fairly often, he identified her as
someone who taught him many lessons. She taught him "the responsibility of
surviving at any length, at any cost, survive."

He had one younger and five older siblings who all looked out for each other and took care of each other. In addition to his mother, Kevin also identified his brother, who was a cross-dresser, as a role model in his life.

Kevin reported being an angry child, and, during the third grade, he stuck another student in the eye with a fork. This incident was a turning point in his life; he became more alienated from his mother and his school. Kevin's relationship with school always seemed tenuous: "I just remember in my elementary days going to school, getting into trouble, running away from school, running home, and the school people coming back and getting me. . . . [I] had a whole lot of discipline problems there." One of his worst memories was flunking fifth grade.

When he was in junior high school, at the age of thirteen, he started "wearing dresses and working the streets." Other worst memories included "just the sex thing. The first time I had sex and all the beatings that I used to get." At the age of twelve or thirteen he was raped for the first time: "I just remember somebody on top of me, and I was holding my eyes closed." Later, he was raped by an older man the first time he went to a gay bar: "I was being fast and went around the corner with this guy, the old JC Penney building that used to be downtown, and he made me do things that I didn't want to do." The next day, Kevin's brother returned to the club and beat up the man.

In junior high school, Kevin met a lesbian teacher who mentored him and helped him to stay in school:

> I related to a teacher that was gay, and I used to talk to her a lot
> about my problems, and I hung out mostly with her. . . . I was
> working the streets then, too, [at age thirteen or fourteen] on the
> weekends. . . . In high school, I was kind of lost 'cause she wasn't
> there, so I started getting into trouble again. Started fighting more.
> Plus, people calling me queer, faggot and all that. So I got in a lot of
> fights.

Kevin did not experience much homophobia in the projects where he lived. He recalled that people in the projects did not pay any attention to anyone's sexuality: "We grew up in the projects, it was okay. . . . Didn't nobody pay us no attention. . . . Back then when I was coming up and I hung out with the girls, the girls wouldn't have sex unless I had me somebody to have sex with too."

Kevin encountered racism and a lot of hostility when working the streets in the midsized military town that he grew up in: "Just when we used to be standing on the corner and stuff, the white guys used to ride around in their cars and throw eggs and say, 'You fucking black whores . . .' They used to say 'black whores,' throw eggs and sometimes shoot, and stuff like that." Kevin believed that much of the abuse he endured while working the streets was simply part of the job. He was beaten and raped repeatedly while working on the streets.

In eleventh grade, Kevin decided to try his best to fit in at school. He applied for and got the position of school mascot, but soon trouble started again:

> I had a lover at that time, and I had a football game. He got into some trouble with the police; police was throwing him against the fence and stuff, and I got out [of] my uniform, just to try to help him. And the next day, they called me to the office and took my mascot position. I walked out of the office and wrote a note saying that my mother gave me permission to drop out of school, and they accepted that, and I dropped out of school. And for three months, my mother didn't know I was out of school.

Kevin joined the military in 1980 but left shortly after because of his homosexuality. Eventually, Kevin did receive his GED and also a cooking certificate.

One of the more violent events in Kevin's life took place in 1990, when he and some friends (all of whom were drag queens) traveled out of town "to have a good time." While out of town, the group ran out of money, so Kevin had to go work the street in order to support the group. To prepare himself, Kevin got drunk and then went out in drag. The first man he met on the street offered him $100 but also wanted to get high. Kevin bought him $100 worth of crank, but told the man it was worth $200 in order to pocket $100 for himself. The customer then wanted another woman to join them, so Kevin found a woman working the street. Kevin told her that she would receive $100 while telling the customer that she cost $200, allowing Kevin to pocket another $100. The customer then wanted $100 in liquor, so Kevin bought $20 worth in order to keep another $80 for himself. Swiftly stealing more money from the customer, Kevin returned to his friends' hotel room to find that they had left. Then he returned to the customer and the woman: "So I was ready to go ahead and do what I had to do, but she wanted to get totally undressed and dance around the room. So he wanted me to get totally undressed, but I couldn't . . . and still be a woman. So I told him I couldn't do that, [but] that I could go ahead and do what I had to do, so he said no; he wanted me to dance like she was." Kevin tried to leave the room, but the customer said he would kill Kevin if he tried to do so. Kevin "turned around to cuss him out" and was shot. Kevin woke up with four bullets in him.

His brother came to visit him in the hospital "crying and all this shit," so Kevin told his brother to get his money and clothes from the hotel room.

> He went to the hotel, [stole] my money and [stole] my clothes, and came and told me that he didn't get nothing [from the hotel room]. . . . So my brother came in, and he said, "Well, you need to get up off your ass and start trying to walk, 'cause we ain't going have nobody wipe your ass for the rest of your life. . . ." So after then, my brother never did come back to the hospital. After he found I was walking a little bit, he never came back to the hospital. So then they got ready to discharge me. They didn't know that my brother had a place, or what I was going to do, so they called my mama, and she said I could come home.

Kevin explained that he was very upset that his brother betrayed his trust by taking his money and clothes and, more important, by not returning to the hospital.

ROB

Rob was the youngest of four children. He was very close to his brother, who died in a car crash when Rob was nineteen. His parents were not married, but he was able to see his father a lot because they lived in the same midsized North Carolina town. His father, a brick mason and an alcoholic, was not allowed in his mother's house. His mother was a house cleaner. He reported that his father, who died when Rob was thirteen, used to try to beat up his mother, but "my mama whoop his butt, more than he whooped her." Rob said that his parents were very loving toward him, and that his mother worked very hard.

As a child, Rob liked playing softball, baseball, and football and going to the park: "We used to go down to the swimming pool. We used to clean the swimming pool up and stuff and stay at the swimming pool all day and go home in the evening and then go play softball or play baseball. You know how you have Little League baseball. We would go get our uniforms on and go play baseball. We had a good time, you know. . . . This was all at the park, man, I'm telling you."

Rob also enjoyed the freedom of making his own way in life: "We used to go sell pecans and stuff. We always had a little positive thing going on. We would go out there early and make a little hustle, go sell pecans, during Christmas-time mistletoe; summertime, everybody had bicycles in the neighborhood. We used to go and, you know, they were tearing down houses; go get copper and sell copper, so that was a little change in our pocket. Yeah, we kept money in our pockets."

SAM

Sam was in a rural Pennsylvania town until age six, when he moved to a small North Carolina town. Sam described his childhood community as "hell without a fire." Sam's parents were not married; his father was an "alcoholic," and his mother "drank a lot." Their house was always run-down, and there was little food. Sam, as the oldest of five children, became the "protector" of his little brothers. At a young age, he began stealing food from grocery stores for his brothers; Sam was later diagnosed with kleptomania. When asked about childhood aspirations, Sam said: "I never made any aspirations for myself. I just made sure that my brothers were okay. I did what I had to do. Made sure that they [my parents] didn't harm them."

About his father, Sam said: "But my father, like I said, was an alcoholic. Sometimes when he sexually abused me, I felt like he didn't. Looking back on it now—I can honestly say that he probably didn't realize I wasn't Mom. Because he was a lot of time disoriented. Does that make sense? He was very vicious. In other words, he should have been neutered before he had children. But I don't love my father. I have no emotions whatsoever towards him. I can't honestly say that I hate him."

His mother would lock the children in the basement when she went out or wanted to be alone. There was no bathroom in the basement, so the children urinated and defecated in the corners of the basement. Sam was sexually assaulted by two male "sitters" when he was young, and he attributes his being gay to that experience. When Sam was asked at what age he knew that he was gay, he responded by saying: "I never knew it was wrong because of the way I was treated as a child. It was programmed. I suffer from, I have been diagnosed as, programmed behavior. It was programmed into me."

When Sam was eight, one of his mother's boyfriends poured kerosene on his little brother and set him on fire. This younger brother was taken out of the family by Social Services and eventually adopted, while the other three children entered separate foster homes. Sam was placed in a home with a Baptist preacher who repeatedly made Sam feel very bad about himself by saying that homosexuality is a sin. In tenth grade Sam realized that not everyone was out to get him, and so he made friends and graduated from high school. Sam also left the foster home as soon as he was able—at age sixteen. Sam further reported:

> My whole life was a traumatic experience. . . . I guess the only thing
> that was good was when I was placed into a children's home, but
> then the molestations occurred there. We were put into a foster
> home, which threatened the hell out of me. I didn't understand that.

You just don't take children and throw them wherever the hell you want to throw them without explaining what's going on, and that's what happened. I resented it. So yes, I was hell on wheels. I sincerely let everybody know not to fuck with me. . . . Peace didn't come to me until I graduated and moved back here; then a whole new trauma began. Now that my sickness is here, I just look at it as a resting period from it all.

Of all his family members, Sam felt closest to his aunt: "My aunt's been more than a mother to me, and I will respect her to this day. We get in our little fights here and there, over my sexuality and shit, but she's always been there because I've talked to her about it."

Sam, unlike most of the participants, frequently used mental health services, where he was diagnosed with posttraumatic stress disorder and was told that his sexuality was "programmed behavior." Sam seemed to work hard to keep his own anger contained. As an adult, Sam both entered into abusive relationships and engaged in violence. He would speak only generally about the "violent organization" in which he and his last partner, who died of HIV, were involved. He reported that he had seen at least one person "seriously injured or violently killed" as part of his involvement with the group. During different interviews, he repeatedly alluded to the group but would then explain that he could say nothing more about it: the group wanted him dead because he knew too much.

Because he loved to watch the force and violence of hurricanes, Sam always remained in his home near the ocean when they hit: "I was running out there at the Sheraton and watching all them boats bang up against each other. Slapped in the face with hard rain and wind. I thought it was a trip. . . . It's my way of looking at God as being a bitch. Personally, I think it's His way of unleashing maybe just a little bit of anger towards us for some of the stupidity that we cause each other, and so I enjoy it because I know that we deserve it."

THESE VIGNETTES ILLUSTRATE a few of the hardships and the joys that participants experienced. When patients walk into a provider's office, they walk in holding all their past experiences in their beings. Yet these memories are almost always hidden from the provider's view.

Chapter 4

Interpretation of the Pre-HIV Histories

If you knew the history of my life, you would shoot dope too.

Did I deserve any of this shit? Am I innately—am I just bad?

INSIGHT INTO THE complex and intricate histories of clients assists policymakers and providers to create accessible systems of care by illuminating the roots of problems and taking the focus away from the symptoms. Current behavior is often a symptom of past events. Health policymakers can utilize life histories to create an infrastructure that takes into account the needs of the population to be served, including support services such as appropriate HIV case management, mental health provision, and substance abuse services. Their understanding can help providers discover new ways to work with patients by increasing patients' trust of formalized services. Providers may become more empathetic to patients' seemingly illogical behavior when they understand the context of that behavior. This understanding may also reduce the feelings of frustration that providers report.

Because so many case study participants experienced childhoods that were marked by chaos, harsh/erratic discipline, benign neglect, abuse, poverty, and deprivation relative to peers, the first part of this chapter reviews the current research on the impact of childhood conditions, particularly trauma and subsequent behavior. The second section revisits the narrative within the context of the reviewed research. Unifying approaches thus allows for a transition to the third section on providers and preliminary health policy implications, which we explore further in the final chapter.

The Literature

SOCIOCULTURAL STATUS, PARENTING/CAREGIVING, AND PEER REJECTION

Childhood experiences influence adolescent and adult behavior. By the age of five, it is possible to predict the likelihood of childhood behavior problems, including hostile and aggressive physical behavior toward others, impulsivity and hyperactivity, and noncompliance with adult and peer limit-setting (Deater-Deckard et al. 1998). Such behaviors in adolescents and young adults can lead to engagement in high-risk activities that increase possibilities for HIV exposure; subsequently these behaviors may also detract from one's ability to adhere to structured medication and service utilization regimens.

Childhood characteristics that predict future behaviors have been divided into four broad categories (Deater-Deckard et al. 1998; fig 4.1). These categories encompass several overlapping, interconnected characteristics that make it difficult to separate and address each one in isolation, but they serve as a good introduction to the effects of childhood experiences and their resulting effects into adulthood. As you read about these characteristics, think back to the lives of the case study participants.

The first category of childhood characteristics that predict future behavior addresses the child's family sociocultural status, including socioeconomic status, child-to-adult ratio, teenage pregnancy, unplanned pregnancy, and stressful life events of the parents (Deater-Deckard et al. 1998; McLoyd 1990). The concept of sociocultural status also relates to race and living environment. As just one of many examples, Howard and colleagues (2000) found large racial differences in mortality rates from accidents, heart disease, diabetes, and homicide and found that much, but not all, the differences were attributable to lower socioeconomic status of blacks.

Others have found that community characteristics, or ecological factors, predict health outcomes above and beyond skin color (see chapter 11 for further discussion of the importance of race). Living in rural areas may create emotional barriers to care and may contribute to the slower recovery from negative childhood experiences. The perception of living in small rural towns is often of calm, moral living, but the case study participants suggest otherwise. Misperceptions that substance abuse and homosexuality are behaviors that do not occur in small southern or rural towns, as well as a misperception that violence and trauma in these areas are not as serious as in urban areas, create a misunderstanding of the patient's situation. In rural towns most people know each other and each others' families; people see each other constantly. The individuals responsible for inducing the trauma, if not actual fam-

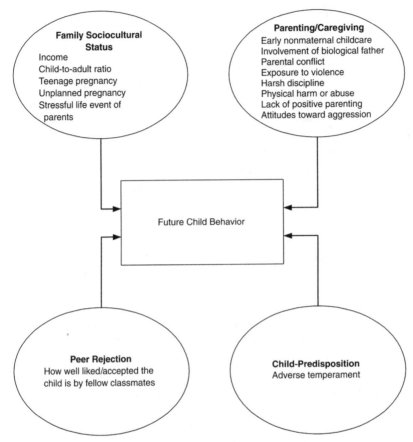

Figure 4.1. Childhood Characteristics Found to Influence Behavior. Source: *Figure Derived Primarily from Deater-Deckard et al., 1998.*

ily members, are often community members; thus, it is difficult and sometimes impossible to fully discuss or escape these interactions without leaving the community.

The second childhood characteristic, parenting/caregiving, covers interpersonal exchanges; these include nonmaternal childcare in early life, involvement of the biological father, parental conflict, exposure to violence, maltreatment, lack of positive parenting, and attitudes toward aggression (Deater-Deckard et al. 1998; Patterson et al. 1989). Failure of caretakers to meet children's basic emotional and psychological needs (including love, belonging, nurturance, and support) have been found to result in adverse adult health outcomes (Walker et al. 1999a; Walker et al. 1995; Heim et al.

2000). Individuals who have experienced childhood maltreatment and a general negative home environment have lower levels of social support as adults from family members and higher levels of distress and parenting stress, all of which result in poor parenting skills (Harmer et al. 1999) and adverse adult health outcomes. Maltreatment includes sexual abuse (sexual contact between a child younger than seventeen and a person at least five years older), physical abuse (bodily assault on a child by an older person that poses a risk of, or results in, injury), emotional abuse (verbal assaults on the child's sense of worth or well-being or any humiliating or demeaning behavior directed toward a child by an older person), physical neglect (failure of caretakers to provide for a child's basic physical needs, including food, shelter, clothing, safety, and health care), and emotional neglect. Adverse outcomes associated with maltreatment include higher rates of physical and mental disability, increased numbers of distressing physical symptoms, and greater numbers of health risk behaviors (Walker et al. 1999a). The adverse relationships remain even when persons who have experienced sexual abuse, which is considered the most severe type of abuse, are not considered.

The third category of characteristics predictive of future behavior is peer rejection, measured by how well-liked and accepted the child is by peers. Peer rejection has been documented even in kindergarten (Deater-Deckard et al. 1998; Parker, Asher 1987). Negative peer interaction and problematic psychosocial adjustment have been found to be rooted in socioeconomic status and may be directly influenced by the primary caregiver's traits. Peer rejection results in bullying and/or being bullied (Nansel et al. 2001).

Experiences of peer relations include episodes of discrimination. Discrimination directed at immutable characteristics with which one is born—such as race, gender, or sexual orientation—tears at one's sense of self-worth. Discrimination can take the form of verbal taunts, acts of hate, or more constant subtle acts that erode people's sense that others can see beyond these exterior characteristics. They fear that others see only the physical characteristics and pass judgment. Such experiences may make it difficult for people to believe that a provider could truly understand them, which may decrease their willingness to explain or advocate for themselves because they believe that no positive outcome can result. Such attitudes may lead to behaviors that providers find irritating or disrespectful. For example, a patient may not call if she is going to miss an appointment because her sense may be that the provider or system does not really acknowledge her existence. Discrimination erodes senses of self-esteem and efficacy. The acts, making the person feel that she has less control in her environment, can cause the person to devalue herself. Persons with a lower sense of self-worth and less ability to control their environments are less likely to engage in health-promoting activities.

African Americans often experience more than isolated incidents of discrimination. They experience repeated acts of violence, verbal harassment combined with "subtle and covert slights, accumulated over months, years and lifetimes, which [have an] impact far more than the sum of individual instances" (Feagin 1991). It may be difficult for white providers to remember that their patients grew up during the time of integration of the school systems and great racial hatred especially in the South. Racism itself may result in diminished health status (Kindig 1997); some theories find racism causes higher levels of hypertension, poor pregnancy outcomes, cancer, and heart disease (Dressler 1991). Dressler also has found a dose effect of darker skin color with greater levels of disease among African Americans, regardless of income.

Experiences with racism as children may directly influence the level of trust that persons of color have within primarily white medical care and social services systems. African Americans are less likely to use appropriate medical care services even when availability of such services, measured in terms of insurance coverage, income, education, and distance, are equal among races, as found in studies of war veterans (served by the Veterans Administration) and Medicare recipients (Gornick et al. 1996; Optenberg et al. 1995). Early positive experiences with persons of other races may indicate that the providers' race will not be important later in life; negative experiences may make the patient more aware of racial differences and increase the potential for distrust.

Research indicates that the race and gender of the provider influences the degree of comfort that the patient has with the provider. Patients in race-concordant relationships with their physicians report that their visits are significantly more participatory (Cooper-Patrick et al. 1999) and, in some studies, have better retention in services (Blank et al. 1994). Although racial physician-patient matching may not be critical over time, such matching may increase initial trust. This possibility is not to say that African American patients who have experienced racism are only comfortable with African American physicians, but it may be easier for them to gain comfort more quickly. Focus groups conducted in the eastern half of North Carolina with African American women concluded that the participants would feel comfortable with white physicians as long as the clinicians were able to listen to them and understand their needs. White clinicians may need to spend more time "proving themselves" to black patients, and black clinicians may have to spend more time proving themselves to white patients.

Just as with race-based discrimination, poorer persons may worry that they are not able to interact positively with a predominately white, middle- to upper-class provider system; after all, the school systems were unable to reach across their poverty. Fears may be heightened in persons who faced socioeconomic status-related discrimination as children. Magnus and Mick (2000) hypothesize that social class concordance with medical providers may be at least as important as race concordance. They argue that emphasis should be placed on recruiting physicians from disadvantaged backgrounds so that they will be better able to relate to and understand their patients. Such matching could increase treatment dialogue between the clinician and the patient and increase treatment adherence.

Not as much research has been conducted concerning experiences of homophobia because it is difficult to obtain adequate and representative sample sizes. Individuals who have sexual relations with others of the same sex are often anxious about seeking medical care for fear of having to divulge the information (Saunders 1999; Ungvarski, Grossman 1999). Such individuals are afraid of negative reactions and consequences from the provider and of breaches in confidentiality (see chapter 9).

The fourth category of childhood characteristics related to adult behavioral difficulties is a child's predisposition to adverse temperament, which includes such characteristics as hyperactivity and irritability (Caspi et al. 1995; Deater-Deckard et al. 1998; Johnson et al. 1999; Rothbart, Bates 1997; Rubin et al. 1995). Adverse temperament has been measured through observation of the child combined with parental surveys regarding the child's temperament.

People who experience multiple types of childhood maltreatment have the worst self-rated and physician-rated health. When combined, these four measures have been found to explain approximately 35 to 45 percent of the variation in behavior problems. In addition, further studies have found that when a child has three of the four risk categories, approximately 40 percent will have significant conduct problems in the sixth and seventh grades (Dodge 1996). The number jumps to 57 percent when all four risk factors are present.

Effects of Trauma

A traumatic event is defined by the American Psychiatric Association (1994) as an extreme "stressor involving direct personal experience of an event that involves actual or threatened death or serious injury, or other threat to one's physical integrity; or witnessing an event that involves death, injury, or a threat to the physical integrity of another person; or learning about unexpected or violent death, serious harm, or threat of death or injury experienced by a family member or other close associate." Experiencing a traumatic event can have long-lasting effects. Childhood trauma is associated with more risk-taking and aggressive behavior in children and adolescents (Patterson et al. 1989; Cunningham et al. 1994). For example, approximately one-third of adults who experienced childhood trauma, abuse, or neglect suffer from lifetime Post-Traumatic Stress Disorder (PTSD) (Widom 1999), which is estimated to affect 10 percent of the U.S. population (Kessler et al. 1995).

PHYSIOLOGICAL IMPACT OF TRAUMA ON CHILDREN

Recent research indicates that physical childhood trauma can negatively affect brain development (Ito et al. 1998) through long-term effects on the structure of the brain (Bremner 1999; Bremner et al. 1999; Bremner, Narayan 1998; Teicher et al. 1993). Various medical techniques have been used to confirm such structural changes. For example, magnetic resonance imaging (MRI) shows reductions in volume of the hippocampus in victims of childhood abuse with PTSD (Bremner 1999), which may be particularly problematic for individuals because the hippocampus is an area responsible for declarative memory (e.g., recalling recent events or facts) and any structural changes may result in memory deficits. In addition, because the hippocampus is responsible for accurately assessing the degree of danger or threat in a given situation (McEwen et al. 1992; Sapolsky 1996), its decreased ability likewise decreases the ability of a person to react appropriately to danger.

Dysfunction also occurs in the medial prefrontal cortex, which contains the dopaminergic system, one of the most sensitive areas of the brain to even mild stressors (Roth et al. 1988). Dopamine is released by the dopaminergic system in response to stress and serves to calm the brain and body. If the dopaminerigic system is not functioning correctly and a person enters a stressful state, then the person will have difficulty remaining calm or returning to a calm state (Vogt et al. 1992; LeDoux 1993; Devinsky et al. 1995).

Moreover, dysfunction is found in the visual association cortex (Bremner et al. 1999), which mediates the visuospatial processing critical to survival in life-threatening situations (Vogt et al. 1992; Devinsky et al. 1995). The excessive vigilance seen in persons with PTSD may be associated with increased demands on brain areas involved in visuospatial aspects of memory function and immediate response to potentially threatening stimuli (Bremner et al. 1999).

Women with a history of childhood sexual abuse have dysfunction in several parts of the brain (Bremner et al. 1999). Similarly, Heim and colleagues (2000) found that women who had experienced childhood physical or sexual abuse reacted to stressful situations with as much as a sixfold increase in the adrenocorticotropic hormone that regulates stress when compared to women who had not experienced abuse. Patients with lesions in the medial prefrontal cortex show dysfunction of normal emotions, which causes an inability to relate to others in social situations that require correct interpretation of the emotional expressions of others (Damasio et al. 1994). Furthermore, animals with damage in this area are not able to stop their fear response following a stressful situation (Devinsky et al. 1995).

IMPACT OF TRAUMA ON ENGAGEMENT IN RISK-TAKING BEHAVIOR AND ON GENERAL HEALTH STATUS

Childhood trauma, including abusive discipline, has been directly linked to greater HIV-related risk behaviors such as substance abuse and unintended pregnancy (in both adolescence and adulthood) as well as homelessness (Adams, East 1999; Dietz et al. 1999; Goodman et al. 1997). Substance use and abuse act as forms of self-medication for the PTSD-related symptoms, such as heightened and chronic anxiety. The rate of HIV infection among trauma victims of violence and accidents was found to be high (Tardiff et al. 1998).

Past sexual and physical abuse history, often in childhood, in adults of both genders and different races is predictive of increased sexually transmitted diseases, risky sexual behavior (e.g., unprotected sexual intercourse, multiple partners), likelihood of having a partner who is physically abusive (especially when he is asked to use a condom), substance abuse, use of alcohol, and needle sharing (Duncan et al. 1996; Lenderking et al. 1997; Bartholow et al. 1994; Wingood, DiClemente 1997, 1998; Thompson et al. 1997; Strathdee et al. 1997; He et al. 1998; El-Bassel et al. 1998; Epstein et al. 1998). A large proportion of intravenous drug users have experienced childhood trauma and abuse (Clarke et al. 1999). Additionally, witnessing domestic or community violence as a child significantly predicts post-traumatic stress disorder, which then leads to higher risk taking in adulthood (Kilpatrick et al. 1997; Ensink et al. 1997).

For HIV-positive persons, engaging in continual substance abuse can further damage the immune system, while the use of unclean needles and engagement in unsafe sexual practices can infect the person with different strains of HIV, which causes still further health declines. Other plausible, but not tested, risk-taking behaviors may include nonadherence to medications or routine ID clinic appointments.

Although extensive literature shows the detrimental impact of trauma in a variety of populations (Felitti et al. 1998; Springs, Friedrich 1992; Leserman et al. 1996), few studies have examined the health effects of trauma on HIV infection. One study found that HIV-infected women with sexual or physical abuse histories reported more physical symptoms and were diagnosed with higher rates of AIDS-defining conditions than nonvictims (Kimerling et al. 1999). Sexual and physical abuse have also been related to more psychological distress and consequently poorer quality of life among HIV-infected samples (Kimerling et al. 1999; Bartholow et al. 1994; Harlow 1998).

There is a growing literature documenting the negative impact of sexual and physical abuse and other trauma on health status, particularly in female populations. Women who experience four or more types of abuse during childhood are one and one-half times more likely to have an unintended first pregnancy in adulthood (Dietz et al. 1999). Among low-income, HIV-infected urban women, childhood sexual abuse predicts adult drug use, assault, and prostitution, while childhood physical abuse leads to alcoholism and physical assault (Goodman, Fallot 1998). Adverse childhood events most strongly predicted future physical illness (Andrews et al. 1978). Women with sexual and/or physical abuse histories have been reported to have more current functional disability (Leserman et al. 1996; Scarinci et al. 1994; Golding 1994), somatic symptoms (Scarinci et al. 1994; Golding 1994; Walker et al. 1995; Felitti 1991; Springs, Friedrich 1992; Briere, Runtz, 1988; Moeller et al. 1993; Walling et al. 1994; Drossman et al. 1990; Lechner et al. 1993; Leserman et al. 1998), pain (Leserman et al. 1996; Golding 1994), and psychiatric illness (Scarinci et al. 1994; Walker et al. 1995; Browne, Finkelhor 1986).

With respect to dollar costs, women who report any childhood abuse or neglect have been found to have median annual health care costs that are $97 higher than those who do not experience maltreatment, and women who report childhood sexual abuse have median annual health care costs that are $245 greater than those who do not report abuse (Walker et al. 1999b). Persons who experienced childhood abuse are more likely to have PTSD in adulthood as well as other personality disorders (Johnson et al. 1999).

In one of the few studies examining abuse and other childhood trauma in a large representative sample of both male and female HMO patients, Felitti and colleagues (1998) reported that those with more adverse childhood experiences were at greater risk for diseases such as heart disease, cancer, and chronic lung diseases (Bartholow et al. 1994). Adverse experiences during childhood included sexual, physical, and psychological abuse and household dysfunction (e.g., substance abuse, mental illness, violence, or criminal behavior by someone in the childhood home).

IMPACT OF TRAUMA ON SERVICE UTILIZATION

Experiences of trauma increase health services utilization (Hidalgo, Davidson 2000). Conversely, adults who have had histories of severe childhood trauma have been shown to have difficulty with interpersonal trust. Lack of trust is associated directly with decreased health service utilization (McCracken et al. 1997) so that health services are sought only on an urgent-need basis. Lack of trust inhibits a patient's ability to form close social support systems (Saunders, Edelson 1999). Fewer social supports in turn further decrease the likelihood of a patient's attending to both medical appointments and medication regimens (Fahs et al. 1994; Penning 1995). These individuals, who may also have more difficulty in trusting their case managers and their clinicians, may be the very people who most need supportive relationships.

In non-HIV-positive adult samples, both childhood and adult trauma are independently associated with greater utilization of mental and physical health services and hospitalizations (Bartholow et al. 1994; Switzer et al. 1999). Salmon and Calderbank (1996) found that childhood abuse was related to a greater number of hospital admissions and surgical procedures in college students. In a study of HMO patients, Sansone and colleagues (1998) also found a significant relationship between five types of trauma (sexual, physical, and emotional abuse; physical neglect; witnessing violence) and increased telephone contacts with physicians, physician visits, ongoing pre-scriptions, and acute prescriptions. Furthermore, abuse symptoms (i.e., chronic depression, sexual compulsivity, revictimization, and substance abuse) block potential effects of HIV education and intervention (Allers et al. 1992).

The Participants and the Raw Numbers

A standard Traumatic Events Checklist (see appendix C), measuring incidents of traumatic experiences, was added to the interviews because of the strikingly high number of reports of such events being disclosed during the case studies. These include experiences of rape, other physical trauma, seeing physical abuse, seeing someone killed, death of a parent or loved one, verbal abuse, and witnessing family-specific violence. The twenty-four participants who completed all the interviews retold more than 175 traumatic events. (Joanna did not complete the final interview and so is not included in the tally.) These events were categorized into the Events Checklist. A participant may have experienced more than one event in a category (for example, more than one rape as a child), but these multiple incidents are included in the Events Checklist as one event. Condensing the experiences resulted in 166 events. Each of the five women who were sexually assaulted or raped as children were also assaulted or raped as adults. All but one of the participants who were physically abused or assaulted as children (ten of eleven) were physically abused or assaulted as adults. Twelve of the fourteen participants who reported assault or abuse by a partner in their adult life had also either been assaulted, raped, or witnessed family violence as a child. As defined by this instrument, twenty-one of the twenty-five interviewees described events that would be considered traumatic childhood experiences.

In terms of caregiving and child/adult relationships, six of the twenty-five respondents were raised in two-parent homes, while the other nineteen participants were raised by single parents, other relatives, institutions, and/or foster families. Thirteen of the participants spoke of caregivers who abused alcohol or other drugs. As children, fifteen of the participants experienced the death of or permanent separation from a parent or someone like a parent before the age of eighteen. Almost half, eleven participants, experienced physical assault or abuse as children. Thirteen witnessed people hitting or harming one another in their family while growing up. Thirteen had seen someone seriously injured or violently killed, and all but four of the participants witnessed someone being physically assaulted or abused outside the home. Nineteen experienced the death of a spouse, partner, or loved one. Fourteen had been physically assaulted or abused by a partner (nine of the women and five of the men). Fifteen had experienced a natural disaster (usually a hurricane) that the participant felt was traumatic (although one participant reported that he enjoyed violent hurricanes). White participants experienced a mean of one more trauma category compared to African American participants (7.4 versus 6.6). Men and women experienced similar levels of traumatic events (6.8 and 6.9, respectively).

When asked to list "other traumatic experiences," less than half reported that being diagnosed with HIV was a traumatic event; men were more likely than women to report their HIV diagnosis as being traumatic (six men vs. two women). Other studies of persons with life-threatening diseases, such as cancer, found that the patients usually include their diagnoses on the traumatic events checklist. This lack of perceived trauma among interviewees, given all the other trauma, may be integral in determining the importance, or lack thereof, that HIV plays in the lives of patients.

Most events formally reported during the final interview, using the list of traumatic experiences, had already been discussed throughout the interviews. An exceptional category was rape or sexual assault as children: only one male participant told of sexual abuse as a child during the interview sessions. However, when using the Events Checklist, five of the twelve male participants stated that they had been raped or sexually assaulted as children. This increased reporting may be a result of multiple interview sessions with the same person for a total of six to eight hours spent talking together. At the time the list was read, the participants were asked if they wished to elaborate on the traumatic events that had not been mentioned previously; the four who had not previously mentioned the childhood and sexual abuse stated that they would rather not elaborate.

In contrast, during the general interview, five women recounted times when they had been raped or sexually assaulted during childhood, but, when asked in the checklist format, one did not want to answer the direct question, and another did not list a previously mentioned sexual assault. The latter woman may have interpreted sexual assault as implying penetration, which she had said did not occur. The gender-specific reporting styles, particularly for the question of rape or sexual assault, may have implications for how related survey tools are used in the future. Although the sample of participants is too small to conduct statistical tests, no trend differences in average number of events emerged between men and women. Women reported on average 6.9 event categories (of fifteen possible categories) while men reported a mean of 6.8. The minimum number of traumatic experiences was two, and the maximum was twelve for women and eleven for men.

The Narrative Tapestry

While describing their childhood home lives, the interviewees focused on the most basic human necessities: love, stability, housing, food, and clothing. With the exceptions of Joy, Clark, and Dean, the sociocultural situation of the participants was low, and needs were often just barely met, if at all. The respondents lived in or near poverty for most of their childhood years. Poverty, by placing stress on the parents, may be an indirect cause of some neglect, abuse, and trauma, which concurrently made healing more difficult. Albert remembers, "We were living in a house just back of Granddaddy's. Mother had one of them white kerosene stoves that you cooked on, you know one of those old timey ones that you cooked on and you had a glass container for it. We had to use an outhouse for the bathroom because we didn't have no facilities. The only thing we had, we had to bring waters into the house and all that stuff." Respondents slept in beds with multiple siblings. The participants were often responsible for helping their parents care for their siblings (Amy, Betty, Joni) and with household chores, including gardening before school (Amy, Joni).

Participants lived in houses that were unsafe. Damon's stove exploded, and Bill's house burned down. For participants such as Gina, the neighborhood in which she grew up was "bad, terrible. Lots of gangs, fightin' going on. People gettin' killed on the step where you live at." Some of the individuals moved frequently, creating a feeling of dislocation: either the foster care system required the move, or the participants were forced to move as places were condemned, houses were sold, and rent was unpaid.

Caregiving was also problematic. The stories from childhood are full of instances of parental neglect and abuse; in some cases, the very primary caregivers created traumatic experiences for children. Respondents such as Albert and Lori felt that their caregivers neither loved them nor even liked them.

Small communities and family ties did not provide a network of support for the participants, and, in fact, seemed to exacerbate some problems. Lisa's rapist, for example, was a close family friend, and her husband was incredulous that she could continue to see this "cousin" at family functions and not feel outrage. Lisa explained that she had to let it go because he was family. The story of Amy seeing one of her rapists at the grocery store many years after the event also illustrates the difficulty of experiencing trauma in rural areas where you might continually confront the attacker.

Socioeconomic status, parenting, and location are only some childhood characteristics that increased our participants' likelihood of later engaging in high-risk activities. Discrimination also played a role in defining their lives. Betty stated that "black people stayed in their place, and the white people stayed in their place." Joey, Kevin, and Joni each described growing up in towns where racism was palpable. Although Damon did not report being teased for being gay in high school, Kevin reported chronic episodes of taunting and discrimination due to his sexuality. Sam left his foster family because his foster father constantly told him that he was a sinner for being gay. Other forms of teasing were mentioned in the participant interviews, including negative peer interactions, embarrassment over physical appearances (e.g., Gary's teeth, Lori's weight) and invalidating comments made by the adults (either noncaregiving or parental) around them. Several female respondents had a strong sense that their inability to wash regularly and lack of acceptable clothes caused their peers to ostracize them.

Peer relationships are important predictors of behavioral outcomes, yet few participants spoke of having or maintaining childhood friendships. Among other positive attributes, friends provide a support system outside the family and can help people be accepted in school settings. Some respondents had positive school experiences, such as when Albert won the award and when Bill won the track meet. Betty and Christine found school a welcome relief from chaotic home life, and Dean and Clark both did well in high school. However, other respondents, such as Amy, whose mom frequently made her late to school and who did not have adequate clothes, did not feel supported in the school systems. James, Joanna, Rhonda, and Teri associated junior high and high school with the beginning of their drug use and recalled causing trouble.

Because of the living situation at home, small acts of validation such as gifts made a large impression on some of the respondents. For Joey, it was the five dollars given by a stranger. For Lori, it was a small toy she had in one foster home. The children did not have much so providing what may seem like a small gift left a large impression. Many children did not expect much from their environment. As Joni stated, everybody was poor, but her family was always the poorest.

Other participants recalled positive peer interactions. Amy reported that her only happy memory was shooting marbles with other children. Bill found that being part of a gang protected him from some emotional damage from the surrounding abuse. He said that he "wasn't that intelligent of a speaker" so he had trouble defending himself verbally. When he was picked on in school or beat up, he had people to go to. The gang was Bill's best support system, willing and able to protect him.

The holidays, important happy events for some respondents, were times of respite when the tension was lifted from their lives, if only for a little while. Joanna remembers, "All of our Christmases were good. Thanksgiving was good. Any holiday that came and it pertained to children or family together: ours was good."

In addition, some reported adult caregivers who made a positive impact on the participants' lives. Lisa's close relationship with her aunt was very important to her. The teacher who had believed in Albert gave him a rare feeling of self-worth. Because parents were absent or abusive, simple acts of love created lasting positive memories. Joni, who was raised by her sisters after her mother died, remembered her mother "actually sewing a dress on me." Joanna's father, who was often drunk, demonstrated his love for her by being willing to fight her abusive boyfriend to help her. Grandparents provided love and relief from immediate family situations for Dean, Lisa, and Betty. Betty reported, "My grandmother, she had me spoiled. . . . Everywhere she went I went."

SUPPORT SYSTEMS

Often in the stories of traumatic experiences shared by the participants, the part of the incident that an outside observer might categorize as the worst aspect of the experience did not correspond to the participant's designation as the worst aspect. Angel's mother's refusal to believe Angel's story felt worse than actually being chased by the boyfriend. For Lisa, the puppy's death was worse than the gunfights. Even though Joni's sister knew that her fiancé had raped Joni, she still married the man, which for Joni felt worse than experiencing the rape itself.

Christine felt worse about her neighbor's distrust or lack of affection shown in not allowing her into her house when she arrived at her door, stabbed and bleeding, than she felt about the stabbing itself. For Kevin, his brother stealing his belongings and not returning to the hospital left long-lasting scars. Part of the tragedy of the traumatic events was that they magnified the lack of true support and love in their lives; even when the participants were at their lowest, most injured, and defenseless states, loved ones, friends, or onlookers would not come through for them. That neglect was the participants' greatest shock and loss.

The participants seemed to accept the unexpected and terrible, or at least they could handle the distress, if only they were shown some support and respect. The slow loss of trust in others led the participants to feel unloved; they were not priorities in the lives of those in their support systems.

Adding to the problem of inadequate support systems, death of loved ones was common in the participants' lives. Fifteen of the twenty-four participants who completed the final interview had experienced the deaths of parents, siblings, or caregivers. Eighteen participants shared that as adults they had experienced the death of a close family member or friend owing to drugs, violence, and chronic and acute diseases. As Joey stated simply in one interview, "I have seen a lot of death."

EXPERIENCE WITH SYSTEMS AND PERSONS OF POWER

Through their environment children learn to interact with structured systems and persons in power. The primary large system with which a child interacts is the school, and the most important persons in power for children are the adults in their lives. Experience with systems and power relationships predicts their later interactions with health care services.

Many case study participants experienced abuse, neglect, and trauma at the hands of systems and persons in power. As Sam stated, "My whole life was a traumatic experience." The school systems, where the participants brought their frustrations from home, did not know how to deal with them.

Angel and Lori both had experiences with social services that hurt them more than helped them. Angel's confiding in a social worker about her molestations only worsened the situation. Several participants had their children taken from them by social services. Lori lost custody of her son when she tried to commit suicide. Teri lost custody of her two children when she lived on the streets. Wendy's husband and mother-in-law wrestled her child from her arms, but she did not receive help when she turned to the local sheriff.

While these actions may have been in the best interest of the children, the good intentions do not negate the experiences and emotions the participants felt toward the system, which further complicate their later relationships with any formal power structure.

The traumatic events experienced by the participants would require long periods of physical and emotional treatment. However, in the case of the participants, there was repeatedly no time for healing after an event. As children, participants frequently did not have people to turn to because the traditional support systems were absent or had even caused the trauma. As adults, the traumatic events repeated themselves and often led to more instability and chaos. Sam was the only participant who successfully (measured only in terms of satisfaction and not quality) used mental health services. The other participants lived with their memories of neglect, abuse, and trauma and the possible brain functioning changes that occurred without necessary help.

ANGER AND VIGILANCE

Participants such as Joni, Sam, and Teri expressed a great deal of anger about their childhood injuries. Participants discussed the difficulty of keeping their anger under control on a daily basis. Bill also described how being sexually assaulted as a child influenced him:

> You might say that it affects me because I think about it sometimes and I get disgusted. If I seen somebody do it, I would probably hurt them before I would even go call the cops; I probably would hurt them if I seen somebody else doing it to somebody else's child. Because I know how bad it is. That is something that child is going to think about all their life. It has kind of made me scared of people because I don't know what they are gonna do.

Several participants, such as Joey, expressed the need to heighten awareness of their surroundings because they never knew what would happen next. Angel also explained how her traumatic experiences influenced her daily life: "I always try to be very careful and listen to try to figure out the person that's trying to con me because of living with one for so long. I guess that's one thing that is really, I guess, still really strong. I don't want anybody to try to pull anything over [on] me. . . . I don't know how to explain it."

Sam reported similar feelings to Angel's; he said that he would never again get close to an individual: "There's always that part of myself that I'll always reserve for myself because it keeps me from being hurt." He said that, on occasion, he lets that barrier down but usually with the wrong person. Sam further reported that, while he does not intend to hurt people, he sometimes is accused of trying to hurt others because he isolates himself; then he will not harm them verbally: "I figure if I keep my distance, then I can judge and can't hurt."

Damon has not tried to kill himself, but he does engage in periods of self-harm. During those times of anger and frustration he does not eat, drinks lots of liquor, and smokes cigarettes: "I don't know, sometimes I just go through it. I don't know if it's inner side, suicide or just I don't want to be bothered; it's my way out from you all, leave me alone." Many female participants had attempted suicide as teenagers and young adults.

In light of the past experiences and the participants' expressed desire to control emotions that arise from the past, it is possible that the participants' high rates of past substance abuse were types of self-medication to help forget the past, reduce chronic feelings of anxiety, and deal with the present. Researchers have found that illicit drugs temporarily decrease feelings of anxiety resulting from past abuse and trauma. Teri stated that she used drugs to deal with her mother's death, while Christine was provided illicit drugs by neighbors to help her cope with the death of her son.

SHUTTING DOWN

Damon had bouts of indecision that he ascribes to the violence that he has experienced:

> [In] life, which way to go. One be right, the other be wrong, but I
> didn't want to do half right, half wrong. Tired of this, sick of that. I
> didn't know which way to go. Every time I go a way, it was the wrong
> way, so I just stood there, stood there in time, folded in light, didn't
> know what to do, and everything just shut down. I just, like
> everything, everyday, everything else, walking around like everyday
> was Monday . . . didn't know when my head hurt, didn't know when
> I was hungry, just shut down.

Several participants reported that they avoid talking or thinking about the events. As Angel said:

> I try not to get too deep on the subject because it's just, it brings up
> stuff I try not to. I mean, really, I could really sit down and tell you
> inch for inch about my life completely, but I try not to dig in little
> details because it really makes the aggression that I'm already [feeling
> come up]. Last couple of months I been more demanding on things my
> way. I want, I want to be the boss. I want to be in control and I've
> been tryin' to do two households. And if I dig in my past then that
> makes it worse because it makes me a little bit ill and I just—the things
> that people done to me that when I grew up, I'm out for revenge.

In summary, socioeconomic and cultural status, one's care as a child, peer rejection, and child predisposition influence one's likelihood of participating in high-risk activities later in life; some high-risk behaviors, such as intravenous drug use, put one at risk of exposure to HIV. When HIV is contracted, the ability to engage in structured and continuous care, as is necessary with HIV, is deeply influenced by these particular childhood experiences. HIV-positive patients with negative childhood experiences are more likely to live chaotic lives; have difficulty trusting others, which might include doctors, insurance companies, case managers, and medications; have additional medical complications; and have a need for mental health counseling. Childhood experiences of an adult patient therefore are relevant to disease treatment if our goal is to promote good health habits.

Relevance to Providers and Policymakers

Several environmental factors should be taken into consideration when formulating and applying policy. In meeting their case managers, mental health professionals, and substance abuse counselors, patients bring with them a host of past experiences. Because childhood experiences have the greatest long-term impact by teaching us how to judge and interact with our environment, personal histories are particularly important. Only when these issues are factored in can policies and care moderate the internal decision-making process, service use, and adherence; thus, ultimately childhood experiences influence patients' health status and engagement in high-risk behaviors. Directly influencing the environmental realm means supporting and enacting changes inside and outside the health care field: educational, family, and community interventions.

Past literature has shown that the number of years of formal education is often a significant predictor of health care utilization and outcomes (Powell-Griner et al. 1999; McManus et al. 1990; Rask et al. 1994; Roberts et al. 1997; Scholer et al. 1999). In analyses even when income is controlled for (education is often assumed to act as a proxy for income), schooling is still frequently a significant determinant of health status and related behavior (Evans et al. 1994; Wilkinson 1992). Researchers often assume that the dependent relation between education and health care utilization corresponds to educational achievement; this dependence signifies the degrees to which patients are inquisitive about their health and can learn from educational materials. Evidence supporting this theory is, however, mixed. Some studies find that health education presented to patients in a way appropriate for their literacy level is effective in changing their behavior (Chesson et al. 1998), while other findings show that such educational techniques are still not able to change behavior (Moon et al. 1998; Powell et al. 2000). One randomized study conducted in a low-income clinic using a pictorial health education message (versus a written sheet) found no difference in recall of information (Powell et al. 2000).

We put forth a supplemental theory concerning the role of education in service utilization: school experiences predict how the individuals feel about structured systems and influence their techniques for interacting with such structures in the future. Drawing from individuals' past experiences with institutions, we find that their longest and most consistent interaction with formal systems of care is within schools. The framework of the classroom teaches the individual about the trustworthiness of large social structures. Through peer and adult interactions, children may see school as a place for growth and learning. Positive experiences with authority figures representing formal systems may make individuals more inclined to trust others, such as physicians, case managers, social service providers, or government agents. Conversely, children may learn that such systems can neither understand nor handle their complicated lives and emotions, thereby creating a feeling of being outside the formal structure. Because the degree to which children are welcomed and understood may set their expectations for later experiences with social services or health care systems, those who did not complete high school, which indicates a negative experience, may have less effective use of service systems.

Other confounding factors may complicate an individual's engagement in the school system and subsequently later regimented schedules. Family life, childhood trauma, and peer relations all influence a child's successful completion of education and a positive perspective on structured systems. The more difficult the individual's home life, the more likely it is that the individual will not finish high school. For individuals who grow up in families whose daily lives are characterized by trauma and chaos, having completed or not completed high school may indicate only the skill to maintain a routine through difficult situations, not the person's ability to comprehend a health education message. Additionally, if family members did not graduate from high school or if education is not highly valued, then the motivation to graduate while living in a stressful environment may make it too arduous for a child to attempt graduation.

Outside the home, peer relations and community serve as significant factors as well. The degree of acceptance and belonging predicts the student's development of self-esteem, interpersonal skills, and possibly integration or satisfaction with society. Experiences of negative peer relationships, such as past incidents of discrimination, affect how clients approach interactions.

Perhaps most significant is the role of trauma in a patient's life, which may cause complications in the above-mentioned areas. Research already shows that traumatic experiences, particularly sexual abuse, lead to increased high-risk behavior. The literature also indicates that childhood and adult trauma negatively influence a person's ability to function effectively in families, groups, and society and to negotiate complex systems (Himelein et al. 1994); Alexander, Lupfer 1987). Because trauma and abuse influence mutable personal and behavioral characteristics, health status, and internal decision-making processes, the authors hypothesize that childhood and adult trauma decrease utilization of health services and adherence to medications. Substance abuse, often associated with trauma, may be a coping mechanism for individuals who see no other way for experiencing pleasure in life. The literature indicates that persons dually diagnosed with addictive and mental disorders experience high rates of hospitalizations (Drake, Wallach 1989).

REVIEWING THE COHORT IN LIGHT OF THE RESEARCH

In a nationally representative survey of persons living with HIV in the United States 25 percent had not completed high school (Zierler et al. 2000). Nine of the twenty-four case study participants for whom we have education information did not finish high school (38 percent). The low levels of education already put the participants at risk for poor health outcomes because of reduced earning potential, educational messages not geared toward lower reading levels, and the patient's poor interactions with past systems.

In our study we documented an average of seven traumatic events per person. This rate of trauma raises concerns about its effects particularly given that the sample of participants comes from a population of rural-living, HIV-positive people, who, having HIV case managers, were already engaged in a system of care and were willing to talk about themselves. The number of traumatic events per individual in this study leads us to believe that this statistic is conservative and that those representing the new wave of the HIV epidemic, including those who would not feel comfortable talking about themselves, experience much more trauma than we have previously realized.

Possible Interventions

Without detailed life histories, providers do not know which of their clients have experienced discrimination, difficult school years, difficult home lives, or trauma. Given time constraints on practitioners, it may be prudent to treat all patients as if they had experienced difficult childhoods and faced great discrimination. Although the participants may appear to be of the same ethnicity, race, gender, or nationality as the providers, the health care worker may have to make an extra effort to prove to their patients that they are able to understand, respect, and address their concerns. Providers should not expect patients with these experiences to volunteer their concerns or desires even as they relate to treatment structures; training may be needed to help clinicians act in a way that elicits the best response from patients. Providing medical students with opportunities to work extensively with disenfranchised populations both in the hospital and throughout their communities, in clinical and social settings, could further increase understanding.

In addition the authors hypothesize that recruiting more physicians from less advantaged backgrounds would improve access to health care. Using similar reasoning, Magnus and Mick (2000) argue that affirmative action in medical schools should be extended to account for social class as well as race. Training programs have been demonstrated to be effective for physicians to learn and improve their interpersonal skills (Curtis et al. 1999) It is important to remember that providers include not only physicians but also case managers, substance abuse counselors, mental health counselors, and nurses, among others.

Adequate services to aid people in finding healthy ways of coping are supposed to be available, but we find that the existence and accessibility of such services are limited in resource-poor rural areas. The only mental health services available for poor individuals are from the county mental health centers, but the staff counselors are often not trained in HIV-specific issues. Even basic knowledge is lacking: they cannot explain how the virus is spread, let alone summon the necessary unique skills needed to provide adequate counseling. Furthermore, they are not trained in PTSD care or issues of substance abuse unless the counselors themselves decide to further study this area. Obtaining mental health services elsewhere becomes problematic because North Carolina Medicaid will only pay for mental health services provided by the county mental health centers or a physician. As part of our work in North Carolina, we have documented more than twenty cases where the Medicaid-funded mental health system has either failed to admit or created barriers specific to persons with HIV. Mental health professionals can use both prescription medications (Heim et al. 2000) and therapeutic approaches that have been shown effective in improving, for example, anxiety disorders and post-traumatic stress disorder (Foa et al. 2000). In addition, clients often hesitate to use mental health services because not only are the staff members living in their communities but clients also perceive the stigma related to mental health needs. With proper training, mental health service providers could offer PTSD therapy by structuring care in a way that best facilitates utilization by people who have experienced trauma. Such a system would provide treatment for PTSD and other mental health counseling, which has proven effective at lessening signs and symptoms (Foa et al. 2000).

A new model of care for HIV-positive people who have PTSD and are active substance abusers is being tested at Boston University (SAMHSA, HRSA, NIH 2000). The outcome measures being examined are cost, adherence to medications, and health outcomes. Similar studies are being conducted at seven other sites around the country, including North Carolina, to evaluate integrated HIV medical care, mental health counseling, and substance abuse treatment. If the studies find positive outcomes, policymakers should consider funding and actively promoting such integrated models, particularly in light of research showing that appropriate mental health service utilization reduces costs of care (Gabbard et al. 1997), improves health status, decreases stress (Mulder et al. 1994), and increases medication adherence (Kelly, Scott 1990). Furthermore, integrated treatment is effective when provided in HIV primary care settings in urban areas or in other integrated care delivery formats (Drake et al. 1996; Osher 1996).

Directly influencing the environmental realm means supporting and enacting changes outside the health care field such as promoting good relationships through community, family, and educational interventions. The Conduct Problems Prevention Group has initiated a ten-year study of children who are at high risk for conduct problems. The program encourages peer relationships by matching high-risk children with "cool" children, provides mentoring though an intensive long-term tutoring program that also decreases the likelihood of school failure, and works with parents to improve parenting skills (Conduct Problems Prevention Research Group 1999). The intervention is proving effective at reducing conduct problems; we would hypothesize that similar programs could reduce chances of HIV infection and increase health promotion activities. Because many of our participants were not encouraged to engage in schools or to seek regular health care, prevention of trauma should include working with parents to build their own self-esteem and teaching parents how to talk with teachers or doctors; that is, we must focus on the family unit as well as the school system.

HIV did not occur in the case study participants as isolated negative experiences. Any combination of childhood trauma, familial complications, or peer conflicts led to infection and continues to influence health care behaviors. For policymakers and practitioners, the goal is to create a system that is flexible and patient enough to care for all the needs of the individual by recognizing the interplay that experience and emergent behaviors have with each other. This recognition means looking at all aspects of system structures and care, providing both postdiagnosis and prediagnosis interventions and, most important, treating each individual's concerns with understanding and respect.

Part III

Life Following the HIV Diagnosis

Chapter 5   Enter HIV

*[HIV is] like a death sentence, but it brings
some good out of it. You don't actually start
living until you find out you got the virus.*

*You've got one foot in the casket and the
other foot on a banana peel.*

It's just icing on the cake.

The HIV DIAGNOSIS IS one event in the continuum of the HIV-positive person's life. As we learned in chapters 3 and 4, the life course preceding their diagnosis for many participants was difficult. Many of their lives were filled with loss, pain, and violence. As predicted by previous research on human behavior, participants with difficult childhoods often entered into abusive adult relationships, were abusive toward others, used and abused drugs (possibly as a form of self-medication), lived on the streets or in substandard housing, and lost custody of their children. Yet they survived it all, even finding moments of happiness. Into this life mix comes a deadly player: the Human Immunodeficiency Virus.

This chapter explores the entry of HIV into the participants' lives. Participants share both the circumstances surrounding their diagnosis and how they learned to live with the disease. We begin with a review of the literature related to how people react to their HIV diagnosis and the impact of their reaction on health outcomes, including disease progression. Most of the literature comes from urban settings because few studies have been conducted on coping with HIV in rural areas, and nothing targets the South.

Literature

For many people, being told that they are HIV-positive is completely unexpected; others may have guessed that they had HIV, but testing positive was still a shock. In the first wave of the epidemic, an HIV diagnosis was a relatively quick but painful death sentence, allowing for an approximated six months to live (Schiltz, Sandfort 2000). Now, in part due to new HIV therapies, earlier detection and a possibly less virulent strain of the virus, the life expectancies of people living with HIV have been extended. HIV changed from a quickly crippling disease to a chronic, manageable disease (Deeks et al. 1997; Freedberg et al. 1998; Marwick 1998; Palella et al. 1998; Stephenson 1998). Nevertheless, a diagnosis of HIV is still life-threatening and life-altering. To live, major lifestyle changes must take place—from the food one eats to the relationships in which one engages (e.g., family, friends, and significant others). "The social prognosis may seem as problematic as the medical one" (Adam, Sears 1996).

Initially, these necessary behavioral changes seem so daunting that some HIV clients consider them equivalent to a death sentence (Adams, Sears 1996). However, the way in which the HIV diagnosis is initially relayed to the patient, as well as the follow-up contact and education, can influence the reaction and subsequent behavior of patients. Studies have found that providing a patient with more information and skills-based training (e.g., demonstrating how to properly use a condom or properly clean the equipment needed for injection drug use, such as needles and cotton) strengthens the potential for decreasing risk-taking behavior (Pinkerton et al. 1997).

Participants' HIV Diagnoses

When the participants were interviewed, they had been diagnosed with HIV for about four and a half years. Of the twenty participants for whom we know why they were tested for HIV, seven did not get tested for HIV until they became severely ill, two discovered their HIV status while donating blood, and three women were tested only because they were pregnant and sought prenatal care (table 5.1). Only two of the participants had been tested regularly. When participants were asked whether they suspected that they were HIV-positive before receiving the test result, half said that it had not occurred to them that they might be HIV-positive. Six male and two female participants identified being diagnosed HIV-positive as a traumatic event and/or an important event in their life. What is perhaps striking is that more than half of the participants did not identify their HIV diagnosis as a major event.

Table 5.1
HIV Diagnosis

Client	Mode of HIV Transmission	Age at Diagnosis	Years since Diagnosis	Reason for HIV Diagnostic Test
Albert	Hetero	37	12	Blood donor
Amy	Hetero	35	7	Pregnant
Angel	Hetero/IVDU	22	10	Friend got tested
Betty	IVDU	52	1	Pneumonia
Bill	Hetero/IVDU	Unknown[a]	—	Suggested during regular physical
Brad	Hetero	29	5	Regular doctor's visit
Christine	IVDU	35	8	Unknown[a]
Clark	MSM	42	1	Unknown[a]
Damon	MSM	34	5	Was regularly tested and had a friend with AIDS
Dean	MSM	26	1	Blood donor
Gary	Hetero	28	2	Illness
Gina	Hetero	26 or 32	5–11	Doctor stuck himself with a needle while treating Gina; doctor had her brought back to hospital for testing
James	Hetero/IVDU	Unknown[a]	—	Illness
Joanna	Hetero	36	3	Pneumonia
Joey	IVDU	47	4	Unknown[a]
Joni	IVDU	38–39	4–5	Unknown[a]
Joy	IVDU	35	7	Post-quitting drugs, part of rehabilitation
Kevin	MSM	35	1	Illness
Lisa	Hetero	18	7	Pregnant
Lori	Hetero	26	6	Pregnant
Rhonda	IVDU	40	1	Was tested at the health department and immediately became severely ill
Rob	Hetero/IVDU	38	1	Illness
Sam	MSM	Unknown[a]	—	Illness
Teri	Hetero	38	1	Substance abuse treatment center
Wendy	Hetero	27	3	Unknown[a]

[a]"Unknown" denotes that the authors do not know the age at which the participant was diagnosed or the reason for the participant's diagnostic test.

NOTES: MSM = men who have sex with men. Hetero = heterosexual contact. IVDU = intravenous drug use. Hetero/IVDU = either heterosexual contact or intravenous drug use.

Given their life histories of terrible events, the bland reaction to their HIV diagnosis becomes more understandable.

There was an array of reasons that participants were tested for HIV. When the test results were provided, two of the three pregnant women were asked by their providers to consider abortions, including Amy, who was asked quite forcefully. Amy ultimately decided to have an abortion and asked God to forgive her for her sins because she did not want the baby to be born with HIV.

In retrospect, Gina thought she should have been diagnosed earlier in her lifetime. Her husband was in a car accident and tested for HIV in the hospital. The clinicians encouraged her to be tested also, but she was too scared. She was tested two years later, in 1993, only because a clinician stuck himself with a dirty needle that he had used on her. Knowledge of the needle stick apparently either happened after she left the clinic or the clinician only began to worry about the possibility of HIV after she left: "So then, after that, I had a whole lot of police cars to come in the house . . . and that scared the life out of me because I didn't know what was going on. They told me that I needed to go to the hospital, and they escorted me to the hospital. I thought I had done some kind of crime or something." The manner in which Gina was brought to the hospital for HIV testing and Amy was forced into having an abortion indicates the environment of ignorance in rural communities, where people often react from fear and without understanding the issues of confidentiality and patients' rights.

Several participants reported that they were notified of their HIV status in an unsympathetic manner. Some participants reported simply being left alone after being told, while others were given inadequate information about the virus and its effects. Most participants knew very little about HIV: they believed only that they would soon die, leave their children to grow up alone, and never be close to anyone again. They feared rejection and did not want to share the HIV diagnosis with their family or friends. Some participants were indeed viewed as a "disgrace" to their family once they told their family about being HIV-positive. Most participants were diagnosed just as antiretroviral therapies were slowly coming into the market. Lacking sufficient information to understand the virus's biological mechanisms and the new medications to treat it, participants thought an HIV diagnosis meant immediate death.

When diagnosed, Joni did not know what to do with herself because she knew little about the disease and was not told much at the time of diagnosis. She became very depressed and was "waiting to drop dead." Similarly, Joanna smoked an eight-ball of cocaine after being diagnosed "because when I heard 'AIDS,' I said 'Okay, I fixin' to die, so I'm going out like I want to go out.'" Even when providers take the time to talk with clients about their diagnosis, clients are often in a state of shock or rage, and they cannot comprehend, as Angel explained:

> I was twenty-two [years old], and I just felt like, you know, my life is
> over, I really did. I just felt like that any time I was gonna get sick
> and die. . . . I had no idea. . . . I found out through the health
> department, and they gave me a free test and counseled me at the
> time, you know, which wasn't much help, but I'm not sayin' it

wasn't—that it was their fault. It's just that, you know, when you're twenty-two years old and you find out news like that, you know, I don't think anything can help!

Albert wanted to throw himself off a bridge. Damon stayed in bed for days until he decided he wanted to have sex with someone in order to give that person the virus: "Anybody. I didn't care who it was, because 'Fuck me, you going to die with me.' That was my state of mind that I was going with." Two days after being diagnosed with HIV at the health department, Rhonda went to a school event to run a three-legged race in order to win a prize with her son. Instead, during the race, she collapsed with "full-blown AIDS" and thought that her life was over: "Signed my children over [to my sister], arranged my funeral and everything."

Like Rhonda, people diagnosed with HIV often immediately think of their family's needs, particularly their children's, as Wendy discussed: "When I got diagnosed: big hit, like, in the face. First thing I got thinking about was my kids and what's the future for them, and I been going through it ever since '95." Lori, who was also a mother, continues to perceive a "ten-year limit" on her life: "They said within ten years that is usually when you die. I have been sick for six, so I keep looking for that tenth year."

The magnitude of HIV-related stigma in their small communities caused some participants to feel that they put their very lives at risk when telling others of their HIV status. Some "chose" to live in silence, bearing the burden of HIV alone. When a man pulled a knife on Joey because he was HIV-positive, Joey learned all too well the risks of living in a rural community. "All they care about is you got it. They don't care about how you got it. They don't think about how, but you got it. . . . They just be afraid because you got it. . . . Once you get the stigma on you that you're HIV-positive, you in trouble. . . . I told two of my closest friends; they don't care about that. But shit, people that I don't trust, I don't tell them." Between interviews, Dean was evicted from his apartment because of his HIV status. (While such discrimination may not be legal, few feel sufficiently empowered to bring a lawsuit; see chapter 10.)

Besides feeling pain and despair, people often feel anger when they are diagnosed with HIV. Some interview participants were angry with themselves, while others wanted to lash out at the ones they believed had infected them. When diagnosed, Lisa was enraged with her boyfriend from whom she contracted the virus. Already very upset, with no one to support her, she became more distraught when he told her that she could not tell anyone about her HIV status: "I gotta tell my mama! He said, 'Don't you, don't you tell nobody! She'll hate you for the rest of your life!'"

Fear of rejection and humiliation can stop people from sharing their HIV status. The level of secrecy is particularly high in rural areas, where informal information networks are strong (Heckman et al. 1998a,b; McKinney 1998; see chapter 9). After a while though, some people find ways to rebuild the support network that they need. Social support is associated with feeling less helpless after an HIV diagnosis (van Servellen et al. 1993). Damon educated his family about HIV before telling them of his diagnosis. In time, Damon found his HIV status "a blessing" because it got him off the streets and was a "real nice [reality] check." Being diagnosed with HIV motivated Damon to reexamine his habits and activities, which allowed him to change his lifestyle to live a healthy, stable life.

Adhering to Medical Advice

Due to the advances with antiretroviral medications, people now are truly "living" with HIV and not awaiting death. The change of HIV from an acute disease to a chronic illness has forced many people to rethink their lives and prepare for the life they had once given up on. Clark promotes his new outlook:

> There is a great possibility that this medicine that I take may work, may help me, and just may put it in remission for a while . . . which would be wonderful. I don't want to be reinfected, so I changed my lifestyle. Changed my lifestyle of hanging out. I've started getting proper rest, eating properly—three meals a day. I take good care of myself. I continue my activities as far as going out and socializing, because I feel like that's one of the biggest downfalls you could do is when you withdraw yourself from people.

At the same time, though, the medications also cause numerous types of negative side effects. Christine and Joni spoke of medication side effects, such as skin color changes and bumps on their skin. Other participants spoke of how sick the medications made them feel and how difficult it was to take so many pills so many times per day. Joni describes the physical pain and lethargy that were at times unbearable: "Sometimes I just lay in there like my bones aching. Skin is changing. I got this constant cough. . . . I always got a sinus infection. It is affecting my vision. Seems like my ears hurt. My whole body hurts. I just don't feel well ever, and I told you I stopped taking the pills, right. The pills don't make me feel no better."

While some participants were afraid of the physical changes that they might have to endure as the disease progressed (e.g., the associated pain and unsightliness), others primarily feared that the physical changes would be identifiable to the public as HIV-related. Thus, participants decided on their own what to do with the medication information and advice given by their providers. The fear that others would be able to determine their HIV status by looking at them haunted some participants and influenced some of their health-related behaviors. Joni and Christine were worried that others would notice the visible body changes (that they ascribed to the medications) and figure out that they were HIV-positive, so they stopped taking their medications. As another example, Gina's infectious diseases physician wanted her to lose 130 pounds in order to improve her health. She was fearful, though, of what such a noticeable physical change would mean to people around her:

> I got this theory if you lose all that weight, then everybody is gonna know you are sick because they are going to say, "Ooh, you done lost all that weight; you must be sick with the AIDS virus." That's another reason why I am too skeptical about trying. I guess when I get that mental block out of my head and thinking about what everybody is going to be thinking I'm sick, I probably could lose this weight. That sticks right there in the back of my head.

Instead, she decided to stop seeing the doctor who wanted her to lose weight. Dean had a similar reaction to his own potential weight loss: "I had two friends die of AIDS . . . and I saw the way they changed, how they got real small. I don't want to get small."

The participants did not contact their providers to express their medication- or weight loss-related concerns so that an alternative plan could be made; instead, participants did what they had done all their lives—they tried to interpret the information given to them and then make their own decisions. Their childhood experiences taught them that systems and decision makers are not able to understand their needs and cannot provide useful consultation. Most participants took drug holidays without informing their providers.

Teri was "scared of that disease." It makes her sick to think of what people living with HIV have to go through, and she anticipates a horrible future for herself. "When I go to the clinic, just looking at some people, some people have those big sores. No, I don't want know nothing about it, just let me go through it if I have to go through it."

RURAL SUPPORT

Rural areas are often thought of as being supportive, close environments in which to live. The majority of the case study participants' life histories indicate their families or caretakers were most likely not part of the backbone of the rural communities. They were neither community leaders nor respected by those community leaders. Some families behaved in ways that most likely put them outside the norms set by the community, and others were of the wrong race. For the most part, the participants did not enjoy close peer relationships as children. In addition to weak supports external to the families, many families themselves were dysfunctional structures and so offered little support to their children. The participants, for the most part, had not felt loved, nurtured, or supported by their caregivers. The availability of support networks, particularly given the lack of HIV-specific networks in rural or mid-sized cities in the South, may be as weak as or weaker than that in urban areas. In urban areas, people can divorce themselves from one group and start again with a new group. In rural areas, people cannot move from group to group.

Some participants learned to turn to service and care providers for support after being diagnosed, in part because their families turned against them. Even though participants' family members tried to remain supportive, they showed through their actions that they were still fearful. For example, at a picnic, one participant witnessed her mother bringing out a fresh bag of ice to immediately replace the bag from which the participant had scooped a cup of ice because of fear of spreading the disease through touch. But even when participants felt that their support network was at its worst when family members avoided contact, some found that their situation could and did get worse, such as when their relatives told neighbors and friends about their HIV status. Lori, whose aunt told the community of her HIV status, explained:

> I want to sit on the porch. I couldn't 'cause the people would come by and they say, "She got AIDS," and even after I had [my son] and I started walking and getting out, it was like that. So I'm more of a person that stays secluded in. You don't see me out anymore, I don't party no more. I used to drink, get high. I don't do nothing no more, I just—it's like I'm secluding myself.

Wendy's mother also turned on her. "The only thing she said now with the HIV [is] that she can take my kids over and she can take my possessions and she can control me, and I told her that's not so. She said she [would] go to [the Department of Social Services] and take my kids from me, and I told her she can't do that now." After being diagnosed, Wendy also had a friend going around their town telling people about Wendy's HIV status.

Gina was able to share her HIV status with her family, who rallied around her and wanted to beat up her husband, who gave her the virus. She was actually mad at herself for allowing herself to "catch it." But she said that she mostly stays in denial about her diagnosis: "I told [my brothers] that I wasn't sick at all, which today I still don't believe [that I am HIV-positive]. It is in [my] mind that I don't believe I got it. I just don't look like I'm sick, and I stay in denial about that because sometimes I think they made a mistake or something. But every time I go up there to that doctor's office, I know it is reality, but in my mind, I say no."

Other participants wanted to talk to their families about the effect of HIV on their lives, but they found that the family members avoided the topic. Sometimes, not only did family members and friends turn against the participants, but our participants felt that medical and social service systems also turned against them. Gary noted: "It's shit like [this] that kills us. I got AIDS; they'll rip my child away because I got AIDS, but your parents are sitting there beating the kids every day, and they'll let the kids stay with the parent who's beating them every day."

A REASON TO LIVE

Several participants believed that they are not meant to die, saying that if God meant to kill them, they would be dead already. Instead, being HIV-positive is a reminder to them that they should use their time on earth to benefit others. Christine wanted to help others with HIV and/or substance abuse problems to keep a positive attitude and find services that they need. Christine reported that the only effect HIV had on her life is that it made her tired. Joanna had worked previously as a nurse and said that her work with AIDS patients helped her deal with her HIV status: "They just lay there like there is nothing [else in] the world . . . 'Good gracious! God put you here for a reason, why you gonna lay there and do that? Just let yourself waste away, you ain't trying to help God or nothin' [when you just lay there],' you know."

Some participants found ways to continue with their lives, as if not hindered by their HIV status, such as Lisa: "We just talked to my doctor and asked them for permission to have a baby. And, because my health is doin' excellent and he said if we were gonna have one, it was best to do it now. . . . I said it's time to make a family settled." Lisa wants her daughter, who was five at the time of the interview, to have a sibling to be with and take care of when Lisa passes away. She is afraid to leave her daughter alone in the world, and, in preparation for her death, she wants to have another child.

Several participants noted that HIV had actually prolonged their lives because it caused them to reduce their drug intake and got them off the streets. Betty and Joey noted that most of their old friends from the streets were dead, but that they were still alive due to HIV.

THE MEANING OF HIV AND DEATH

When asked what HIV meant to them today, participants responded in a variety of positive and negative ways.

- "It means that I should not try to hurt no one else knowing that I have this illness." (Amy)
- "Fear of dying. I feel like sometimes I will never have friends." (Wendy)
- "It means you're going to die if you don't do the right thing. Death. Get your insurance ready; you're going to die." (Rhonda)
- Being HIV-positive means being "damned," but because of it "I mean to live. The things I took for granted [previously], I take them more seriously [now]." (Damon)
- "HIV always turns to AIDS. HIV is only HIV for a little while, but when it turns to AIDS, that's when you crapped out." (Joey)
- "It's like a death sentence, but it brings some good out of it. . . . You don't actually start living until you find out you got the virus." (Gary)
- "It's just I've got to take certain amount of drugs every day." (Rob)
- "It's just that I have to be more responsible with things that I do." (Kevin)
- "If I could change anything about HIV and AIDS, I would just have to leave the babies alone. But if you think about HIV and you know in the Bible it says something is going to come to the world that is going to be like the plague spreading, taking everything. I believe to myself that this is the plague because from the time I first heard about it, it has spread so much. This is just something that you have to be able to really deal with . . . you got to be strong." (Joanna)

Most participants noted that, for everyone, death can come in any form, whether from old age, another chronic disease like diabetes, or an accident. With that in mind, some participants were able to focus their lives on what can still be accomplished in life in order to enjoy each day. Gary explained that people living with HIV usually cannot focus 100 percent of their energy on their future: "I will live a couple more [years]. It would be nice to live another five years, but I don't look that far ahead, because like I said, you can go any time: a simple cold, chicken pox, something stupid that [my son] is gonna give me."

WITH THE DIAGNOSIS of HIV, a new relationship with the health care system is formed. Even though we are entering the third decade of the AIDS epidemic, people continue to experience gaps in education, support, and guidance related to their HIV diagnosis. Sometimes patients, unaware that they are being tested for HIV, are abruptly given the news that they are HIV-positive. In some instances, participants were notified of their HIV status without being given information on either current available treatment or prevention of secondary transmission and infection. The case study participants were linked with HIV case managers, but the referral process is long, and, as we show in chapter 10, even HIV case managers lack substantive HIV training and are often not aware of available local resources for HIV-positive persons.

Educational trainings have revealed that many health departments and mental health centers in the South have minimal HIV knowledge and maintain stereotypes about transmission and care that were seen in urban areas in the 1980s (Whetten-Goldstein et al. 2001a). These public health centers often serve as individuals' first contact with HIV-related care and, as such, can influence how people cope with discontinuity in the health care system. After notification of an HIV-positive status, people may feel cheated out of a long, healthy life, while others feel guilty. Some patients have thoughts of suicide after being told of their status, while some want to spread the disease to others out of anger at having been infected. Adequate support and counseling systems are critical.

A large proportion of HIV tests are performed in local health departments and in private physician offices. In rural areas, there must be more basic HIV training and information on how to give the diagnosis to the patient, counsel the patient on issues related to childbearing and risk reduction, and activate immediate support systems.

In rural communities, people living with HIV may want to leave their family and friends; they believe that they will be ostracized from an entire network because being HIV-positive is considered taboo or a sin. Given the ignorance about HIV in their neighborhoods, they may feel obligated to hide their status and may avoid seeking care or support so as not to risk their confidentiality. HIV case managers report anecdotally that patients have refused case management because their communities know who the case managers are and what their job means. Neighbors assume that if the HIV case manager or her car is seen at a person's house, then someone in the house is HIV-positive. Clinicians report that patients are also known to hide their medications in unlabeled bottles so that family members will not know what medications are being taken. Sometimes HIV-positive persons will not take their medications with them when they leave the house for fear that people will either know why they take pills or ask about the medications. Social workers in infectious diseases clinics report that, frequently, rural patients immediately throw away HIV-related educational material given to them in the clinics. This perceived and oftentimes actual lack of support and understanding from HIV patients' communities and families can lead to negative physical, mental, and emotional effects for the patients. In chapters 6 and 10, we review the current literature that provides evidence of the positive effects that social support networks can have on patients' mental and emotional status, as well as on their biological markers.

Additionally, some cultural and ethnic beliefs about the disease become barriers to learning how HIV works in the body and what effective treatments exist (Flaskerud, Calvillo 1991; Phillips et al. 1995). For example, some people use herbal remedies because they avoid or cannot access medical treatment (McVea 1997). Although not discussed by the participants, at least one HIV-positive community leader in southern North Carolina is advising HIV-positive persons that HIV medications harm the body and that only herbal medicines can save them.

Coping with HIV

How a person handles the diagnosis psychologically has implications for health outcomes. Individuals cope with illnesses or adverse events differently. Some may try to forget about the illness; that is termed "denial coping." Others may be apathetic about their illness and possibly feel hopeless. Both denial coping and helplessness are associated with faster HIV disease progression (Antoni et al. 1995). Passive coping strategies are predictive of greater immunologic impairment (Ironson et al. 1994). Specifically, denial coping is associated with faster progression to AIDS (Leserman et al. 2000), and active confrontational coping is associated with a lower probability of symptomatic disease progression (Mulder et al. 1995). Furthermore, HIV-infected subjects who became symptomatic after one year have more denial and less fighting spirit (Solano et al. 1993). Alternatively, a person may actively try to understand a disease. Such a person, engaging in "active coping," may look for support networks and resources and try to reinterpret the disease to understand its positive effects on life. Coping with the threat of HIV progression to AIDS by means of active strategies has been associated with less psychological distress, increased life satisfaction, and improved quality of life compared to using passive coping strategies (Carver et al. 1989; Demas et al. 1995; Folkman et al. 1991; Heckman et al. 1997; Leserman et al. 1992; Swindells et al. 1999).

For individuals routinely engaging in high-risk behaviors such as substance abuse, an HIV diagnosis may prompt altered behavior in a direction the patient finds more satisfying. The Transtheoretical Stages of Change model posits that as people become more aware of the negative consequences of their behavior, they are more likely to change (Prochaska, DiClemente 1982). A negative life event, such as a disease diagnosis or injury, that is related to a particular behavior is predictive of a reduction in that behavior. This relationship has been found for many types of health-related behaviors, including substance abusers where a specific loss (Blume, Schmaling 1996) or regret for behavior actually reduces substance abuse (Blume, Schmaling 1998) and smokers who quit smoking following diagnosis of an acute health condition (Carosella et al. 1999). Specific to an HIV diagnosis among gay and bisexual men, suicide ideation and attempt following diagnosis have been found to provoke a process of coping with HIV disease (Siegel, Meyer 1999). Their coping included redefining the meaning of HIV, enhancing their sense of control over life, promoting a renewed effort at self-help, seeking a new commitment to life, and reappraising their personal goals.

A qualitative study of HIV seropositive and seronegative injecting drug users indicated that the most common styles of coping were seeking social support, substance abuse, and mental disengagement (Demas et al. 1995). Some individuals with HIV have coped by forming positive perceptions of life because of their illness (Carver et al. 1989), turning to religion (Carver et al. 1989; Demas et al. 1995), or utilizing active strategies such as researching new treatment and illness information (Folkman et al. 1991; Heckman et al. 1997). In terms of seeking care, women have been found to initiate HIV-related care later than men (Siegel et al. 1997). Several reasons for such delays have been reported: cognitive distortions of the reality and significance of HIV; paralyzing fear and anxiety about having HIV (i.e., physical symptoms, stigma of HIV/AIDS, and fear of dying from HIV/AIDS); turning to substance abuse to blunt the emotional impact; actively abusing substances; being incarcerated; suffering financial constraints; possessing limited HIV related knowledge; and experiencing problems with medical personnel (Siegel et al. 1997).

Identifying coping mechanisms and their effects on emotional distress is important because of their potential effects on depression and treatment adherence (Caplan et al. 1976). Research on the effects of coping strategies on therapy adherence and risk reduction by HIV infected patients showed that adherence to medications was associated with less avoidant coping, less hopelessness, and more active, problem-based coping (Singh et al. 1999). Additionally, it has been documented that interventions can modify an individual's coping methods and social supports, which can in turn be important elements in altering her psychological health, perceived locus of control, and quality of life (Antoni et al. 1991; Chesney, Folkman 1994; Ell 1986; Fawzy et al. 1989; Hoffman 1991; Kelly et al. 1993; Lutgendorf et al. 1997; Lutgendorf et al. 1998; Mulder et al. 1994; Siegel, Krauss 1991).

Participants expressed a range of coping strategies from denial to active coping. Some participants showed evidence of using HIV to turn their lives around. The HIV diagnosis acted as the pivotal point to enhance the person's readiness to change risk-taking behaviors. Being diagnosed with HIV was a wake-up call signifying that there was one more chance in life to reduce substance abuse and, as we see in chapter 6, to form stronger supportive relationships. For some participants, HIV provided a deeper life meaning.

Care-seeking hiv-positive individuals undergo a series of changes that can affect their perception of themselves and the life that they live. They enter a system of health care and social service that, in rural areas and for the disenfranchised population, is not always friendly, is at times discriminatory, and can be difficult to navigate. Changes to their physical state and lack of energy can exacerbate feelings of being out of control. Having to initiate and maintain a daily routine of taking many medications can add to one's sense of constraint. Envisioning that dramatic changes will occur can accentuate the belief that being HIV-positive is a death sentence because the life that a person has always known is ending and an unknown replacement, without preparation, is beginning. Within this realm policies can be developed to ensure that necessities such as basic HIV information and coping training are immediately available for all individuals who provide care after diagnosing someone with HIV. As well, standards should be developed to maintain confidentiality and enable provision of information regarding local peer and professional support. HIV providers in rural areas must work harder to assist clients in creating supportive networks given the constraints and biases of families and communities; for example, support groups may need to be formed in discreet ways via telephone, for those with access.

Chapter 6

Support Systems

Proposed singles advertisement: "Horny, single, and diseased. Need mate."

Partners, Family, Community, Religion, and Support Groups

GARY'S SUGGESTION FOR a classified ad reflects the difficulty and frustration that HIV-positive persons have in negotiating sexual relationships. This chapter explores post-HIV diagnosis sexual and emotional relationships and support from families, communities, religion, and HIV support groups. Relationships with children are explored separately in chapter 7. Although some HIV-positive people choose to isolate themselves or are isolated from family and friends, many studies document the benefits of social support in mortality and morbidity, psychosocial adaptation, and adherence to treatment (Ell 1996). As a coping strategy, a means to stabilize one's life, or a helping hand, a support system can reduce a person's level of stress. Support systems not only enable people to share the burden of their fears and doubts but also offer patients a wider network of information and greater access to sources of assistance in times of need.

Social support systems may differ for rural-living persons. Communities are small; it is difficult to maintain confidentiality. The stigma of HIV, which can be strong in rural areas (Heckman et al. 1998a,b), and fear of confidentiality may result in HIV-positive persons' either not telling anyone of their HIV status or telling a small and select number of people. Alternatively, a whole community may quickly learn of a person's HIV status and react to the news (Whetten-Goldstein et al. 2001c).

Following a review of the literature, this chapter examines actual support of the case study participants and their potential sources of support identified in the Southeast HIV Patient Survey (SHIPS). In discussing participants' relationships with partners, we examine the emergence of love in the years following their HIV diagnosis. Many studies undertake the study of sexual behaviors preceding and following an HIV diagnosis; few, however, explore the inception of new significant relationships.

Literature

For infected persons to seek support, they must trust that disclosure of their HIV status will not result in further ostracism. Often the primary concern of HIV-positive people is the negative effects the stigma of HIV will have on their children and personal relationships (Demas et al. 1995; Moneyham et al. 1996). While people usually develop support systems that suit their needs, living with a stigmatizing condition that is associated with socially unaccepted behaviors limits an HIV-positive person's choices in creating her support network, particularly in rural areas. HIV-positive persons are concerned that disclosure of their HIV status will result in discrimination and breaches in confidentiality (Moneyham et al. 1996) (see chapter 9).

Strong support networks among persons with chronic diseases can result in positive health outcomes (Stanton, Snider 1993). In addition to providing a greater array of resources to draw from, social support appears to buffer people from potentially pathogenic effects of stressful events (Cohen, Wills 1985; Sorensen et al. 1998). Support systems are associated with behavioral changes such as adherence to medical regimens, successful smoking cessation, and diet changes (Sallis et al. 1987; Stanton, Snider 1993). Social support positively affects self-efficacy, which is correlated with fewer HIV-related, high-risk behaviors (Montoya 1998) and greater use of health services. Additionally, support of friends and family early in the course of HIV has been found to be associated with good coping skills (Brook et al. 1997). The combination of an available social support network and lack of conflict within these networks has been found to be related to healthier psychological status (O'Brien et al. 1993) and higher quality of life (Friedland et al. 1996; Heckman et al. 1997; Pakenham et al. 1994), while poor social networks lead to combined physical and psychiatric illness (Andrews et al. 1978). Furthermore, unsupportive social interactions have been found to increase depression in HIV-positive persons (Ingram et al. 1999).

In a study of HIV-infected gay men Leserman and colleagues (1999) found that less cumulative support is associated with faster disease progression. In a small study of hemophiliac patients, those with less support had faster deterioration in CD4+ lymphocyte counts during a five-year period

(Theorell et al. 1995). In another study with HIV-infected persons, those with low initial CD4+ lymphocyte counts were more likely to become symptomatic after six months if they had less social support (Solano et al. 1993).

Past research does not explore differences in social support networks between rural- and urban-living, male and female, and African American and Caucasian people or how these differences in social support structure might influence HIV progression. Most studies of HIV and social support have been conducted among white men. However, at least one study showed that women living with HIV are less likely than men to seek social support as a means of coping, to be less socially integrated, and to have fewer places and people to turn to for guidance (Catalan et al. 1996).

Partners are an important source of support for patients. HIV-positive people may live with partners whom they were with when they became infected and were diagnosed. Others find significant relationships after their diagnosis with both HIV-positive and -negative people (Adam, Sears 1994a,b). SHIPS found that only 17 percent of the respondents were in steady relationships where they were living with their spouse, partner, or had a regular partner (table 6.1). Yet, maintaining a steady relationship is associated with lower mortality rates and more appropriate utilization of health care services, particularly for men (Stansfeld 1999). Similarly, poor-quality relationships can have negative health effects. For example, major depression is associated with less care from a current partner and an unsatisfactory social support network (Boyce et al. 1998).

Care-seeking people living with HIV are in contact with their case managers, medical clinicians, and other health and service providers who

Table 6.1
Marital Status and Living Situation of Respondents of the Southeast HIV Patient Survey (in percentages)

Marital Status	Percentage
Legally married and living with spouse	9.5
Legally married and not living with spouse	4.4
Living with someone as though married	6.3
Regular partner and not living with the partner	1.3
Widowed	3.5
Separated	4.8
Divorced	14.3
Single and never married	56.3
Living with another adult in the house	43.6
Had multiple living/housing situations in the twelve months prior to the survey	47.9

NOTE: Total N = 555.

offer specific support. This support, however, is limited in its type and quantity. Even within these paid support systems, trust must still be built with the caregivers so that appropriate support can be provided. (We discuss relationships with providers specifically in chapter 11.)

Support of Participants

LOVE, PARTNERS, RELATIONSHIPS

Most case study participants were not married at the time of participation in the study. The initiation or continuation of romantic and sexual relationships and wanting children after being diagnosed with HIV involved some complex issues, including fear of transmission, negotiating safe sex, fear of rejection and discrimination, and changes in levels of sexual desire due to changes in health status (Adam, Sears 1996). On the following pages, nineteen of the case study participants speak about negotiating relationships, partners, and love. We hear first from the women.

AMY (DIAGNOSED WITH HIV SEVEN YEARS EARLIER). Amy has been sexually involved with one person after her diagnosis. She has found having relationships difficult and is never sure how to tell people she has HIV. She worries about infecting people. She also has a hard time connecting with others; she feels she has "no love for nobody."

> You don't know how to tell no one that you're infected with the virus. You won't know how to approach them about it. And there's a friend that likes me, right. And I haven't told him nothing. . . . He acts like he likes me a lot, but you know, I told him to find somebody else . . . because I don't want to hurt him. I don't want to pass it on, like that. But it's hard, and it's hard for me. I do want a friend.

ANGEL (DIAGNOSED WITH HIV TEN YEARS EARLIER). Angel contracted HIV through either shared needles or sexual relations with a man she had seriously dated for nine years. They were together for more than two years before Angel discovered her HIV status. Before Angel learned of her HIV status, she had wanted to marry him, but he had always declined. Once they learned of her HIV status, he told her that he wanted to marry her. This sudden change of heart hurt Angel:

> But what really bothered me more than anything is that before we found out, we had talked about getting married and, ahmm, he said no. I'm like "Well, okay," and we had been together like two and a

half years, and that really hurt. After we found out [about my HIV
status], then he wanted to marry me. And I'm like, "Now you feel
like you're trapped, now you wanna marry me?" Y'know, I was like, I
don't think so. [laughs]

Angel had stayed with this boyfriend for the six and one-half years following
the HIV diagnosis in part because he had her convinced that no one else
would want her due to her HIV status: "Here I am with this deadly disease,
and I don't want to give it to anybody else, y'know, I don't want to go through
the rejection, y'know the pain of all that. I don't know. Like I said, he had me
where I felt like I couldn't get anybody else."

When Angel left this man, she started to date a man who did indeed
reject her because she was HIV-positive. Angel felt obligated to tell all potential partners about her HIV status. About nine months after being rejected,
Angel met an HIV-negative man whom she married just a couple of months
before her first interview.

He's not like anybody else, y'know. He doesn't try to control me,
y'know. He doesn't try to make me do more than my share of,
y'know, of things; he helps me out. He's very good with [his son],
matter of fact, there's a lot I don't know about kids, y'know, I still
have a lot to learn about kids, especially a three-year-old. I'm
learning. . . . He's wonderful, he does his share of the housework,
y'know, and when I told him [about my HIV status], he said it was
funny because ahmm, he said he would never have dated anyone in
my position. . . . I know that, y'know, how he still has his fears,
y'know, because he, he doesn't wanna get it and he doesn't want [his
son] to [get it], and that's completely understandable, y'know. [About
my HIV status] we take precautions, y'know, and I've even talked to
him. I said, "Y'know, if I get sick, y'know, it's gonna be, it's gonna be
a very hard road, y'know." I asked if he's gonna be able to handle it,
y'know. And I hope he will, y'know, but I feel like that as long as
God's Number 1 in both our lives, that He'll work it out for both of
us and maybe [my husband will] never even have to worry about that.
And even if he did have to worry about it, I'm sure that God will
give him his strength to deal with it 'cause He wouldn't give you
more than you can handle.

For Angel, HIV did not stop her from entering into a significant, positive relationship with an HIV-negative man.

CHRISTINE (DIAGNOSED WITH HIV EIGHT YEARS EARLIER). Christine often
lived on the street, where she had mostly abusive relationships with men. She

has never been married: "I am really not interested [in relationships] 'cause I got hurt so many times when I was out there in the world, and I done had enough of men right now. It wouldn't bother me if I didn't see none for five more years. I mean I was good to them, you know. I worked, and if they needed anything it wasn't a one-way street; they helped me, I helped them. . . . I done had my share of men." At the time of the interviews, Christine did not want to enter into either short-term or long-term relationships with men, but she did not rule out such relationships for the future.

GINA (DIAGNOSED WITH HIV FIVE YEARS EARLIER). Gina had married some-one she had known since ninth grade. During hospitalization after a car acci-dent, he discovered his HIV status. Sensing that she was already positive but not wanting to be tested, Gina and her husband did not use protection during sex. Gina discovered she was HIV-positive only after being tested several years after her husband's car accident. She then separated from her husband in 1993 or 1994, and he died a few years later.

After Gina left her husband, she refused to enter a relationship with an HIV-negative man who was interested in her because she did not want to be responsible for infecting anyone. When interviewed, Gina had been dating an HIV-positive man for three years, and she reported being very happy:

> I aggravate the hell out of him, but we still get along fine! I aggravate 'im just to be doin' somethin'. But we get along great. I ain't never thought—'cause after stayin' married to my husband, and we fought, fight and kick and scream and holler—And I didn't actually think, if I could ever get into another relationship without having an argument. We'd do more laughin' and playin' than—I ain't never played so much before in my life! Just like I'm a little kid!

Gina and her boyfriend are attracted "like a magnet." HIV did not stop Gina from having a serious relationship, but she only wanted to be with someone who was already HIV-positive. Gina would like to marry her boyfriend, but he was worried that if they got married, then the amount he received from his disability check would be decreased.

JOANNA (DIAGNOSED WITH HIV THREE YEARS EARLIER). Joanna began dat-ing an HIV-negative man around the time that she was diagnosed. They mar-ried two years following her diagnosis, and he went for HIV testing every six months. Her husband was an illicit drug user, and Joanna tried to help him get off drugs: "The only way he got clean was through me. I became clean first and just like I told myself, [I told him] 'I will give you an ultimatum: you said you love me so much, the only way this is going to work is that you abstain from drugs too, because I'm still weak.' I have been clean now for a year." As it turned out, Joanna and her husband were not married for long and had separated about six months before the interview. Her husband was not able to stay clean.

JOY (DIAGNOSED WITH HIV SEVEN YEARS EARLIER). Joy was married to an HIV-negative man, whom she called a "knucklehead" because he refused to use condoms: "I don't have no desire for that mess no more, girl. I'm too old! I go, '[name of husband], you need a new wife!' He's full of firecrackers! That's why I'm old, I don't want no sex. I ain't givin' it [HIV] to nobody." Joy's husband also refused to be tested for HIV, saying (according to Joy), "Nothing wrong with me." Joy even made an appointment for him to be tested, but he did not go. Joy's husband's refusal to use condoms or recognize her HIV status created stress in their relationship and guilt for Joy; she did not want to be responsible for infecting her husband.

LISA (DIAGNOSED WITH HIV SEVEN YEARS EARLIER). Lisa became HIV-positive through sexual contact with her husband. He was emotionally and physically abusive to her. He had tried to convince her that no other man would want to be with her and that even her family would ostracize her if they knew of her HIV status. Lisa ultimately left her husband.

At the time of the interviews, Lisa was dating a man named Noah. She described in detail what it was like for her to enter into significant relationships post-HIV diagnosis. Lisa met Noah in a park. He was only seventeen at the time, but he was very kind to her. On their third date, they were going to pick up a friend of his and had thirty minutes to wait: "So we was sitting in the Pizza Hut parking lot, and I said, 'I need to tell you something.' I said, 'Lock the door. Don't get out. You need to tell me what you think before you move.' I said, 'Whatever I tell you cannot leave from this car because . . . it will ruin my life!' He said, 'What are you talking about?' I said, 'I've got AIDS,' and [it was like] that was the most common thing he could realize."

Soon after Lisa's disclosure of her HIV status, Noah moved in with her. He helped Lisa to raise her daughter. Noah's relationship with her daughter was very important to Lisa; Lisa would wake in the night to find Noah asleep in the rocking chair with a bottle in his hand and the baby asleep in his arms. He was the "perfect dad," and Lisa had found this "dad" after her HIV diagnosis.

Lisa felt guilty about being HIV-positive, in light of Noah's HIV-negative status. The guilt drove Lisa to make sure that Noah knew that he could leave at any time and she would be okay. Sometimes she would try to push him away, but he "just would not go." Noah and Lisa loved to go to the beach, walk in the park, and sit home and watch television together. Lisa did not want to marry Noah too quickly because she worried about Noah having to pay for her medical and funeral bills. She also worried that she would not qualify for Medicaid if she got married. Lisa and Noah were hoping to have another child, and, if she got pregnant, then she hoped that she and Noah would get married.

LORI (DIAGNOSED WITH HIV SIX YEARS EARLIER). Lori had dated five men since becoming HIV-positive. One rejected her when she told him that she was HIV-positive, but the other four stayed with her. At the time of the interviews, Lori had a boyfriend, Tim, living with her. They had started dating six years prior to the interviews, but Tim spent four of those years in prison. During the time that he was in prison, Lori entered into other relationships while keeping in touch with Tim.

At the time of the interview, Tim and Lori were together for more than one year. Tim is HIV-negative, having been tested several times. They did not always use protection when they had sex: "He gets in the mood and he says that he'll die right along with me, which I don't like, because I feel like I'm responsible. If he gets sick, it's going to be my fault, which it is 'cause he's negative." Lori had tried to refuse to have sex with him unless he used a condom, but this did not work. They stopped having sex: "I don't know, I just—I don't have no sex life. I mean we have—not like I used to. I think about me being sick, and my life is a lot different now."

Tim constantly worried that Lori was having affairs while he was at work. He also had a "drinking problem" and had been fighting with Lori a lot at the time of the first interview. While Lori was not satisfied with her relationship with Tim, Lori did not want to leave him because she did not like meeting new people and having to reveal her HIV status:

> If I have intercourse, I tell [the person] I am positive. That's why I don't want to meet people or meet a new man. Because I go through a lot of wondering if I should tell 'em, or what should I do, how they going to react. I don't like meeting. But when I do, I'll be with them for awhile before I have sex with them. You know I tell them before that. You know if I feel like I'm going to have sex, I tell them, "You know it's on you now, you do what you want to do, but I'm HIV-positive." So, whoever I been with knows.

Although she feels that she could live financially without Tim, Lori said that she could not survive emotionally.

TERI (DIAGNOSED WITH HIV ONE YEAR EARLIER). Teri married Jon between the second and third interviews. Jon attended Teri's substance abuse treatment center and was also HIV-positive. He was a very calm man who could handle her anger. He and Teri were good friends: "Me and my husband, my husband-to-be, you know, sex is not everything; we talk; sex isn't really in us. We don't do so much sex. There is other things to do without having sex." When they did have sex, Teri and Jon did not use condoms even though the doctor had told them that they should. Jon had other sexually transmitted diseases that he could pass to Teri: "I never did like a rubber. You know, but I gotta learn how to start usin' 'em like [the doctor] told me! [laughing] Well we, you know—we don't have—I don't have the desire for sex much like I used to. We don't have sex much, you know. We talks a lot, go out in the evening and have fun, kind of. . . . Sex ain't really our thing. Make me think we had enough sex out there in the streets [laughing]."

WENDY (DIAGNOSED WITH HIV THREE YEARS EARLIER). Dave, Wendy's live-in boyfriend from whom she contracted HIV, died from AIDS between interviews. Soon after Dave's death, Wendy started a new relationship with Nate, who had been a friend of Dave's. Nate was aware that Dave died of AIDS, and Wendy told Nate about her own status: "[Nate] understands [HIV] enough that he uses a condom, and he understands that if I get cut not to touch me, and he understands that I am dying. Well, I don't mean to say it like that, but you got to face it."

Wendy was wary that Nate would really want to have a significant relationship with her. She told him: "'If you [Nate] want to come back, you can come back, and if you don't want to come back, I don't blame you after I told you [about my HIV status].' But, honey, he came back last night after I told him. He wants to buy me a trailer. He wants to get married in December. I telling you, girl, I don't know what I have gotten into. I said, 'Married?' I said, 'No, no, no, I just got out of one.' He wants to get married." Wendy told him that she wanted to wait at least one year before they could get serious, but he wanted to spend what time she had left with her and her children.

ALBERT (DIAGNOSED WITH HIV SIX YEARS EARLIER). Albert had been separated from his former wife for four or five years. He did not think that she was HIV-positive because she had not lost any weight, but she also did not plan to get tested because they felt that she would be fired from her job if she was HIV-positive. Albert, who lived on the streets, was not in a relationship during the time of the interviews.

BILL (DIAGNOSED WITH HIV SIX YEARS EARLIER). Bill, who was in the middle of a divorce, acknowledged that the situation was probably his fault because he "had done some things wrong." At the first interview, he seemed to have some hope that they would get back together but was prepared to tell his wife that he would not be able to get together until after December, when he would receive temporary disability payments. Between the second and third interviews, his wife visited. They almost had sexual relations during her visit, but Bill used an old condom that broke as he put it on. His wife got mad and left. Bill said that he had not really wanted to have sex with her because he knew that all of his condoms were old. He had first told her that he could not have sex because he did not have any condoms and then said that he had some but they were all old. Bill said that he really does not want to have sex any more with anyone, explaining that he is "paranoid" because he does not want to get any more sexually transmitted diseases. He befriended a woman who was homeless and frequently stayed with him during the summer, but he had not had sexual relations with her and had no desire to do so in the future.

BRAD (DIAGNOSED WITH HIV FIVE YEARS EARLIER). Brad had not had sexual relations since he found out that he was HIV-positive.

> I wouldn't take the risk of having sex without a condom. That's exactly what I did [to get HIV], and I blame myself for that. I wish I would have took it more seriously. But you don't know, when you think about stuff like that, you don't think there's a chance that you will contract stuff like that, and I guess that's how a lot of people contracted it too.

> I'm not going to say that I wouldn't [enter into a relationship]. But there probably would be a time when things did get to a point where if [a potential partner] were very serious about me, yes, I probably could sit down and try to tell them. This is one of the reasons why I don't want to get in a relationship. I will [have to] go down and explain my medical history and what happened.

CLARK (DIAGNOSED WITH HIV ONE YEAR EARLIER). When asked whether he had post-diagnosis relationships or sexual contacts, Clark stated: "Yes, I'm not dead. I'm not dead yet. Hopefully, it won't carry me to my grave, either. I have, I've had protected sex several times since [the diagnosis]." Over the course of the interviews, a man asked Clark to be sexually active with him. Clark's response was: "You told me that you were not HIV-positive at all. Why would you jeopardize your life know[ing] that I am and you're not? Well, rubbers . . . they are not 99 percent protection. They can bust or anything. Why would you want to take that chance?" This attitude led Clark to believe that the man must already have been HIV-positive but was just not admitting it to himself.

DAMON (DIAGNOSED WITH HIV FIVE YEARS EARLIER). After Damon found out that he was HIV-positive, he stayed in bed for six months and did not date for two years. Since then, Damon has had sexual relationships with several people, not always telling his partners that he is HIV-positive. Damon tries to use a condom as often as he can, but sometimes in the "heat of the passion" he does not. He had a "bad experience" where, just before a man was about to penetrate him, Damon asked him to put on a condom. The man was very upset and thought that Damon must have requested the condom because he was HIV-positive. Since then, Damon had found a fairly regular HIV-positive partner with whom he often did not use condoms. Damon did not like to use condoms for oral sex because he did not like the feel or taste. He had not had a long-term committed relationship since he was a teenager and stated that he had probably had sex with more than five hundred men in his lifetime. Since becoming HIV-positive, he had been with four or five men, indicating a significant change in lifestyle. "I don't have any other man. I had my share. I lived my life. I did it my way. I had everything I wanted my way. And at the end, I was blessed with HIV." He saw the change required in his lifestyle behaviors as a blessing rather than a burden.

GARY (DIAGNOSED WITH HIV TWO YEARS EARLIER). Gary learned of his HIV status on Valentine's Day, one week before he was to get married for the third time. He and his fiancée decided to go ahead with the wedding even though she was HIV-negative. "But I believe there's someone out there for everybody. Even if I had AIDS and if I was single, there's gotta be someone out there that's single with AIDS and they ain't going to worry about catching the disease from somebody who's got the disease. You'd be able to find a mate. You need to have an AIDS classified ad: 'Horny, single and diseased. Need mate.'"

Like other participants, Gary worried that he might transmit HIV to his current fourth wife:

> I didn't want her using my razor because if I nick and cut myself, you know. I don't know, I worry about her catching it, but she doesn't worry about it. At least she doesn't tell me about it. That's what kills me. 'Cause I wonder how she thinks sometimes. I'd be thinking about it. Am I throwing my life away? Am I jeopardizing myself, with my

kids, this and that. She don't talk about it, though. All she does is bitch.

During the third interview, Gary said that he and his wife had been fighting all month about "bills, sex, whatever. . . . We have no money, gotta fight. . . . The other day, I say, at least I don't offer you money to do things [e.g., for sex]. That pissed her off. Then the other day, I told her I wished she'd hurry up and catch the AIDS and die. That really set her off for a week. It was just a joke."

JAMES (UNKNOWN TIME SINCE DIAGNOSIS). James started having fevers and night sweats when he was with his first wife. These ailments prompted them to be tested for HIV: James's result was positive, and his wife's was negative. They decided to stop having sexual relations and then divorced.

James met another woman with whom he had been engaged for five years. His fiancée was HIV-negative and knew of James's HIV status. The woman lived a few hours away, but she visited frequently and cared for him when he was sick. The couple had not set a wedding date at the time of the second interview. They fought regularly because she interpreted his frequent travel and lack of sexual desire as meaning that he went out with other women. James explained that he was not seeing other women and that the medications had made him impotent. He said the impotence made him feel bad and complained that his doctors never asked him about this aspect of his life or whether he "could handle it."

By the last interview, his fiancée had left him for another man, which made James very sad. "She's been a good companion. She stayed with me in the hospital, go to the hospital, took care of me, did my med box, did all my washing and cleaning and stuff. Then it just didn't work out."

JOEY (DIAGNOSED WITH HIV FOUR YEARS EARLIER). Joey had been married for twenty years. He left the relationship after being diagnosed with HIV because he felt that he was not good enough for his wife. He felt that his wife always knew when he messed up and that he could not stop messing up. His daughter was about fourteen and his son was about three when he left. Joey did not like to visit his family because he worried about them finding out about his HIV status. He worried that they would reject him and think that things like shaking hands could give them HIV.

KEVIN (DIAGNOSED WITH HIV ONE YEAR EARLIER). Upon discovering his own HIV status, Kevin started trying to protect himself and others by using two condoms at once when having sexual relations, which he did not know was an inappropriate technique. Between the second and third interviews, Kevin had a friend, Don, ask him to spend the weekend. Kevin explained to Don that before their relationship could go further, they needed to have a sit-down talk about HIV. Kevin knew through a mutual friend that Don was HIV-positive, but Kevin had not told Don about his own HIV status; he felt no need to disclose it unless they were going to have sexual relations. Kevin also wanted to wait to see if Don would tell Kevin himself that he was HIV-positive.

ROB (DIAGNOSED WITH HIV ONE YEAR EARLIER). When Rob found out that he was HIV-positive, he did not know how to tell his wife, and they had unprotected sex. When she learned of his status, she felt that Rob was trying to kill her or put her in the same situation that he was in. They stayed together for a while after the disclosure of his HIV status, but eventually she left him. In addition to Rob's HIV status, financial concerns placed a great deal of strain on their relationship. When his wife left, Rob lived with no income while trying to obtain disability assistance.

THE CASE STUDY participants did not receive counseling or advice regarding how to negotiate sexual or emotional relationships. No couples therapy was offered. HIV changed the nature of the relationships in which participants engaged. HIV made Angel, Lisa, and Lori stay in relationships that they might not have stayed in otherwise because, although the relationships were abusive, the women were afraid to start over. They did not want to have to disclose their HIV status to new people and were afraid of being rejected. The women did not want to put others at risk. Amy and Brad found it very difficult to enter into new relationships. Other participants, like Damon, greatly reduced their number of sexual partners after their HIV diagnosis or no longer found sex appealing. As was found in the work of Adam and Sears (1996), participants did not seem to differ in their reactions to HIV and relationships based on whether they were homosexual or heterosexual, male or female.

Several participants (Gina, Joy, Lori, Teri, and Gary) were in relationships with HIV-negative partners. These participants shared a concern about infecting their partners and had mixed feelings about their partners' occasional ambivalence to being infected. Some women were unable to convince their male partners to use protection, which left the women with feelings of loss of control and guilt.

Brad, Teri, Lori, Joy, Christine, and Damon expressed feelings of not wanting to have any sexual relations after their HIV diagnosis. They explained this reaction by saying that through sexual relations they became ill and it is how they could infect others. They seemed to reevaluate their lives and did not want to repeat past mistakes. Some said simply that they were tired of sex, even those who were entering into significant relationships at the time. Clark, James, Kevin, and Gary also expressed a desire to protect others from HIV.

HIV acted as an agent for change for some participants, allowing them to enter some of the least abusive and most supportive relationships they had ever had (compare with chapter 3). For these participants, HIV allowed them to take their relationships more seriously and to choose partners carefully. Joanna even found the courage to tell her partner that he had to stop using drugs if he wanted to be with her.

A fear of the loss of federal financial benefits kept at least four of the participants—Bill, Gina, Rob, and Lisa—from getting married. In North Carolina, calculating Medicaid eligibility for adults takes into account a spouse's income as well as one's own income. Federal law dictates that married people are responsible for one another for Medicaid purposes. Therefore, some North Carolina residents, as exemplified by the case study participants, prefer not to marry so that their partner's income is not considered into the financial eligibility formula, thus qualifying them for more aid individually than if they were married. In North Carolina, common law does not exist, so two people can live together and still not be considered legally married. Furthermore, if a married couple legally separates for more than a year, then each is counted individually for Medicaid purposes.

OTHER SUPPORT SYSTEMS

When the SHIPS participants were asked who they turn to most when in need of help or support approximately: 11 percent reported spouse or partner; 37 percent a family member; 11 percent a friend; 14 percent a counselor or case manager; 9 percent God or other higher power; 6 percent a health care professional; 1 percent a religious leader; and 5 percent reported that they turn to no one (see table 6.2).

FAMILY. Participants differed in their perspectives on sharing their HIV status with family members and relying on family for emotional support. Participants struggled with the decision to tell family members about their serostatus. Brad felt:

> You don't have any aunt or uncles that would probably respect your
> wishes unless they really, really care about you. But that's one of the

reasons I mainly kept it to myself, because it's a demand, a respect of
my wishes that I don't want [my HIV status] out. And trust me, you
got relatives that don't know how to keep their mouths shut,
especially about personal stuff.

Clark too had not told his family about his HIV status, but not because he
lacked trust. When asked who he would contact first when he needs help,
Clark responded: "Yeah, I call my family first. I told you, we were a very close
family. We real, real close. It's just [my HIV status] that I can't discuss with
them right yet. I got my own time to sit and discuss with them about it. But
yeah, I call my family." Clark, diagnosed only one year before the interview, felt
the importance of closeness to family and friends in his life. At the same time
he had not shared his HIV status with many of those people close to him: "No
I don't like lying to people, and I don't like hiding things from people. [HIV is]
something you don't tell everybody. Our family . . . I really don't like lying
to them, I really don't, but they never question me." Clark finds support in

Table 6.2
Social Support for Respondents of the Southeast HIV Patient Survey

Questions	Percentage
Whom do you turn to the most when you need help or support?	
Partner or spouse	10.5
Family member	37.2
Friend	11.3
Priest, minister, rabbi	1.3
Social worker, counselor, case manager	14.1
Doctor, nurse, other health care professional	5.9
God or other higher power	9.4
Nobody	5.3
Other	3.4
What is the total number of adults, that is people over 18, including yourself, in the household?	
1	15.7
2	54.6
3	20.4
4	7.31
5+	2.1
Did someone help you because of a disability or health problem in the past week?	12.2
In the past month, did someone remind you, or help you in some other way, to take your medications?	37.4
Do you currently have an HIV/AIDS case manager—someone who is assigned to help you get services?	67.1

NOTE: Total N = 555.

religion: "When I want to escape or something is worrying me, I just pick up the Bible and read it. I listen to Gospel. Just something relaxing and soothing."

Sam, however, lost hope that anyone could adequately understand and support him. Sam distrusted humanity in general because of the abuse he suffered:

> I don't think anybody can ever understand me as an individual or a person ever. . . . When I walk out that front door, I feel like I'm walking into a disaster area because I feel like I'm above it all as far as spirituality goes and the way I look at life. When people like this [neighbor] over here wants to get in my face and all, I won't back down to him. . . . I don't think there's anything else that could mutilate me anymore ever. I've been there, done that. It can't affect me anymore.

Participants with children worried about the reactions their children would have to their HIV status (see chapter 7). Teri said, "I don't want to make [my daughter] feel sorry for me like that. They might not want to be close to me, you know, 'cause people think funny ways about this HIV stuff." But Joanna felt that because her sons knew that she was HIV-positive, they were able to better support her. Both were adolescent men who were still "so clingy" to her. The boys worried about their mother, constantly asking about her health, reminding her of her medications and appointments, and even shaking her awake when they thought she was sick or had died when she had just fallen asleep. Joanna expressed throughout the interview the love she shared with her sons and the support that they gave to her, all of which contributed to her positive outlook and willingness to survive. She also found joy in speaking to young people about her experiences, in teaching them not to repeat her mistakes.

Seeking and accepting financial support from family members and friends concerned the participants. For example, Rhonda lived with her sister during the first two interviews. She did not have her own transportation and felt guilty about having to rely on her sister. She also felt badly for eating her sister's food so Rhonda's case manager helped her get food vouchers so she could contribute to the household. Participants uniformly did not want to be dependent on others, particularly family members. Even when dependency was caused by an illness, it was embarrassing and/or shameful to the participants, and so some tried to avoid relying on others, even when it meant living without emotional, financial, or medical support.

Support can be evidenced through simple positive acknowledgment of a person. For Betty, her aunt's support was a treasure: "She told me I could make it, don't give up praying. I get a letter just about every week." Betty told some family members about her HIV status, and they were accepting: "Sometimes it is good to tell somebody. I know it ain't nothing to be ashamed about because a lot of people have it." Her family tried to cheer her up after she discovered her HIV status, but after that they no longer talked to her about it. "They don't act like they are scared of me because I don't let nobody drink [my drink], but I know you can't catch it like that, but I still be careful."

For the participants, family members were occasionally a source of support and occasionally a cause of fear and hurt. Although some participants could tell family members of their HIV status, others felt they could not. Lori had hoped to be able to rely on her aunt for support, but her aunt both ostracized her and told the community about her HIV status.

FRIENDS. Friends can be another source of support for people. Dean viewed himself as a private person, unwilling to discuss his HIV status with most people. When asked to participate as a case study participant, he said that he surprised himself by agreeing. Dean wanted to participate because he hoped that the interviews would allow him to release some of his pent-up emotions by confiding in someone unrelated to his life. "There's a lot of people out there right now that will never ever discuss things like I'm talking to you about [this]. I'm glad I'm talking about [this] because I have these things I can't talk about at all."

However, Dean did tell a couple of his friends of his HIV status, and their support of him was important. If not for his friends and their encouragement, he may have given up on life.

> They give me a hope that I'm longin' for, that some day something's going to happen and someone's going to find a cure for this disease— also give me encouragement each day. It's a lot of hard work. Because I was about to give up work, and I said, "Just move away and be by myself," and they said, "Stay at work. Don't give up there, because you'll give up the fight against the disease as well," and it's true, you know. So they give me more or less my backbone when I don't have my backbone.

In general, the participants did not have a lot of friends to support them.

COMMUNITY. A breach of confidentiality in a rural area can result in rapid spread of the diagnosis news throughout the community (Whetten-Goldstein et al. 2001c). The interaction of rural-living, HIV-positive persons with their communities is vitally important because it is not possible for people to hide within their small communities. Participants, such as Lori, were ostracized by their communities when the word was spread that they were HIV-positive. Lori could not sit on her porch without being heckled, and she worried about the safety of her son.

HIV providers have begun to describe HIV as a chronic disease, but, for many respondents, HIV has always been a "cancer" to them, an illness that they would fight for a long time in order to live a full life. Because of the promise of new medications, people have begun living with HIV, finding mechanisms to reinvigorate themselves to become members of their communities. But many clients found that the systems around them were not yet ready to reinstate them.

Amy has tried several venues through which she could possibly feel active again by working. Not wanting to sit around and give in to her illness, she wanted to find a way to be with people and to help them again.

> I feel like, you know, ain't nothing wrong with me. Though I know something's wrong with me, you know, but then I'm ashamed. I try to call places. I say, "Maybe they don't want people like me working," you know, like that, "Maybe they don't want nobody like that." Because they don't have to know, you know. . . . And it's hard for me. I do want a friend. And I want to do something to better myself, you know. I don't want to be doing nothing, sitting here [in special housing] just like I'm sitting now in a prison zone. And doors have to be locked at eight [p.m.], open at eight [a.m.] and stuff. It's bad. I feel like I need to go on and get my GED, do something, you know, do some type of work. I'm lonely.

By understanding HIV and the people living with the virus, individuals in the communities in which HIV-positive persons live can help people with HIV feel accepted. When Christine fell ill with pneumonia, her pastor visited her, and she told him of her HIV status. "And, see, I didn't feel bad about it because, see, he had talked about it at church one Sunday. He had a nephew or somebody that had tested HIV, and he said anybody that needs to talk to me in confidentiality, they could come and talk to him. He said, 'And I will hug you or whatever, because you can't catch it.'" For the most part, the community supports for case study participants were lacking.

RELIGION. Eight participants expressed the importance of God, religion, or church in their lives. Albert had wanted to be a gospel singer. At the time of the interviews, he regularly attended church, although he reported that he did so only because they handed out free food to the homeless. Christine attended church occasionally and felt that a weight had been lifted from her when her pastor talked about AIDS in church. His openness gave her the courage to tell her pastor that she was HIV-positive, and her pastor visited her when she was sick. It was a relief to Christine to know that HIV was not God's way of punishing her. Amy was proud to have a son and daughter-in-law who were "saved." Amy believed that God had saved her by giving her HIV so that she would take life more seriously. Angel reported that God helped her to be more positive in her outlook, and she regularly attended church. Lisa was planning on getting her daughter and boyfriend to regularly attend church; she saw this as a way to further stabilize her family. Bill wanted to start studying the Bible more and going to church, and Joy was waiting for the Lord to call on her. Clark and Kevin also spoke of the importance of God.

Not all of these participants regularly attended church, but religion was important to them. Many when young had found church to be an escape from their families. Participants viewed the church as a place attended by people with stable, hopeful lives, and the participants wanted to join this group. Acceptance from the church, such as Christine's pastor, was important.

SUPPORT GROUPS. Support groups can be important places to talk about the disease and gather information. Rural areas often do not have HIV support groups, and when they do exist, there is no choice of group type that one would find in urban areas. Patients cannot choose among groups for women, or gay men, or African Americans. The lack of choice leaves patients either having to fit into the one group that exists or not participate. Thirteen participants had at one time participated in an HIV support group. A different subset of thirteen knew of people outside of support groups who were living with HIV, but only nine were willing to talk with the individuals about their HIV-related problems.

Lori stopped going to the support group in her area because it was held in the hospital, where everyone knew that people were going into the "AIDS room." She tried to go for a while but then became too fearful of disclosure. She could not go to another support group in a nearby town because she lacked transportation. Lori knows one other woman who is living with HIV, but, because that woman leads a lifestyle that Lori does not agree with (the acquaintance does not disclose her HIV status to the men she sleeps with), Lori chooses not to speak with her.

Lisa relied on her support group as a source of friendship: "See, I don't have many friends." Angel had participated in a support group in the past but no longer sees the group regularly. For her, meeting people with HIV afforded her different perspectives on living with the disease. People living with HIV often are not given sufficient time with their physicians to ask questions about the virus and the symptoms they feel. Therefore, support groups can be the source of camaraderie that people need to know that they are not alone and that their HIV-related illnesses are common.

> [The support group] helped me to see a little bit differently about other people and how they are dealing with it because I had only dealt with my own life. And, actually, I hadn't been sick much, so I didn't have a whole lot of knowledge of what other people were going through, and their struggles and their pains and going to the doctor and having [to] spend all this time going to doctors or the different cocktails and stuff that people get on. So it did actually help me learn more about other people and what they were dealing with instead of just reading something or just what I was told.

Rural-living participants were often quite isolated from others with HIV. Support groups that could have served to support isolated patients were ineffective due to fears, like those expressed by Lori, of community members identifying the participants as being positive because they quickly learn why a group of people are meeting at a certain place and time. Other participants said they did not want to attend a support group that had gay men in attendance, and some women expressed a desire for a women-only group. Such group divisions are not possible, given limited numbers of providers who donate time to organize them and limited numbers of patients who live in any one geographical area.

Networks and Support

Positive social support networks can improve quality of life, health outcomes, and adherence to medical regimens (Fahs et al. 1994; Penning 1995). There were some participants who did not want to talk with their families about the everyday problems that they faced, even when the participants had disclosed their HIV status with family and friends. These participants reported feeling that talking about their problems would place unnecessary burdens on the family and friends. Overall, though, whether a respondent had a strong network of people to rely on for support, participants felt that it was up to them to make a difference in their own lives; to face HIV or AIDS, they had to find strength within themselves. It is possible that the respondents expressed this self-dependence because they had nowhere else to turn.

With all the past research and examples provided by the case study participants, we find a dire need for people living with HIV to feel comfortable in disclosing their HIV status to obtain access to appropriate medical and social services. Lack of disclosure can lead to a lack of a support network, which research has shown to negatively influence a person's physical and mental health; in contrast, the existence of a support network can positively assist people. Yet with the tremendous amount of stigma about HIV still prevalent in rural areas, disclosure can be dangerous.

In general, participants were not offered many supports from either family or friends or the health care or social services systems. For HIV-positive persons, barriers to creating a social support network could be reduced in several ways. First, education on several levels could clarify misperceptions that raise barriers for people living with HIV. For example, basic education of all medical and social providers, specifically in rural areas, regarding HIV prevention, transmission, and confidentiality could deter the possibility of inappropriate behavior and disclosure in, for example, emergency rooms, clinics, and offices. Education throughout communities, including religious leaders and teachers, may better inform people about HIV so that they can learn to support and care for HIV-positive people without fear. Educating religious leaders and asking them to speak publically of HIV, as Christine's pastor did, could open community dialogue.

Beyond education, providers and policymakers can still act to improve the lives of people living with HIV in areas related to support. Coordinating regular support group meetings that are held in safe environments and within accessible distances creates the opportunity for HIV-positive people to talk and learn from others. In rural areas, support groups are sometimes seen as a threat because people do not trust others with the confidentiality of their HIV status. If a person cannot travel to a support group outside the immediate community, then that person may not be willing to attend a group at all. Medical and social providers can create alternatives to face-to-face support groups such as telephone groups or one-on-one buddy systems. Several case study participants spoke of wanting to marry but expressed fear of doing so because they might lose their income supports. Policymakers should be aware of such barriers as they look for ways to strengthen family structures. The SHIPS results illustrate that the majority of those with HIV in the rural South do not have spouses or partners; however, they do have other adults in their lives with whom they live and turn to for support. Care providers would not usually expect or invite these individuals to participate in the patients' care in the way that a spouse or partner might be. Therefore, providers may want to investigate ways to incorporate these other family members and friends into the care system. If policymakers were to uniformly allow HIV case managers to provide behavioral adherence counseling (e.g., how to organize one's life around taking medications), they could incorporate appropriate family members and friends into this counseling.

Counseling regarding the negotiation of safe sex should be offered and should go beyond how to put on a condom. Participants struggled alone with negotiating relationships with HIV-negative partners who refused to use condoms. Couples counseling should also be offered.

Chapter 7

The Importance of Children

NATIONAL DATA REVEAL that more than one-quarter of HIV-infected adults who seek health care have children and that women are more likely than men to have and live with their children (Schuster at al. 2000). More than two-thirds (approximately 70 percent) of the women in SHIPS have children living in their homes (Whetten-Goldstein et al. 2001b) (table 7.1). Not only are increasing numbers of HIV-infected persons the caretakers of children, but data suggest that persons with HIV have children after their HIV diagnosis (Sowell, Misener 1997). One national study found that 12 percent of all women with HIV conceived and bore a child after HIV diagnosis; an additional 10 percent conceived before but gave birth after their HIV diagnosis (Schuster et al. 2000). Although the risk of transmission of HIV from mother to child during pregnancy and childbirth has declined dramatically with proper maternal HIV medication during pregnancy (Davis et al. 1995), there are other consequences to having a child when one or both parents have a life-threatening and stigmatizing condition. Sowell and Misener (1997) examined the reproductive decision-making process among primarily rural-living and African American HIV-infected women in Georgia and South Carolina, half of whom had been pregnant since their HIV diagnosis. The women based their decision to have children on spiritual and religious beliefs, knowledge and beliefs about HIV, previous experience with childbearing, attitudes of families and sex partners, personal health, and intrapersonal motivation to have a baby.

In this chapter we examine the role children play in the lives of our respondents; the decision to have children; the decision to disclose their HIV status to their children, and the concerns about, and benefits of, such disclosure; whether care of children interferes with care of self; fears around future

131

Table 7.1
Patients with Children: Results from Southeast HIV Patient Survey
(in percentages)

Question	Percentage
Have you ever had any children by birth or adoption?	49.5
If you have had children, how many natural or adopted children have you had?	
1	39.4
2	24.3
3	17.0
4	9.7
5	4.3
6	3.1
7+	3.3
Do you have children under the age of eighteen living with you?	33.8
Women only: Do you have children under the age of eighteen living with you?	68.6

NOTE: Total N = 555.

guardianship of the children and grief after the parent's death; the importance of being a grandparent; and the importance of stopping cycles of abuse. Probably owing to the predominant demographics of the HIV epidemic in the United States to date, issues around parenting have been largely ignored by HIV researchers, providers, and policymakers. Current research evaluates differences in the quantity and quality of childcare provided by mothers and fathers with children at home and the effect that such care provision has on health-related behaviors of the parents. But research does not focus on the similarly important role that children can play in the lives of HIV-positive caregivers who are not the parents, such as grandmothers, uncles, fathers without custody of their children, or people who want but do not have children. These individuals' feelings about children affect their sense of well-being, social support, and self-esteem. Therefore, it is important to hear the voices of people who have or want children in their lives. Case study participants conveyed strong feelings about children, whether they had children of their own or in their lives.

Literature

Women are more likely than men to delay seeking HIV care; furthermore, having a child in the home is associated with delaying care further (DeMarco et al. 1998; Stein et al. 2000). Although previous studies found no difference in adherence to HIV medications between men and women (Haubrich et al. 1999; Kaplan et al. 1999; Holzemer et al. 1999), data indicate that physicians are less likely to provide highly active antiretroviral therapy (HAART) to women (General Accounting Office 2000).

The role of caregivers is often explored in terms of their burden in caring for someone who is ill or elderly. But there is little research on how providing care for a family affects an HIV-infected parent. A major theme in one study of mothers and grandmothers was the centrality of children in their lives (Roberto et al. 1999). When diagnosed with HIV, parents must undergo several decision-making processes in terms of children they care for: whether to tell their children, when and how to tell them, and, most important, how to prepare for the children's care when the parent passes away. Interviews with mothers living with HIV indicated that they were concerned about the stigma associated with HIV/AIDS and the resultant discrimination that their children would face. Mothers were also concerned about guardianship for their children (Hackl et al. 1997) and about infecting their children and the impact of grief on their children (Faithfull 1997). Such findings suggest that specific interventions addressing women's needs within their family systems are necessary.

Often, parents, especially mothers, forsake their own care and well-being to ensure the safety, nourishment, and care of their children, even though their intent is to live as long as possible to care for their children (Demarco et al. 1998; Lima et al. 1998). This maternal instinct may interfere with the treatment and rest that she needs to survive HIV. However, some might argue that caring for their children is the therapy that mothers need. Past literature has shown that women tend to remain silent about their illnesses and needs, but other studies have shown that mothers with HIV can progress from silence to action if their family is threatened (Demarco et al. 1998). Even for those who are not parents, the presence of young nieces, nephews, or grandchildren can provide a therapeutic joy and sense of peace.

The financial resources available to the family affect the environment in which parents raise their children, and those representing the new wave of HIV are poor. Recent studies show that financial strain negatively influences the parent-child relationship and the sense of adequacy as a parent (Gutman, Eccles 1999). In urban areas fathers who were employed had children with fewer behavior problems (Black et al. 1999). In a sample of rural, single-parent, African American families, the families' financial resources were related to mothers' childrearing efficacy, which was further linked to the children's developmental goals and academic and psychosocial competence (Brody et al. 1999).

Few studies have examined the effects of parents' HIV status on their children. It is estimated that eighty thousand to one hundred thousand children and adolescents have been orphaned in the United States after the death of their HIV-positive parent(s) (Wilfert et al. 1999; Joslin, Harrison 1998). One study examined predictors and outcomes of children or adolescents assuming adult roles when one or both parent(s) had HIV. Mothers with AIDS who used drugs often had daughters who would undertake a parental role (Stein et al. 1999). Greater parental AIDS-related illness was also linked to the assumption of an adult role by a child. Taking on this role increased the children's internalized emotional distress and problem behaviors (i.e., sexual behavior, alcohol and marijuana use, and conduct problems).

Voices of Participants about their Children

FORCED ADULTHOOD: JOY

Children whose parents choose to tell them about their HIV status must learn ways in which to deal with the realities of their parents' illness. Joy was a single parent with four children—ages twenty-three, nineteen, and sixteen-year-old twins. One twin is female, and the other three children are males. Joy made the decision to tell all of her children about her HIV status so they would be prepared when she became ill and to have them tested for the virus (the children all tested negative). She also wanted to be able to teach her children how not to follow in her footsteps.

> When I told my kids, my daughter just knew I was going to die tomorrow. [My case manager] came in and talked, got all my kids together, and sat and talked with them, and now, they don't even think of it. And I tell them, I said, "You know, you need to go out there and cut that grass 'cause you know I might not be here tomorrow" [laughs]. . . . My son . . . said, "Mother, let me tell you something. I'm not feeling sorry for you no more; this is over. I'm going." And he just goes. He says, "I felt sorry for you one time. I don't feel sorry for you no more. You're healthier than me."

The manner in which Joy sometimes expressed her outlook on her life to her children might have had a lasting influence on her relationship with them as well as on their own lives. Joy tried to instill in them an understanding of what other people living with HIV face. "I take my kids to the support groups to see how some of these people look that got AIDS." When asked if she talks to her children about safe sex, Joy responded:

Oh, definitely. . . . We're really open . . . because, you know, life is so short and I don't know when the Lord is goin' to call me. But I just want to be open with them, you know, somethin' that they could look back on . . . [to say], "Mommy, she was cool," you know, and stuff like that. 'Cause if your parents don't teach you, who, who will? If I don't be honest with them, if I sugar-coat the truth and sugar-coat life, they'll never know. 'Cause that's what happened to me.

Joy worries about what will happen to her children when she passes away: "They lose their mind because I'm not here with them. . . . And since they learned about my illness, they got close. They help support each other. . . . And [the female twin is] like the mother now, you know. They look to her. . . . I believe if anything happens to me, [she] is going to take control." Having an HIV-infected mother brought the children together, but it also forced the sole female child to take on the responsibility of parenthood for her older siblings.

Joy's children encouraged her to continue with her medications. This support was important to Joy because she felt that her children were all that she had left: "So I take my medication because . . . my kids, that's all I have. . . . And I'm not ready to check out yet. So I gotta take my medication."

FEELING GUILTY: LISA AND GARY

As difficult as parenting is, people living with HIV face additional emotional hardship in wanting to eliminate the effect of their HIV status on their children's lives. Lisa wanted to raise her daughter differently from the way in which she was raised; she felt that she was deprived of certain things that could have changed the course of her life. She also felt guilt for the life she had created for her daughter by having a disease that may kill her while her daughter is young. It may seem illogical then that at the time of the interviews, Lisa and her live-in boyfriend were trying to get pregnant. Lisa wanted to leave them with a baby to care for who would be in the same situation as her first daughter. She wanted the siblings to support each other:

My young'un has been through hell and back with havin' friends, havin' cousins and everything taken away from her, between her papa and her grandma actin' stupid. I said it's time to make a family settled. . . . This—the baby—[my boyfriend and daughter] are the only reason I'm havin' another baby; it's not for me. I'll take care of it, look after it and love it, but it's not for me; it's theirs. [My daughter] will take over this baby. When I get pregnant, she'll take over.

Lisa made clear throughout her interviews that she blamed herself for the isolation in which her daughter lived. She did as much as she could to provide for her daughter, but she felt that the best thing she could give her daughter was the love and support that Lisa herself never felt while growing up.

> I want things to be easier for her in life. I want her to be able to have things I didn't get. . . . [My daughter] can't have them things [referring to excess toys and electronic equipment], but she can have the quality time that . . . I can give. . . . It might help her better in life, it might not. But she can't say her mother ever turned her away. That's the key I'm lookin' at. Because my mother turned me away many a times.

Lisa is one of several parents we interviewed who were trying to make changes in their children's generation by raising their children better than they felt they themselves had been raised. The parents did not always succeed, as is seen in the words of Lisa below. Lisa explained that compared to the abuse she had experienced, the experiences of her daughter were minor and should be treated as such:

> So me and [my boyfriend] had a fuss here one day, and we was just pushing each other around. [My daughter] went and told the Day Care, and they told me about it, and when they did, I pull [my daughter] off to the side, and I said, "Look—what happens at home, stays at home. Unless I beat you, that's the only thing you come back and tell them." I said, "Unless I break your arm or try to kill you, that's the only thing you tell them." I said, "You do not spread nothing that happens in this house. . . ." Because she is mine, and I know you're not suppose to whip your children. But if you don't show them some authority, then they are going to run over you when they get older. . . . But my mother didn't spank me, when I was growing up, enough. And I know she didn't. If she probably would have, I probably would've not done some of the stuff I have come into. So what she didn't do for me, I'm going to reverse and change it for [my daughter].

Lisa said these words with no indication that others might view her actions as wrong. She was struggling with how to discipline her child without being able to draw on past experience or other support.

Lisa felt that her mother wanted to take Lisa's daughter away because Lisa was HIV-positive. When her daughter grew older, Lisa agreed that it would be her daughter's decision as to whom she would live with. Lisa believed that "if [my daughter] has a sister or brother, I know where she's gonna stay. [My boyfriend will] keep 'em. They'll be [my boyfriend's and daughter's]; he'll keep them. And I'm hopin' and by chance, maybe we can get married and [my boyfriend] can adopt [my daughter] and . . . be his, and then he have legal rights to her." Lisa spent a lot of time planning for the life her daughter will have after Lisa passes away. Lisa wanted her daughter to feel secure by having a parent figure and a sibling to whom she could attach herself. Lisa had not told her daughter, aged five at the time of the interview, about her HIV status, but said that she would "once she gets older and realizes, when her mouth calms down some."

Lisa's daughter's isolation from family was not the only loneliness for which Lisa blamed herself: her HIV diagnosis, she believed, had also isolated her daughter from school-aged friends. One of Lisa's neighbors down the street worked in Social Services. Both women were pregnant with their daughters at the same time and delivered their children at almost the same time.

> But do you think her daughter comes to [my daughter]'s birthday party, and even though she is invited? Do you think she invites [my daughter] to her birthday party? We are right down the street. So you tell me. So that is what gets me, is how close you can be to somebody, and then if I just open my mouth and say, "Hi, I've got such and such [referring to AIDS]," what would people really do?

In a similar situation, Gary had a stepson and daughter from a previous marriage and a son from his current marriage. He, like Lisa, worried about what his HIV status meant for his son, the only one of his children who lived with him:

> I want my kid to grow up hoping that he won't have to go through [AIDS], but he's going to have to go through it, because I'm dying of AIDS. He's going to be marked as "His daddy died of AIDS. . . ." I hope he don't have to deal with it. I know it's going to affect him. That's just make him a stronger person, I hope. Either that or he'll kill himself and he'll be with me. . . . I hope somebody can learn from what we got, deal with it. Don't make the mistakes I made.

Lisa and Gary spoke of their struggles in being HIV-positive parents, having both present and future concerns for their children.

PREPARING IN ISOLATION FOR THE END: WENDY

In addition to worrying about facing HIV and death alone, parents also have to think about the effect their death will have on their children. Wendy planned to leave her two sons, ages six and ten, to her sister, who had seven children of her own. Wendy's live-in boyfriend, who was also HIV-positive,

was not the father of her children, but the children called him Daddy.
Wendy's younger son seemed to be mildly retarded: "He's slow. He's not growing right, and stuff. Then they found something on his head . . . something
like calcium deposits. They waiting [to see] if it's going to grow. So now, you
know, I got my hands full." Wendy's older son had been tested for HIV and
was negative, but Wendy had not yet tested her six-year-old, even though she
was concerned that some of his health problems and weight loss may have
been due to HIV.

Wendy did not tell her children of her HIV status because she did not
want them to worry about her or inform others in the community. Her ten-
year-old son asked her one day if she and his daddy had a sickness. She
responded that their daddy did but that she only had female problems. "But
they're at the stage now, I feel like if I was to tell them they would go spread it.
None of my family knows. Nobody knows but [my boyfriend]." One day, her
older son said to Wendy that he did not want her to die because he loved her.
"You know, he asks me from time to time. I think he suspects it, you know.
Kids are smart." Wendy said that she would do anything to defend her kids
and give them what she could to make them happy: "I take my last dollar, if
my youngun wants a piece of candy, he gets it. I mean, I've always been like
that because me and my kids been down a rough road together." Wendy valued her children's lives more than her own.

LETTING GO: RHONDA

Rhonda separated herself from her children while maintaining a role in their
lives. She had three children: a girl, eight; a boy, ten; and a girl, eleven. Her
children learned of Rhonda's HIV status when she was so sick that the doctors
thought that she was going to die quickly. At that time, they informed the
children of their mother's HIV status, and Rhonda gave custody of her children to her sister: "We cried together, and we just try to make my last days
pleasant. We have good times. Now they know that I'm strong, I can beat
their butts, so now everything is back to normal. I told them, and my sister
and I, we talked, and she agreed to take custody of my children until I'm well
enough or if something was to happen, not to separate them."

When it turned out that Rhonda was not going to die, she did not try to
regain custody of her children. She knew that she was going to die at some
point and believed it was probably best for the children if her sister maintained custody rather than waiting until her death. When given difficult situations regarding her children, Rhonda would tell herself that the children
were her sister's responsibility: whatever her sister wanted to do would be fine.
For example, Rhonda had not had any of her children tested for HIV; she said

that her sister was in charge of the children now, and if she wanted to have them tested, she could, but Rhonda insisted that she would not want to know the results of the tests. When asked what she envisioned for her children's future, Rhonda said, "They'll be happy. They're all going to school. They'll reach their goals."

During the interviews, Rhonda moved to her own place, but only the youngest daughter moved with her. The older daughter stayed with Rhonda's sister to remain in the same school, and the son stayed to continue going to a school that provided special aid. Before the move, Rhonda's son frequently looked in on Rhonda to make sure she was all right. Once he asked, "Mommy, Mommy, the day before you leave, can I sleep with you?" When Rhonda asked why, he replied it was because he would miss her.

Rhonda said she believed that the custodial arrangement was the best way to help the children cope with her potential early death from AIDS. Rhonda's love for her children had provided her the necessary motivation to stop using drugs in earlier years. When dealing with illicit substances, Rhonda had the power to change her lifestyle and eliminate anything that would harm her children, but with HIV, she could not rid herself of the disease so it seemed she tried to protect her children from it by removing herself from their lives.

LOST DREAMS: ANGEL AND GARY

Parents often dream of the good lives that their children will lead. They want to watch their children grow. Living with HIV further influenced participants' lives by interfering with their hopes to raise and be with their children. When Angel was growing up, she wanted to have children because she enjoyed being with her young relatives and babysitting. Angel also wanted someone to love and be loved by:

> Why I wanted to have kids? Because I wanted to have kids at a very early age. I wanted to have kids when I was fifteen, and I got married at fifteen, so I wanted to have kids then, even then, you know. It was very strong on my mind. Even every month, my period would come around, and I'd be like, "Oh, am I pregnant this month?" . . . It was just having that child to love, to take care of. It was an unconditional love. . . . I guess I had a lot of love in me that I wanted to give, and this was one way I could give it, by raising a child.

During her previous nine-year relationship with a man who had a preteen son, Angel grew to dislike children. When the son was twelve, he came to live with Angel and her boyfriend. The son was very aggressive, angry, and sometimes violent with Angel. She slept with a knife under her bed when the boyfriend was away because she was scared that the son would try to harm her in the night. "That child really did a number on me. He had even went on probation because of threats that he had made at school and threats that he had made to me. We went to his probation officer and told him. He was almost thirteen." The chronic stress of living in fear created in Angel an "anger and hate toward" the son and a general wariness of children.

At the time of the interview, Angel was learning to open her heart to children with her new husband, who had a young son, Adam. Angel struggled to reconcile her feelings toward the previous boy so that she could become close to her new stepson: "I had built up such anger and such hatred with [the other son] because of the way he was treating me. I mean, I was so scared for even my own life with him that I had blocked my heart towards him."

> With a three-year old, it's very hard sometimes to remember he's a three-year old. Sometimes that, that anger and hate towards the other child, you know: I see myself holdin' back, keepin' from, keepin' my distance from [Adam] you know. But yet I want to love him and I want to show him love and affection that he's missin' from his mom. . . . Very stressful because I want to do more.

Angel was so worried, and "it hurt me so bad, I even went to the pastor one day. I said, 'Pastor, I really need to work on this. I need the Lord's help on this because I want to love that child like he needs to be loved and taken care of.'" Adam began to call Angel "Mommy" during the course of the interviews and started referring to his biological mother by her proper name. This change made Angel feel good because it meant to her that the boy saw her as his primary mother.

Angel and her husband discussed ways that they might have a child even though she was HIV-positive. They knew a couple who had taken in a young woman and her newborn. The couple were the baby's primary caregivers and the young woman served as a housekeeper in their home. One evening Angel's husband asked if Angel would like the woman to carry a child for them.

> I'm like, "No, No, No." And it made me feel like he didn't want me to [give birth to] my child because I was HIV-positive, possibly. And maybe not. And we haven't discussed it further. He knows that he upset me very badly because if I have a child, I want my own. I told him, "You already have your own child." I said, "It's not mine, it's yours." And I love Adam to death, don't get me wrong. But still, I want my own child. I don't want somebody else's child. And I don't want you to go get somebody else pregnant with my child. . . . That's

one thing I feel that as far as HIV-positive, we just really are careful, if I bleed or anything. . . . We're very careful as far as having sex. But anything else, it's basically normal.

While keeping up with the demands of living with HIV, Angel was balancing life as a newlywed and the mother of a three-year-old while both yearning and fearing to give birth to a child of her own.

In addition to the son living with Gary and his fourth wife, Gary had a step-son and a daughter he helped raise during a previous marriage even though the son was not biologically his and he was not sure if the daughter was either. He no longer saw the children because of geographical distance and his former wife's reluctance to have contact. Gary's current wife was in a car accident with a drunk driver, and Gary wanted to but did not use the money from the settlement to fight for custody of the two children just to see them. Most times, he tried not to think about them.

HAPPINESS IN BEING WITH CHILDREN: AMY
Amy loved having children and had endured separation from her children and an unwanted abortion, given her HIV status. Initially, the two children that Amy did have lived with her. Their father sent support checks on time and tried to help them through school. In time, her two children went to live with their father because "he talked to me and he said, 'Now Amy, you can't seem to keep them in school. Let me take them.'" Her daughter graduated from high school, but her son did not. Amy was proud of her son, who married the minister of a local church in which he was a deacon: "Both of them are saved, so I know that family is gonna be all right, at least I hope it goes all right." As for Amy's daughter, "I always stuck by her because I have seen so many parents that don't stick by their children like they ought to. You know, so many are getting killed."

For a period of time while her daughter was in jail Amy was the primary caregiver for her grandson. She took much pride in caring for the baby and found great happiness in having him with her. When her daughter was released, she took back the baby. "I miss him. You don't know what can happen nowadays. We are living in dangerous times, and I love [my grandson], and I don't want to see nothing happen to him. I pray for him and stuff. You know when you have something and then you miss it and stuff. I loved [my grandson]."

Amy felt an incredible responsibility for her grandchildren: "Be strong with the grandchildren and teach them what we didn't have because that's how I feel. I wasn't taught anything. I wasn't learnt anything. I had to copy off others. I had to go through that."

Amy's son lived in a nearby apartment so he checked on her regularly, and when she did not feel well or safe, she had him spend the night. When Amy disclosed her HIV status to her children: "They just said, 'Oh.' They didn't react none. They don't talk to me. They just check on me a lot." When Amy broaches the subject of HIV, her daughter tells her to stop talking.

Her son had stepchildren through his marriage to the minister. Amy, like other parents and grandparents we interviewed, tried to stop the cycle of neglect and abuse that she and/or her children had once endured. One day, Amy's son "spanked [his stepchildren] and stuff, and [the son] is only twenty-three, and he is not the father of them kids. And I said, '[Son], don't spank them too much because you are not the father of these kids, and it hurts me. . . .' I won't say nothing to him because he will think somebody is trying to tell him something wrong."

Even though Amy could not turn to her children for emotional support, she felt that the people she was closest to were her children. They provided her with a sense of connection to the world and security in knowing that people cared for her well-being.

THE PROMISE OF DEATH: LORI

Lori had not told her young, biracial son about her HIV status: "I try not to let him know much 'cause I don't want him to be afraid. [In their primarily black neighborhood] he gets made fun of a lot already 'cause I'm white; kids are making fun of him." Lori stopped allowing her son to play outside because she heard neighborhood kids "threatening to take a brick and throw [it] up side his head."

Lori felt that the knowledge of her HIV status was a burden her son could do without for the time being. Having an HIV-positive mother had already affected him in numerous ways:

> He's had it rough. He's seen me sick, he's seen me in the hospital that time they said that I was going to die. I caught the chicken pox from him. If I get sick, he starts crying 'cause he's afraid I'm going to end up in the hospital 'cause there, for awhile, I was in the hospital a lot before I got on all my medication. He's had to go through mental health, and he still does, going through [the phase of] 'mama dying.' 'Cause he thinks mama's going to die. They been working with him. . . . When I get sick, I try not to show it, especially around him 'cause I know how he act. He don't know the label HIV-positive. All he knows is I'm sick.

Lori worried that her son would be the one to find her dead body and was concerned about the effect this situation would have on him. Even in trying to provide her son with the basic need for education, Lori had problems: "'Cause I'm trying to get him, before school starts, back on Ritalin. But I can't get to the doctors, and I don't have the money to catch a cab, so it's hard getting backwards and forward." Lori's son's medications were as important or more important to her as her own HIV-related medications, yet she barely had the resources to travel to get her son's medications.

Lori felt that the energy required to keep up with her son also took its toll on her health:

> I go through [having to go after him] all day, 24/7. He's restless, always getting up and down; he's on the go all the time. And it wears me out. . . . His memories of me, I want to be good. I don't want him to remember mommy spanking him all the time or punishing him all the time. I hate punishing him, or I guess that's why he's like he is now. 'Cause I feel sorry for him in a way, 'cause he has a mommy that's sick, and as he grows up, I may not be here for him. Maybe I shouldn't, but I feel sorry for him. I need to give him all the love I can now, 'cause when he gets older, he ain't going to have it. . . . And he said when he turn nineteen, he going to do this, he going to do that with his money with his mommy and daddy. . . . He was in one of his mean spells, and I told him, which he'll tell you, I said, "I'm not going to live to see that day anyhow." And he'll ask why I say that. Like I say, I get in my stubborn moods. . . . I go through stages thinking I'm not going to live to see him graduate, and I feel that way now.

While often feeling guilty that she may abandon her son through death, Lori's fear occasionally comes out as anger when she "threatens" him with her future death, which makes them both feel worse.

Living with HIV had forced Lori into some decisions that she wished could have been made differently. Lori regretted having had her "tubes tied" after having her son, thinking that now she would like to have another child. At the same time, though, she said it may be better that she didn't need to worry about giving birth to an HIV-positive baby: "So it's better having none at all without worrying about it." Lori had a son from a previous relationship who lived with his father. "I would love to have my son with me. I would love for him to spend time with me. But, which may sound bad, but that's one worry I ain't got. And what I mean by that is, if I pass away, where will he [indicating son living with her] go?" Lori had already documented that, if she passed away, she wanted her son to live with a friendly older neighbor who was like a grandmother to her son.

MAKING UP FOR LOST TIME: TERI

Teri was an alcoholic and used drugs when she became pregnant with her first child nineteen years earlier. Teri's family had disowned her because her baby was a "bastard." She was homeless and delivered the baby in an abandoned house. Shortly after, she was taken to prison so her aunt raised her daughter. She had two more children, from whom she was separated because Social Services discovered her continued substance abuse. "[My children] were very young, you know. They stay in the streets all night long and stuff. And my boyfriend beats my ass."

The younger daughter lived with her father, while Teri's only son was in foster care. Teri saw them both occasionally, and at the time of the interviews they were planning to come to live with her; her daughter would stay only during the summers. Her younger daughter occasionally asked about the period of time when Teri was not in her life, saying, "Mama used to be a crack-head. Mama, you, you going back out there?" Then she asked why Teri left her. Teri's daughter sometimes said that Teri could not tell her what to do because she was not her real mother: "You know, sometimes it hurt my feelings. You know, and sometimes I wish I hadn't been out there using so [Social Services] wouldn't have took them from me." Teri was looking forward to having her children with her again: "That'll be nice. Back to the same old ways, you know. Responsibility, take care of my kids. When they were real young, I wasn't a real mama." Teri planned to "really get to know them" and find happiness that "at least I've got in touch with my children again, you know. That what makes me feel so much better 'cause I got in touch with 'em again, you know. 'Cause I thought I'd never see them no more. 'Cause that was what really kept me alive in treatment—my children."

When Teri's daughter came to live with her for the summer, Teri felt happy and did not feel suicidal as she had come to feel and was feeling after her daughter left. Because Teri was getting married around the time of the interview, we asked her about having more children.

> If I was thinking about having a baby, you know, why are [we] going to bring somebody in this world that is going to suffer, to bring somebody in, there's a chance they won't get [HIV], but there is a chance they will get it. . . . I don't want my child to suffer like that, you know. I don't want my child to suffer like that where all his life, he's got to take all this medication and everything. . . . It would be nice to have some more kids. I want eight children.

BEING HONEST WITH HER CHILDREN: JOANNA

Joanna's two sons, eighteen and twenty-three years old, lived with her. Initially, Joanna's drug use made her unwilling to take responsibility for her children, so her mother took them. Joanna later decided to stop using so that she could raise her children. The two sons had different fathers, whom Joanna described as a "sorry set of men." The last time she saw one of them, "my daddy was running him down with a gun then because he was gonna take my baby."

Joanna stressed sex education with her sons and put condoms in their pockets when she did their laundry. The sons both felt very close to Joanna. When the sons would get sick, they would "jump in the bed with me. . . . I ain't got but two. Mess with them two, you are through, because my children are my pride and joy, and I feel like everybody should [feel] like that about your children." The sons worried about their mother's health: "Every time I go to the hospital, they have a sure fit because they think I'm not coming back, because I left one time and went into the hospital and stayed thirty days."

Her younger son had "violent tendencies"; he hit his uncle once with a brick and someone else with an aluminum baseball bat.

> Because my brother whooped him because he wanted to go out and play with a football, and my brother took it and told him he wasn't going outside because it had been snowing. And he went out there anyway, and when my brother went out there to get him . . . he wasn't saying nothing. And my sister said by the time she opened the door, [my son] hit my brother in the back of the head with a brick. . . . My baby fights; my baby don't play. If you make him mad, you are through. Bad temper. The only one that he won't jump back at is me and my sister. You know those big, gray cinder block bricks? My second husband, he was going to jump on me, and my son took [a cinder block] and told him, he dropped that brick down and it busted, and my son had two big pieces and he said, "You want to beat a woman? Beat a man." . . . I think my son snaps, he goes deep out, he goes out.

Her son's mental stability did not seem to concern Joanna, but his aggressiveness was something she noted and considered when thinking about the future; she was concerned for his well-being and safety after her death. She found happiness in enjoying time with her children or by taking care of other people's children: "Children is a livelihood for me now." She also spoke to young people through schools or churches to provide sex education. She had overcome violence and poor treatment from past relationships with men, as well as the initial pain from her HIV diagnosis, to find peace in who she was and what she could give to other people: "I've always learned this . . . can't nobody help you unless you help yourself. If you just give up, [nothing] that the doctors do in this world will help you. You [have] got to have the inner strength to help the outer."

Joanna believed in being honest with her children about her own HIV status and about behavior that might put them at risk for infection. She counseled her sons about safe sex and the risks of illicit substance use. Joanna also taught other young people about protecting themselves.

STOPPING THE CYCLE OF ABUSE AND NEGLECT: CHRISTINE AND JOEY

Christine believed that her previous abuse of drugs and neglect of her daughter resulted in her daughter's getting pregnant at a young age and without a steady partner. Christine's sister cared for Christine's daughter during the last year of Christine's substance abuse; after Christine became sober, she took her daughter back to live in a halfway house:

> I just try not to be as hard on her as my mama was hard on me. Even though it is paying off from that hard time my mama gave me, I just think eventually it's gonna pay off with her, you know. . . . Yeah, I really do feel like my mama abused me when I was small because I got scars on my legs now from some of the whippin's with the switches that she used that had notches and things in it. I got scars in my knees and stuff. . . . Verbally, it was abuse. Coming up, it was physically. . . . That sort of rubbed off on me and my daughter. I abused my daughter too, because a couple of times, I was high and drunk, and I remember at least these two times that I just smacked her for no reason. No reason. I asked God if He would forgive me and I would never do it again. I think some of that abuse was sort of in [my daughter] because I have seen little small, things that she try to do to her little son, and I . . . want that to stop right here in this generation. . . . I remember when he was very small and she was sitting here on the couch and he was crying, and she wanted to go somewhere and she know that if he cried too long, I would get up and check on him and I would get him, you know. I was laying at the foot of the bed, and I looked around to see what she was doing, and she was blowing [in] his face so that he couldn't breathe. I say, "What are you doing?" and so she stopped. I am trying to let that abuse stop right here at his generation because I was not abusive to her like I was [abused]. It was just a couple of times that I hit her that wasn't called for, and it wasn't the right kind of hit.

Christine had not wanted to disclose her HIV status to her daughter because she did not know how her daughter would react. While Christine was in the hospital, the daughter saw "HIV" written on a piece of paper, but she did not say anything until six months later. She called from a friend's house and asked why Christine did not tell her about her HIV status.

> I said, "Well . . . why don't you come home and let's talk about [it]," you know. So she came on to the house, and I say, "It's not the HIV that's killing me; you killing me. You killing me. I can handle [HIV], you know. It's the things that you do and the way you act that is destroying me and keeping me all torn up and scared and nervous at night. . . ." After that, you know, she hadn't said anything else to me. One time, she did say, "Well, what's all that medicine for . . ." and I say, "To keep me alive, you know." That was it.

For the same reason of fearing rejection, Christine had not told the rest of her family.

Christine tried to ensure her grandson's care by giving "the best love that it can get, 'cause it needs that. A child needs that." Christine acted as her grandson's primary caretaker so that her daughter could focus on her education.

> It is just like my child; I just didn't have him. I try to make it as easy as I can for her so that she won't have to do nothing but concentrating on finishing school. . . . I ain't nothing like my mama was. I try to, you know, encourage her because that is what kids need. They don't need that push back. We already been pushed back enough. We need some encouragement. . . . So that is what I try to do: encourage people.

Joey also wanted to stop the circle of abuse with his children and grandchildren. He stopped using drugs when he had his daughter, who is now twenty-six years old. "I looked and saw her. I said, 'I have got to stop all this bull jiving that I am doing out here.' Yeah, kids will make you change." Joey had two older children, a son and daughter. He also had three grandchildren. He could not wait to be a grandfather because he remembered how well his grandmother had treated him. In reference to his daughter's boyfriend, he said:

> He did a lot of things to her, which I was going to do something to him. My daughter said, "Don't bother with him." I said, "Look, I can't have nobody beating on you. If I didn't do it, don't let nobody else do it." See, I was raised up by [my] mother. When she told us to do something, we did it. She didn't tell us twice, although we didn't

get no whipping and beatings. It is a whole lot kids, they get beatings. Then they go and think they can beat everybody they see. They get a woman, they want to whip on her. I never have hit a woman in my life and never will. I believe if I did, my mom would come out of the grave and then slap the shit out of me.

Joey also talked a lot about his nieces and nephews and had pictures of them hanging everywhere in his apartment, in contrast to the stark homes of other participants.

WANTING CHILDREN: DEAN, BRAD, JAMES

Dean had looked at his lifestyle and said to himself that, because he was gay, he was not going to be able to have children. But he wished that he could:

The whole reason I was thinking about it so hard is because I could die any moment, but I won't have someone to carry on my legacy. If I had a legacy, I would want someone to carry on my legacy, like I would like a child one day, not now, but one day. I always wanted one one day. That's why I hate working in the hospital; you see all the babies all around, cute little kids. I always wanted a child. If everything works, I'll probably still have a child. One day I want one. I want something of my own. I don't want to be like everybody else, have one to claim on my income tax. I want a child, something to carry on my last name, fulfill my future, you know. Everybody wants that, they want kids. Because as soon as you see a little baby with his face all day happy, someone you have to care for. . . . So I want it.

For Dean and for most of the mothers we interviewed, simply having a child in their lives would have fulfilled them in a unique way. Dean's statement above touched upon concerns that people living with HIV have: wanting someone to carry on one's legacy, one's name; hoping to give to a child the life that the parent never had; and enjoying the life that comes from caring for one's own child.

As we mentioned earlier, an HIV diagnosis initially brings with it the promise of death. Feeling that life has been cut short, HIV-positive people may desire the life they never had and the life that never will be. Having children can create guilt and fear, owing to the concern that the children will be left without parents; but children also bring hope that the parent's life will continue through the children.

Brad looked back on his life and saw places where he could have made better decisions. He had already separated from his girlfriend when she found out she was pregnant. It was not until his son was three years old that Brad met him for the first time. "Then I said, 'Well, why didn't you say anything to me about it at that time,' and she said, 'I didn't think it was going to make any difference if you was going to come back.' It wouldn't have because I had found a better job up there." Reflecting, Brad wishes he had a daughter and believes that, if he had stayed with his girlfriend, they would have had a daughter by now, "but I always said I ain't never the type to think about big families, all those kids be running around driving you crazy, not me." However, when thinking about the highlights in his life, Brad saw his son as one of them. His son was thirteen years old at the time of the interviews and lived three hours away from Brad.

> I saw him [recently]; he was so happy to see me. I was happy to see him, and I told him I was supposed to go back [to see him] at the beginning of, at the end of May, but I didn't. So I'm trying to wait and see what days I feel like I can make that three-hour drive. . . . I'm trying to like build up my self-esteem about doing this, and we going to see how things work out.

James adopted a newborn son with his now former wife. When he and his wife divorced, she took all custody rights to their son. When James saw the divorce papers, he did not read them carefully and signed them without knowing that he was giving up legal rights to his son. He saw his son occasionally and presumed that his son knew about his HIV status because he had visited James while James was in the hospital. Looking back, James wished he had read the divorce papers more carefully.

PARTICIPANTS WITH CHILDREN spent much of the interview time speaking of their children. They spoke of past regrets and future aspirations. Parents described the issues that past researchers had found to be important to them: those of guardianship after their death (Lori and Lisa); worrying about the grieving process that the children will endure when the parent dies (Wendy, Lisa, Gary, Rhonda, and Lori); and, in at least one case, forsaking their own care for the non-HIV-related care of their children (Lori). The participants did not speak much of the fear of spreading the virus to their children. Grandparenting was important to participants (Christina, Amy, and Joey), as was breaking the cycle of abuse with children and grandchildren (Joey, Christina, Amy, and Lisa).

Parents of children under age eighteen are less likely to adhere to medication (Whetten-Goldstein et al. 2001b), but, when children know about the parent's HIV status, the parent is more likely to adhere to medications (Mellins et al. 1999). The participants differed in their decisions to tell their children about their HIV status, but generally they did not share their HIV status with young children because they worried that the children would tell others (Lisa, Wendy) and that then they and their children would be further ostracized by such disclosure. Other participants (Wendy and Lori) did not want their children to worry too much, even though the children of these two participants seemed to already worry about their parents' health. Christina and Joey worried that their children would think negatively of them if the children knew of their HIV status. Christina's and Rhonda's children learned of their parents' HIV status when the parents were in the hospital. Both Joy and Joanna did not want their children to be infected, and they felt that telling the children about their own HIV status would help the children both exercise caution and prepare for the parents' deaths. The children also provided the parents with support.

Participants with and without children spoke of wanting to have more children (Lisa, Angel, and Dean). They struggled with issues relating to parenting techniques, how and when to disclose HIV status, and whether to have more children without the support or advice of the provider community (with the exception of one participant, who was working with her physician to have another child). Participants were not counseled on the potential pros and cons of informing their children of their HIV status at different ages. They were not able to learn from the experiences of others who have been in similar situations. They did not speak with providers about guardianship or whether there was anything the parents could do to reduce future grieving.

As the HIV epidemic also affects families, the HIV provider community must begin to address these issues with patients. Providers must learn that the nature of relationships in this population may be different than for the majority of persons with other chronic and deadly diseases, such as cancer, but providers who assist people with HIV may come to understand other disenfranchised persons with chronic diseases. It is important that the patient be allowed to define those who represent "family," which can reduce fear and stress; these designations may improve quality of life and even result in improved adherence to medication and appointments.

Community stigma must be addressed if parents are to feel comfortable speaking with their children about HIV. Parents were terrified that they and their children would face abuse and ostracism if others learned of their diagnosis. When neighbors, teachers, and church members learn that a parent is dying of cancer, great sympathy for the person and particularly for their children is forthcoming. As our case study participants, such as Lori and Lisa, have told us, this sympathy is not similarly forthcoming in the case of an HIV diagnosis in rural communities.

Chapter 8   The Future

I be up the river. I ain't got no future.

*No, I try not to think about the future. I try
to stay within today because tomorrow is not
promised to me and yesterday is gone, so I
try to live within today.*

$\downarrow$

MANY OF US CAN imagine tomorrow; we make plans for the future trying to envision even ten to twenty years from now. We may not know what will happen, but we believe those years are there for us. We were taught to dream of lofty goals and to spend our lives trying to make those hopes a reality. And even as we attain some of our dreams, we create more goals, always building hope into the future. Living with a chronic illness changes this perspective on life, and living with a virus that is sometimes chronic and sometimes acutely fatal alters that perspective even more. Additionally, for some participants like Sam and Teri, difficult life histories complicate this further because they never allowed themselves to hope in the first place. Yet our attitudes about the future are predictive of how quickly our health declines and even of our death (Smith et al. 2001). Fatalism, or low self-efficacy, is predictive of fewer health promotion and disease prevention activities, as well as lower utilization of care services (Allen et al. 1998; Dancy et al. 2000; Dilorio et al. 2000; Hurst et al. 1997; Wehrwein, Eddy 1993).

Participants speak of a range of visions for the future: living one day at time, trying to maintain a positive outlook on life, wanting to work or volunteer, desiring to complete their formal education, focusing their hope on their children and grandchildren, wishing to teach others not to make similar mistakes, and reflecting on life and death. Participants recognized that some of their dreams for the future were more realistic than others. Many participants wanted to fulfill childhood aspirations and complete unfinished business: finish school, find jobs that help others, get married, and have children.

Literature

The period immediately following an HIV diagnosis can feel like waiting for the execution of a death sentence. Then, the time during which one becomes accustomed to living with the disease can be frustrating because there had been the belief in immediate death (Sowell et al. 1998; Broun 1998; Brashers et al. 1999). For some people, being diagnosed with HIV ends all hopes in the future; to reinvest oneself into the possibility of a future is too risky (Broun 1998). Additionally, people cannot be sure how they may respond to medications and how long a positive response may last (Brashers et al. 1999). An HIV-positive person might ask: do I believe in a future that could be taken away from me at any moment? Some people living with HIV allow themselves only to live day-to-day; anything more would instill too much hope.

Other people with HIV see the advances made in antiretroviral therapies as a means to take back the life that had seemed to be snuffed short. They make changes to their eating, exercise, and sleeping habits to accommodate the medications and to help their bodies maintain a steady and healthy status. This newfound life offers opportunities to access the community in terms of relationships and work options (Sowell et al. 1998). Researchers, activists, and providers of HIV prevention would even say that the message of reducing HIV transmission is heard less now because the new therapies have introduced the hope that a sort of cure seems to exist for HIV (Keenan 1998); hence, some young people at risk are not adopting protective behaviors to the same level as their older counterparts (Ward, Duchin 1997–1998). Hope in a longer future may also have been enhanced by religious beliefs, which help patients find peace in their future death because they now believe that their god is not punishing them with HIV, as they once believed, and pray daily (Kaldjian et al. 1998). This spiritual well-being is also correlated with psychological well-being and health (Coleman, Holzemer 1999).

Participants' Futures

ONE DAY AT A TIME

Not wanting to invest much energy or hope in a possibly nonexistent future, several participants taught themselves to make the most of each day. Gina explains:

No, I try not to think about the future. I try to stay within today because tomorrow is not promised to me and yesterday is gone, so I try to live within today. That is the reason I try not to set no goals, because I don't know how far down the line it is going to be. So I just try to stay within the day. Really within the second, because the next thirty seconds ain't even promised to us.

Gina had written her will, maintained her insurance policies, and prepaid funeral costs; her children would not have to worry about anything when she passed away. Seemingly contradictorily, Gina said that deep down, she did not believe that she was sick; she knew she was in denial, but, because she did not physically feel ill, she liked to believe that she did not have an illness.

Christine, too, said "one day at the time and live it to the fullest. Do the best I can to help myself and my grandson and my daughter and other people." Helping her children involved trying to stop the cycle of abuse not only by stopping her daughter from abusing her grandson but also by giving them both love and support. "And that is what life is all about: helping one another and reaching out." Christine was interested in, but had concerns about, returning to school: "I think I'm scared that I might not be able to learn. Because I been thinking about going, and the money is in the computers now, but I'm scared to even attempt it. Because I'm scared that I might not succeed and I'll get real frustrated with myself."

I really don't have a future because, see, I don't know how long my health is going to hold out, and I would hate to have goals and not be able to fulfill them, so I just live day by day, and whatever I can do in that day, I try to do it. For fun, I think about going to college. Then nothing but the devil will say, "What's the use?" You know? I just try to live day by day and try to be there and give my grandson the best support I can give him and to love him, and to push my daughter so she can have something and try to make it a whole lot easier on her than what it was on me, because when I had my daughter, my mama didn't lift her hand to do nothing for my child.

STAYING POSITIVE ABOUT BEING HIV-POSITIVE

On the other end of the spectrum from those who find making future plans too emotionally risky are those who believe that living with HIV is no different from living with any other disease or knowing that one could be killed in an accident at any moment. However, each participant who expressed such positive sentiments expressed despair at other times during the interviews. Joey expressed the positive attitude in saying: "'Cause either way [with HIV or not], I'm going to live until I die. See, it's what got put in your mind about the disease. They get scared. [Others] get afraid. It doesn't even bother me. As long as I keep taking my cocktail, I'm be all right." Gary shared a similar belief: "Everybody dies; you just gotta keep your sense of humor. Not let stuff bother you too much." Rob agreed: "But the world don't stop just because one person stops living. The world keeps on rotating, so you got to keep on living, you got to keep on surviving. . . . If the Lord grant you to be here tomorrow, you have to provide for yourself or whatever, so you got to keep on striving to better yourself or make yourself stronger." Kevin did not pay attention to his HIV status because he was "living the life that God gave me, and I'm gonna live it to the fullest."

Rhonda did not necessarily believe that life simply continued regardless of being HIV-positive. She was scared to try anything different so she continued in her daily routine: "I'm going to make it. I'm going to make this work out. I'll be happy." Clark planned on retiring from the military after the interviews and "never give up, and I don't intend to give up until I can't go anymore." He had been with the military for twenty years and said, "Now, with my problem, I need to just enjoy life. Travel, enjoy, do things I want to do. I can always find something to do two or three days a week dealing in the health profession. . . . My hopes and dreams is to build me a home."

Gary's viral load went up during the course of the interviews, and his response was: "I'm going to die anyway. Oh, you hope your body can fight off this shit on its own. But I mean, I just know it's not true. It's not going to happen. . . . I feel good, and that's what's important to me. I feel good. . . . I'll miss my child. Life goes on. I just know everything in life goes, you just deal with [it]."

Some positive participants, such as Joey, accepted that HIV had changed some aspects of their lives, such as their medication regimen and regular physician visits, but claimed that otherwise their lives are the same as ever. For others, such an attitude could result in denying their disease and reducing adherence.

DESIRE TO WORK AND VOLUNTEER

One negative effect of living with HIV can be its effect on one's ability to work or volunteer because of episodes of illness and general lack of energy. With AIDS Sam could no longer work, which was once the biggest part of his life:

> Oh, of course [being HIV-positive] changed my life. I've worked ever since I was capable of working. Worked—started out after school. Jobs . . . as a maintenance man . . . and then all kinds of restaurants. . . . Then I ended up as a graphic artist, then . . . yarn, I dyed yarn. . . . And then I became a truck driver. That's my ultimate goal in life: to become a truck driver. I have succeeded in doing even that. I miss it. My ultimate goal in life was to travel, and I did that. But I miss it.

I still want to do it, but I'm too—I want to say too sick to do it—not actually sick anymore, but I do suffer. I have my good days and I have my bad days. . . . I am just a laid-back individual, whose life revolves around this house. There are times when I get out. I don't see any drastic change [due to HIV] other than working, 'cause that's all I do, work and come home, you know that was me. I never really allowed anybody to become a part of my life. You know I was very standoffish with anybody, and that's what being a driver is all about. 'Cause you allow people to get in your face when you want them to, and then you tell them to fuck off. Which you didn't really say, you just did it. . . . Yeah, hanging out with [other truck drivers]. And they had their special place that truck drivers hung out together with, and talked, watched TV, you know. Truck stops and shit. Ate together, you know. It was just like being in prison, but you weren't. If that makes sense. I mean, you had your freedom. And it was a lot of fun being out there. You saw the world. And I loved it. That was just probably the major thing that I missed the most. I don't think that AIDS is going to be the thing that kills me, not even the opportunistic diseases. I feel like I'm strong, if I do things right. I feel like this is just a vacation. The sickness and all. I've worked all my life, so maybe I need to take a long vacation. The way I look at it is positive. . . . If it's a negative scenario, thinking negative thoughts is just going to wipe your ass clean, take you out faster than thinking about it in a positive way.

Amy felt somehow that working would alleviate some of her loneliness. Amy's son and daughter visited her at times, but most of the time, as she put it, she would simply stare at the wall: "I wish I was doing some type of work, making money, help out, you know." She wanted to volunteer but had no transportation. Working would also have made Amy feel valuable. One loss she mentioned was throwing away a certificate she received from volunteering once; now that she cannot actively participate in the community, she wished she at least had the certificate as a memento.

For several participants, the sheer lack of energy to do any activity for more than a few hours was the most frustrating symptom of living with HIV. This lack of energy made working difficult. Inability to work or be active in the community left people lonely and diminished their self-worth.

To some participants who were not members of the workforce before their HIV diagnosis, HIV acted as a catalyst to get them to live lives that were more conducive to a work routine but still limited their ability to work. Betty attributed part of this problem to transportation inefficiencies: "Then, if I could get a job, if I could hold a job, because I get out of breath. I don't want to work but three to four hours a day, and we don't have no transportation. You can't get no job, you can't get a ride." People living in larger cities can work or volunteer part-time with greater ease because of accessible transportation and various opportunities that organizations can offer to chronically ill, working people. But in rural North Carolina, where traveling somewhere as important as medical appointments is already difficult, participants know that finding reliable transportation for a volunteer job is nearly impossible.

For other participants, the idea of changing their lifestyles to return to work or enter the workforce for the first time was difficult. Returning to work was difficult to fathom because of both low energy and a pattern of having their days free. For example, Christine worried that if ever a cure was found for HIV, she would have to return to work, which did not please her because "I done got used to sitting here at the house."

Dean appreciated his ability to continue working but also worried that being in the workforce around a group of people placed him at additional risk for a breach in confidentiality:

> Every time I go out of town, I see something totally different, and I'm thankful I do have something to go to every morning, and having income coming in. . . . But keeping that confidentiality is the biggest issue, because you don't want anybody in your business. The wrong thing, and people tend to turn everything around and spread the news. And people [would] want to stay away [from me], and that would stress me out.

CONTINUING EDUCATION

Completing educational training was another interest for the participants. Several participants had lives at the time of the interviews that were stable enough to allow them to dream about finishing their degrees. Those who had not completed high school wanted to get their GED. Others wanted to pursue further education through the local community college. Some felt that their diagnosis with HIV gave them the push to realize that life should be experienced completely and they should try to accomplish their remaining dreams. Wendy was interested in getting her GED because it would make her father proud. Amy too wanted to get her GED. "You don't know what God has in store for us, because he is in control of everything. That's why I thank the Lord; he woke me up because he didn't have to wake me up [by giving me HIV]."

Rob also wanted to "better" himself and "get a lot farther than where I'm at now. Have my own ride—transportation—and my own place to stay." He wanted to go back to school in technology to get a better-paying job. However, some days he did not feel well enough to leave home, and he could not predict when this would happen. He also did not want to affect his disability income by getting a job. "My goal is to fulfill everything I left out. When my

mom had her first heart attack, you know, I put my life on hold to help her. . . .
I want to accomplish, I want to make people proud. . . . It's just this medicine
makes this difficult as hell. I'm going to test it out for a couple of months, and
I'll see how it works with my job."

Brad received disability income but going to school would help him keep
busy. "If I could turn back the hands of time and go back to holdin' down a
full-time and part-time job, I'd do it again. If I had a second chance, I'd do it
all over again. You wouldn't see me like this." He was interested in going to
technical school to advance his career and skills in computers. "Like I said, my
career goal, if I didn't get sick, I would try to go as high as I can as to reaching
my goal. My ultimate goals was to become a programmer, and I still want to do
that; nothing has changed."

Bill would be interested in returning to school as part of his effort to
"become better than what I was, to quit downgrading myself and quit letting
other people speak my mind, telling me that I'm out of my mind because I
don't like when somebody is doing that." If he could go to architecture school,
he would in order to find a job where he could become self-employed: "that
way, if I do take ill, I can't get fired."

Joanna wanted to register at the local community college. "See, with me, I
don't want to be rich. I don't want to be poor either, but I don't want to be rich.
I just want to live on a base level, just a level in life, just straight and narrow."

Some participants saw school as an activity to keep them occupied, and
others saw a chance to fulfill past and present dreams and a stepping-stone for
better jobs. Participants felt more positive about the possibility of being able
to attend classes than to actually hold down a job.

FOCUSING ON THE CHILDREN

For participants who had children in their lives, the children appeared to be
the most important part of their future. Two years before the interviews, Lisa
began antiretroviral medications because her CD4 cell count dropped to 250.

> I was just in a shitty mood all the time. I could've killed myself and
> not thought twice about it. But I, I look at that [pointing to her
> daughter] and that's what I know: what I'm livin' for is that. And
> that's somethin' I just have to remind myself every time I think of
> somethin' like [suicide]. You just have to remind yourself what you're
> livin' for. So it's not my life anymore; it's her life. . . . I can enjoy life,
> I'm goin' through it, but it's all for her.

Lisa hoped to see her daughter graduate, go on her first date, and do "all the
stuff that I didn't get to enjoy in life. I want her to see. . . . At five years old,
[she] has been to the beach more times than I have in my whole entire life."

Moreover, Lisa wanted to be at home for her daughter when she began school, which meant changing her work hours and/or having her boyfriend fully support them. Again, it was important that her daughter get the education that Lisa never did. As well, if she and her boyfriend had a baby, Lisa wanted to be able to stay home with the newborn. Lisa wanted the baby to bring the family closer together, to "fill everybody dreams [and] little holes that we have got in this family." One life lesson that Lisa wanted to be sure that her daughter learned was about relationships: "I want [my daughter] to be [a] nun, really. . . . I really don't want her to ever think about having children. Not until she realizes what life is really about. To let her know what I have and how easy it is to get [HIV], and to know that love is special."

Lisa lived to create a life and future for her daughter. She wanted her daughter to have everything she did not have when growing up, and she worried because she did not know how much she would be a part of her daughter's future. Lisa wanted to be more fully integrated into the church and possibly to marry: "I do believe I want to get married. I want a big wedding. I really do. But like you go back to money again. Don't have the money, I guess you can't."

Amy wanted to see that her children and grandson got more out of life than she had. She felt that education was an important part of being able to accomplish more in life. "I don't think about the future. I think about my children. Maybe one day, I could see them because the things I've been through, I wish they could go through it: finish school and getting a good education. I could show [my grandson] what I didn't get."

Joni made sure that she paid her insurance bills so that she could leave her son some money after her death. Joni also tried to teach him to be self-reliant: "My biggest concern is, though, that I just leave him in a position, you know, a halfway position to take care of himself. You know, I done did the things I did, you know, but I want him to have a chance to live, you know. So I'm planning to hang on to [life until] at least he's about twenty-one. Leave him a good piece of change."

Joy felt that if she died, her youngest child, the only daughter, would take control of the family and encourage them to "do right." Joy felt that her daughter would see to it that some of Joy's goals for the children were met, such as graduating from high school. As for anything else in her future: "All I know, I don't have no goals, I don't plan stuff. 'Cause you never know. Even with, without HIV, you just never know."

Teri hoped to win custody of her son again. "Most times, I worry about my son, that's all. Get him out of that place [where he is living]." Teri was getting married and had a house. She did not have a job, but she received disability, and her fiancé worked. Teri was hopeful about the future: "I think we can do it, we can do it together." She would be pleased to spend her time as a housewife and to care for her children. "At least I know I'm going to live longer. Least I can think, I really can think now [as opposed to before HIV and getting clean]. I know where my next meal is coming from, you know. Most of the time, I know that I'm living now, that's all to it, I'm living."

At times Wendy wanted to leave everything behind, including her boyfriend and children. But she knew that running away would not solve anything. Wendy's children need continual attention. With her comorbid conditions, she was tired of physically hurting all the time, and she worried about how her six-year-old son would live after she passed away. Wendy had made plans for her children's future in case she died early: "In fact, I'm going to leave 'em to my sister when I'm close [to dying]." Her final wish was to find her son from her first marriage. Wendy lost custody of this son to the father when the boy was a baby.

At times during the interviews, Gary reflected on his concern for his son. For example, when asked about the future, Gary discussed wanting a lot of things that required money but would make his son happy, such as going to Disney World. Gary did not believe that these dreams would come true.

> I can't really say life has sucked. I mean, I am only thirty. I feel I have lived a good life, I'm not afraid of dying. I am worried about [my son]. My dad's father died when he was eight, and he never got to know his dad. That's the only thing I worry about him. The way my life goes, I will live a couple more [years]. It would be nice to live another five years, but I don't look that far ahead, because, like I said, you can go any time.

Gary even pawned some personal items to buy a battery for his camcorder so that he could record his son, to give him something on tape for his future.

Joanna said that she made her children and her home her first priority, often without paying attention to her own needs: "My husband gives me money for me, and I put it on the house and the children, and he argues about that because he says I don't buy anything for me."

Whether by trying to make the most of the time with their children, or by making sure that all life insurance and funeral arrangements are in order, parents living with HIV expressed worry about their children's well-being more than for their own medical, emotional, or mental needs. This sacrifice for children, discussed in chapter 7, may result in patients' having less time and energy to spend caring for themselves.

WANTING TO GIVE OTHERS A BETTER CHANCE

As we have learned in previous chapters, many participants we interviewed were determined to give others a better life than the ones they experienced.

Most mothers wanted to provide more for their children than they had possessed, both emotionally and financially. A couple of participants regularly shared their life histories with individuals in schools and church groups in order to teach, especially young people, mistakes to avoid in life.

Lori, while going through stages when she believed that she would not live, was interested in returning to school to become a social worker for children. Living in foster care throughout most of her childhood made Lori believe that social workers today do not know how to make the best decisions for children because these social workers have not experienced foster care. "I lived the life. I know how it was lying, saying everything was okay when it wasn't. I feel that I could see [the lying if I were a social worker]. I think I could do better to help kids in foster homes, and people that are out there saying they know how a kid feels."

Joanna kept herself going by trying to help others in need and to help those who could benefit from hearing about her experiences: "I don't worry about it, I keep on going, and I go right on. I just want to be an asset to somebody else. When I'm gone, I want them to say, 'Well, I learn this from her.' Stuff like that." Sam felt that he experienced the worst in his childhood and wanted to protect other children from having similar experiences: "I know how it is to a child. I've been there. I don't want to go back. If there's anything I can do to improve a child's life, I'm glad to."

Wanting to give others a chance perhaps offered respondents a way to bring good out of all the negative things that had happened during their own lives. They desired that others not suffer as they had; this desire encouraged the respondents to work for others and gave them a focal point outside of themselves, perhaps even outside of their own pain.

RELIGION

Some participants felt supported by their religious beliefs. These beliefs helped them find peace and forgiveness. Bill said:

> I have no use for here. I'm not actually gonna kill myself or commit suicide, I just have no use for here. I'm sick, people don't act right.
> . . . I've told somebody that a long time ago when we're young kids, I told this boy [that] one of these days I'm just gonna find me place all by myself and just stay there and ain't nobody gonna know where I'm at, and then I won't have no problems any more. All you need is God to talk to. You can never get away from Him. He will be on you like white on rice; you can't get rid of God. But really He's all the friend you need if you use it right.

Angel used to think negatively about life, but she now believes that having God in her life helped her to "have a lot more positive to look forward to. He's given me a lot more love in my heart, you know. Forgiveness for things that I may have never forgiven people for."

Believing in a higher power was important for several participants, particularly when they felt there were no people available to support them. The sense of calm gained from these religious or spiritual beliefs was sustaining and sometimes motivating.

OTHER THOUGHTS ON THE FUTURE

Albert, who had been institutionalized for the majority of his young life and was homeless at the time of the interviews, wanted to play in a band one day. He also shared a story of pawning a ring that he wished he had been able to keep so he would have something that "I could say was mine, that I paid for myself." Albert simply wanted to get that ring back.

Kevin was creating his own production company, which would support gay pageant participants. "I'm getting into the pageant scene because I'm trying to find another outlet for something for me to do, something I like to do and that I probably could make a job out of."

If an experimental cure for HIV were discovered, Brad would want to volunteer because it would give him hope. "But, like I said, I wish they had more medical knowledge about the new techniques that's coming up. 'Cause I would be a volunteer; I would do anything to try to live longer."

Joy refused to let stress get her down because she knew that her health was dependent on being calm: "I refuse to let anybody get on my nerves. . . . when I get stressed and have things to worry about, I start getting sick."

Clark had a future goal of preventing further HIV transmission in the world:

> The only good thing about it now is your condoms, proper use of the condoms and using [them]. That is wise word to give you as a young man coming up. Remember what they is; don't make the mistake. Use them. Don't be ashamed to go buy them. Don't be no fool. It's the truth. I'm telling you, don't be no fool. Like I told you, you are my next generation, you are the future.

DEATH

Thoughts of death were frequently brought up during the interviews. Several participants seemed consumed by the belief that they could pass away at any moment. The participants knew many people who died from AIDS, as well as from drug use, violence and other diseases. For example, everyone with whom Betty used to get high with in New York had died.

Others have made peace with the life they led and how they will die. Bill wanted his family and friends to know that he will be quite content when he passes away:

> Don't be crying around my funeral 'cause I'm gonna be glad as hell. I'm gonna be glad wherever I am, I said, because I'm gonna be glad, and I expect you all gonna be playing music and dancing and singing and praising God, and just thank God and hope that I am going to heaven to rest and that I'm not here in this world where God gave you all to mess up, because that is exactly what we're doing.

THE PARTICIPANTS' DREAMS were perhaps surprisingly optimistic given their pasts. At the time of the interviews, they had been diagnosed for an average of four and a-half years, but some sensed that they had been living with the virus for much longer. Many participants were able to think about what they could accomplish in life, even if their goals were limited and less than what they had been before HIV. But scrambled among the optimistic hopes was participants' understanding that their plans had to be contained because they could not be very sure about the length or health of their futures.

Research on the effects of having to plan a future life, as opposed to a future death, has focused on HIV-positive people living in urban areas. The same numerous issues need to be understood in the context of living in a geographically dispersed region where resources are limited; for example, there may not exist psychological counseling for people with fears about having to live again or support mechanisms for reentering the workforce. Because of HIV-related stigma and a dearth of reliable public transportation, people living with HIV in North Carolina have been limited in their search for volunteer or paid job opportunities that might help them to live fuller lives. Additionally, understanding the degree to which spirituality may play a role in patients' acceptance of their future and death may help providers understand their patients' decisions about taking their medications, adhering to appointments, bearing children, attempting suicide, or seeking or avoiding social support. Because locus of control (feeling control over the future) helps predict various preventive health behaviors (Schwarzer, Fuchs 1996), including adherence to medication (Barnhoorn, Adriaanse 1992), optimal treatment may need to include empowering the patient to actively and realistically plan for the future. Patients need to realize that they have some control over their future health and well-being. Job training could be critical in this planning process.

Part IV

Trusting the System and HIV Providers

Chapter 9   Trust

I know how the government works. I have   *Confidentiality*
been in there. [HIV is] just population
control pretty much, plain and simple.   *and Conspiracy*

W ITH SUFFICIENT RESOURCES, systems of care could be created that reduce structural barriers to care, such as transportation and child care. With appropriate funding, training, and support, systems of care could be integrated for those with comorbidities such as diabetes, substance abuse disorders, and mental health diagnoses. With sufficient political will, resources could ensure that communities have well-trained case managers who can help patients negotiate complex social services. However, even with the tremendous resources that would be necessary to reduce structural barriers in rural areas, if patients do not trust the system of care, then they will not use the services offered. When patients do not trust their health care and social service providers, they may not be as likely to adhere to appointment schedules and medication regimens (McCracken et al. 1997). Such patients may be more likely to attempt to decide on their own what their best treatment is without consulting any providers. Patients who do not trust the system or feel the system is not honest with them may have less incentive to be honest with their providers.

    A breach in confidentiality is the experience of losing trust in a person, group of people, or system. Experiencing a breach of confidentiality or even learning of the breaches of others can result in more guarded behavior with providers regarding personal information. Breaches cause mistrust, which leads to suboptimal care. Believing that persons or institutions are trying to harm others in an organized fashion is another expression of system mistrust that could potentially lead to suboptimal service use. In the case of HIV, for example, believing that HIV was created by humans to kill other humans is a concrete expression of mistrust of an entire societal structure.

In rural neighborhoods, generations have raised families together, and support systems consist of family members and friends who work in the local health and social service departments, clinics, and emergency rooms. For people living with HIV, especially in rural areas, confidentiality is perceived by many to be essential to their ability to continue their lives in the communities they know and depend on for support (Heckman et al. 1998a; Heckman et al. 1998b; McKinney 1998; Whetten-Goldstein et al. 2001c). Disclosure of one's HIV status may result in discrimination, reduced quality of healthcare, or the subsequent loss of one's home, job, health insurance, and family (Siegler 1982; Horberg, Schatz 1998). This chapter combines case study and focus group participants' reports of breaches in confidentiality by friends, family members, and providers and their beliefs that HIV is a conspiracy to kill a group of people.

Participants' Experiences with Confidentiality

Of the twenty-five participants fourteen had experienced at least one breach of confidentiality related to HIV. The remaining eleven participants had heard of breaches happening to other people with HIV. All participants but one expressed a desire to maintain the privacy of their HIV status; they discussed the difficulties and fears involved in protecting this information. Most feared the rejection and embarrassment they might face in telling their family or friends about their HIV status; another feared losing his job. When their confidentiality was broken, participants felt angry or were saddened by the withdrawal of the person or people who had discovered their HIV status. For most participants whose confidentiality was broken, the reactions of those around them only confirmed their fears about disclosure.

CONFIDENTIALITY AMONG FAMILY AND FRIENDS

The decision to share or not to share their HIV status with family and friends was important to participants. Participants' reasons varied as to why they did not want family or friends to know. Some wanted to avoid placing unnecessary burdens on people close to them; others, such as Brad, did not trust family to keep the status a secret.

Lori's aunt told one of Lori's former boyfriends of Lori's HIV status, who in turn told others, "and it ended up everybody was looking bad at me." Teri did not want to burden her daughter with news of her HIV status and feared her daughter's rejection: "I don't want to make her feel sorry for me like that.

They might not want to be close to me, you know, 'cause people think funny ways about this HIV stuff."

Some participants' confidentiality was breached when medical papers had "HIV" written on them. Christine's sister and daughter discovered her HIV status when Christine mistakenly asked her sister to read a medical document and when her daughter saw a piece of paper from the hospital. Both documents stated Christine's HIV status. When discussing confidentiality issues participants in the focus groups also combated the same problems and commented that perhaps a numeric code could be used in place of "HIV" on medical documentation.

CONFIDENTIALITY IN THE COMMUNITY

Many participants expressed concerns related to living in rural communities, where information can be passed throughout neighborhoods quickly:

- "It's a little town; I don't want a lot of people [to know about my HIV status]. And I know a lot of people down here." (Wendy)
- "This is a small, small place; if anybody found out, I would have heard something about it." (Betty)
- "So, of course, it ended up getting around the whole plant" after Angel's friend told a few people about her HIV status at their common workplace.

Living in a small community can provide support and comfort, if one is accepted. A small community is also a place where bad news travels quickly.

As Wendy stated: "My problem is I know too many people in [my hometown]. And I go to the doctor's and stuff." Amy's neighbor found out about Amy's HIV status when she visited Amy's apartment and read a piece of paper from the doctor that explained how to take her medications. Amy had put the information on her refrigerator: "I felt kind of bad. I just held my head down. . . . That's why I'm afraid of because I don't talk to nobody about it. That's what scares me, you know, because she probably went and told someone else. And, see, I don't say nothing about it. They just look at me funny." Lisa knew of a girl who was taken out of her daughter's daycare center for being HIV-positive and feared that the same would happen to her daughter, even though it was Lisa, not her daughter, who was HIV-positive.

From the focus groups we learned of a local health department nurse who told her elementary school-aged daughter about the HIV status of one of her patients because she was fearful that her daughter would play with the patient's daughter. This patient had not told her own daughter of her HIV status. Within twenty-four hours, the entire school knew that the mother was

HIV-positive and started teasing her child. The woman moved because she feared for the safety of her child.

Most participants did not want to share their HIV status in their place of employment, for fear of losing their jobs and dread of handling their coworkers' reactions. As Clark explained: "The confidentiality. . . . You see more of [coworkers] than you do your family. . . . .You see more of them than you probably do your parents. You're like a family to them. You know what it would feel like [if they found out]. I guess I would feel like a let-down. I would feel like I let them down." Additionally, Clark knew of others who lost their jobs because their HIV status was revealed so he tried hard to hide his own serostatus from his employer and fellow employees.

Sometimes, though, participants found reasons to tell others of their HIV status. Some participants even disclosed their HIV status to near-strangers in order to help the stranger. When one member of Kevin's Alcoholics Anonymous group spoke of getting drunk all the time and wanting to die, Kevin disclosed his HIV status: "I just broke down. . . . I said that's not reason to give up on life. I said, 'I'm HIV-positive, and there's no reason for you to give up on life. I'm still gonna live life regardless. . . . I'm gonna live life to the fullest.'" Joanna used her life experiences to educate church members, particularly those infected with or affected by HIV. When Christine fell ill with pneumonia, her pastor visited her, and she told him about her HIV status.

The participants experienced various responses when their HIV status was revealed: from a supportive pastor to families pulling away support and even telling others about the participant's HIV status. The fear of not knowing how people would react and the impact of hearing about others' negative experiences caused great stress in participants' lives.

CONFIDENTIALITY AMONG PROVIDERS AND IN CLINICS

When breaches took place in their homes or communities, participants often faced embarrassment or disdain. Breaches of confidentiality involving providers seemed to have had a profound effect on participants because the breaches were conducted by professionals on whom they relied for care and support; participants assumed that the providers worked under an oath to maintain confidentiality to the utmost as part of their professionalism. In a recent study of focus group clients living with HIV in rural areas, more than two-thirds of the clients perceived that they had experienced at least one breach in confidentiality in hospitals, clinics, and health departments that occurred by word of mouth, computers, facsimile, and written materials (Whetten-Goldstein et al. 2001c). Sharing stigmatizing medical information among medical providers was considered a breach. Participants made decisions about where to seek care based on the degree of professionalism of medical staff (which included respecting confidentiality), clinic location, or the level of security of the organization's computer network because they believed that computers increase information access (Whetten-Goldstein et al. 2001c). In an area with a limited number of health care providers, such as rural North Carolina, HIV-positive patients are even further limited in provider choice by fear of going to an infectious diseases clinic or social service office where they might interact with people they know.

Clark preferred not to attend the infectious diseases clinic nearest to his home even though this clinic was in a major academic medical center and, in Clark's opinion, provided excellent care. He refused to use this clinic because he feared that his confidentiality would be broken there. He was afraid he would encounter health care providers or other patients who knew him. Clark also could have crossed nearby state lines to see another doctor, but he did not want his employer to inquire about his reasons for visiting a doctor in another state.

Twice while in the emergency room, Christine had problems with physicians revealing her HIV status to others because "they only have little curtains dividing you. This one doctor, he told me, 'You know, you're HIV' and stuff like that, and anybody could have heard it." Another time, a caseworker who worked solely with HIV-positive people contacted the supervisor of Christine's halfway house to discuss Christine's electricity bill. Because everyone in the community identified the case worker as the person who worked with HIV-positive people, the supervisor immediately knew Christine's HIV status. Christine stopped "dealing with [the case worker] altogether because he was very out there; he always knew what was going on."

As a precaution, Dean went through the back door of his infectious diseases clinic for his medical appointments. Disenfranchised individuals already face tremendous difficulties in accessing care systems, so facing breaches in confidentiality within these systems discourages them further. As Teri explained: "When I first found that I had HIV, I had to go to [a nearby town], I had to go the dentist, right? They found out that I had HIV, so that [dental hygienist], she made me feel bad, like she didn't want to deal with me because I had HIV. She was, like, scared. I understand that, but it really upset me, so I just came on back home."

Clark shared his expectation of care providers:

> I would expect for [my doctor] to keep it confidential because that's the oath that he's taken. You know, I wouldn't expect him to go and tell anyone else about it. Nor his staff. To exploit not only my

personal life, but anyone else's personal life, because this is the oath
that he has taken. His staff should be trained to the point to not go
out and talk about patients that come in, and what's wrong with
them. Because that's a good way to be sued.

Clark knew of a medical provider's transcriptionist who discovered a patient's
medical ailment, about which she told people.

One of Damon's interviews was conducted while he was in the hospital
participating in a clinical study. As reported by the interviewer, one nurse
who had gotten to know Damon came in to the room during the interview to
discuss another patient in the ward: "And the nurse told Damon that [the
patient down the hall] had syphilis. . . . [Damon and the nurse] sat there and
kind of gossiped for a couple more minutes, and then [the nurse] left." The
nurse demonstrated that she did not always keep confidentiality regarding
sexually transmitted diseases. Damon said that he knew neither the nurse nor
the patient they discussed prior to his hospital stay, yet the nurse easily discussed another patient's diagnosis with him. As another example, Dean had
overheard two doctors talk about a patient whose HIV status he did not know
until the doctors mentioned it and said, "Make sure you put your gloves on."
Dean also had a friend embarrassed by a pharmacist who yelled out: "Here's
your AZT" in the drugstore.

Although most participants expected their providers to maintain patient
confidentiality, most anticipated the risks they took in visiting any local
physicians. Joy experienced a breach while visiting her family doctor: "One of
the [assistants] in there—the doctor gave her my chart to put up, or somethin', and she wound up lookin' in it and found that I had [AIDS]. And she
was spreadin' it all around that I had AIDS." Bill had to have blood taken by
a lab worker who was a friend of his wife. The lab worker repeatedly asked Bill
if he had HIV, to which Bill answered that it was not any of her business.

A focus group participant felt that her confidentiality had been breached
when her eye doctor, to whom she had been referred by her infectious disease
physician, inquired about her HIV. The woman had not known that the eye
doctor would have access to this information or why it might be important,
and it surprised and upset her. She refused to return to this academic medical
clinic after this incident. In another case, a patient had to fax proof of his HIV
status as part of his application for benefits. When he had the document
faxed, the person sending the fax read the document.

Breaches in confidentiality also affected the willingness of individuals to
be tested for HIV, as with Lisa's boyfriend:

Then this thing with anonymous testing that they've done away [with] it: so now [my boyfriend] don't wanna go at all [to be tested], because it don't take but just a second to find out, especially in the hospital, because the hospital is not as careful as they should be. I've never had an experience, but they're not as quiet as they should be. . . . Because there's too many family members that work certain places, like [my boyfriend's] got a family member up there. If he was HIV-positive, it would be on his records.

Participants experienced breaches in confidentiality on the part of providers and their staff, and they heard about the experiences of others. At the same time, though, they had not heard of any provider being punished for a breach in confidentiality.

Dean expressed a fear, echoed by other participants, not of providers but of other HIV-positive persons that he might see in a provider's office; these other patients might reveal his status to others: "Yeah, because some of my friends are here . . . and I never knew they were HIV-positive until I went to the ID clinic. . . . If [an acquaintance] does see me when I'm up here, it's going to be spread all over. That's why I stay focused; I don't want my days mixed up with his." Several participants expressed similar fears of knowing about HIV-positive persons who did not feel that confidentiality was important; they felt that such persons could be particularly damaging in spreading the word of their own HIV status.

Literature on Confidentiality

Case study participants experienced confidentiality breaches from friends and family members, as well as the medical community. Health care and social service providers can do little about the breaches that occur because a patient leaves HIV-related material on her refrigerator or decides to confide in a family member who then informs others. However, if the stigma around HIV in rural communities was reduced, then the concerns about breaches generally would not be as great.

Within the medical community, some patients were expecting higher levels of confidentiality from providers than the health care community is accustomed to providing. For example, medical professionals routinely share patient diagnoses among themselves, especially when the clinics are within the same institutions (e.g., infectious diseases clinic located in the same institution as the eye clinic). Other breaches were blatant, considered breaches by all health care and social service professionals. Patients did not consider legal action though because it would have further diminished their privacy.

With both the case study and the focus group participants, patients weighed the risk of a confidentiality breach with the benefit of receiving care. Participants tried to reduce risks by traveling farther to places where providers and patients might not know them. In rural areas, confidentiality is difficult to maintain because of the narrow social networks. In many places, HIV stigma is rampant; concerns about discrimination and ostracism owing to HIV infection are high (Horberg, Schatz 1998). Heckman and colleagues (1998a,b) found that rural-living patients are even more concerned about confidentiality than urban-living patients. When examining a group of rural-living women with HIV from Georgia, Mississippi, South Carolina, Texas, and Washington, McKinney (1998) found that high levels of concern about confidentiality posed a barrier to receiving HIV care. The combination of anticipating and experiencing social stigma is a source of stress.

Although most health-related organizations have policies regarding client privacy rights, agencies often do not consistently train their providers on maintaining confidentiality, nor do they have strict guidelines to enforce those policies (Veatch 1997). Additionally, providers may have an understanding of how blatant breaches in confidentiality are caused (i.e., mentioning a client's HIV status in a waiting room), but they often do not realize that simple mistakes are breaches in confidentiality as well (i.e., speaking about clients in the presence of nonmedical persons, leaving a medical chart open at the front desk) (Ubel et al. 1995). Furthermore, even if rural-living, HIV-positive persons were willing to further expose and possibly further isolate themselves by legally fighting breaches of confidentiality, the protections against discrimination are far from adequate (Woodward 1997; Adams et al. 1998).

Conspiracy Theories: Participants' Beliefs

"Conspiracy theories" about the origins of HIV suggest subversive action and/or nonaction, particularly on the part of the government, medical providers, and other persons of authority. In this section, we discuss the beliefs concerning the origins of HIV held by the case study participants and then offer relevant literature.

ORIGIN OF HIV

Eleven of our participants stated that HIV was created by the U.S. government and/or that a cure for HIV exists to which the participants did not have access. European American participants were as likely as African American participants to hold such beliefs. Participants provided reasons for government creation of this disease. Some said that HIV was designed to reduce the number of minority persons in the nation, specifically for genocide or generally to test HIV as chemical warfare. Some blamed racism, while others blamed classism; all said that the government feels certain people are too expensive because they receive welfare and other government support. Others mentioned HIV being brought to the United States from Africa or elsewhere overseas or through gay men or monkeys.

When Lisa was asked if HIV was intentionally given to certain people, her response was:

> Yeah, to knock people off. Because there's too many people. . . . I mean there's too many people; they can't feed everybody. They figured if they can get rid of these people. . . . What I'm sayin' is the government could have, you know how they like test certain things they're comin' up with? . . . They might've made this virus to like demonstrate it on somethin', and what it done was, they, they either issued it to somebody or somethin' and lost control of it and then it started spreadin'. . . . But . . . they didn't find a cure for it. So they got this, this big wide disease now that they can't control 'cause too many people are sayin', "I don't give a shit. Let's take [out] who we can."

Lisa's remarks indicated her belief that the government, in plotting to kill people, did not anticipate that HIV would spread to so many people, from poor and minority communities to other nonminority and wealthy communities.

Joni also said HIV was part of a plan that went out of control: "They had this [disease], they had that [disease], and they could always find a cure. Now this motherfucker mutates, and then they get some more shit. This will kill your ass overnight. . . . I don't believe that nature made this. I believe man made it. . . . And, also, there was nothing done about HIV until it started attacking rich, white people. Middle-class, white people."

Gary, who had been in the military, held similar beliefs: "I know how the government works. I have been in there. Just population control pretty much, plain and simple." Participants who viewed HIV as a form of genocide expressed a realization that the government plan "backfired on them" because "it don't discriminate. It gets everybody," as Joey explained.

CURE FOR HIV

While most participants expressed hope that there could be a cure, this hope was tempered by continuing governmental and general societal interference.

Three participants stated that a cure existed presently but that the "right" people had not been touched by the virus yet or that the cure was simply being hidden. For example, Gina believes "there is a cure; they just ain't released it yet. . . . I believe there is a cure for it. My doctor told me before he went on vacation, he said, 'Gina, if there was a cure, you could rest assure that every one of my patients would have it.' I don't know; I believe there is one. They just give it to the rich people." And similar to the experiences of men in the Tuskegee Syphilis Experiment (see below), Rob said, "I think they got [a cure] for it now. It's just that certain people ain't getting it. . . . And certain people that they let go on [with the disease] and slip through the cracks [to] try to get more in-depth experiments and details about it."

Several participants spoke of seeing talk shows where the people were stating that the U.S. government created the HIV virus. Information has been passed out on street corners in Raleigh, North Carolina, stating that our government is trying to kill us. In societies where bureaucratic systems of care and service have generally been inaccessible and culturally irresponsible, members of that society or community may initiate and spread beliefs about how the care systems function and why the care systems deny services to some people. Such notions about healthcare and service systems can hinder an individual's pursuance of appropriate services to improve health status.

History of Conspiracy

In a door-to-door survey of 520 African American adults, Klonoff and Landrine (1999) found that fully 27 percent of blacks believed that AIDS was created by the government to kill black people. An additional 23 percent were undecided. Holding an AIDS conspiracy view was not related to age or income, but those who were more educated were more likely to hold such beliefs. Furthermore, a survey of 763 low-income African Americans and Hispanics living in California finds that more than half the sample believe that AIDS is a conspiracy (Mays, Cochran 1996). In a random telephone survey in 1990–1991 of both African Americans and whites in California, African Americans were more likely to distrust doctors' and scientists' information regarding HIV transmission modes, to believe that AIDS is a form of genocide, and to think that AIDS information is being withheld from the general public (Herek, Capitanio 1994).

In news media and academic journals, distrust of the U.S. government and medical systems, primarily by minority populations such as African Americans, has been documented; many people believe that the U.S. government is using AIDS to annihilate African American people (Bates 1990;

Guinan 1993; Herek, Capitanio 1994). For many, the Tuskegee Syphilis Study sets the stage for minority distrust of the U.S. government (Fullilove 1998; Thomas, Quinn 1991). The Tuskegee Syphilis Study, funded by the U.S. Public Health Service, enrolled into a research project, more than 399 black male sharecroppers with syphilis and "studied them" from 1932 to 1972 (Jones 1993). The men were not provided optimal treatment when such treatment became available. African American distrust of the government is at the root of beliefs that AIDS is another form of minority genocide. Whether it be an environmental toxin, an agent of chemical warfare, or some other manmade substance, many believe that AIDS is being used to infect specific communities and that the government is withholding information regarding the virus (Herek, Capitanio 1994). Educating people about "the facts" behind conspiracy theories is difficult because "the facts" are not entirely known (Hooper 1999) and because actual conspiracies against minority populations have taken place in our country. Historical events, such as slavery, postslavery night-riders, medical experimentation on African Americans and prisoners (Fry 1975; Turner 1993), and the Tuskegee Syphilis Study, provide evidence of the untrustworthy nature of a medical care system that has proven itself deadly to minorities (Fernando 1993).

The governing organizations of the United States have demonstrated that, historically, they have been unable to support minority interests. Digging deep into historical documents is not necessary to understand why many people believe that our government is untrustworthy. Consider the following examples:

- On January 5, 1999, the U.S. Department of Agriculture admitted that it had been systematically discriminating against black farmers through unfair credit practices. In 1910, there were 218,000 black farmers who collectively owned fifteen million acres of land. In 1992, there were 18,000 black farmers left owning 2.3 million acres of land. Three thousand black farmers were awarded $375 million to compensate for this systematic discrimination on the basis of race (Glickman 1999).
- In February 1999, the Interior Secretary and the Treasury Secretary were held in contempt of court for the government's failure to produce material in its defense of the largest class action lawsuit in history on behalf of Native Americans (*Washington Post* 1999). The government was charged with being derelict as the trustee of three hundred thousand Native Americans, who alleged mismanagement of $500 million in Indian trust funds.

- On December 8, 1999, a jury consisting of six blacks and six whites found that the killing of Martin Luther King Jr. was a conspiracy consisting of the government, the Mafia, and the military (Associated Press 1999). An eighteen-month Justice Department investigation into the assassination, however, found that the killing was not a conspiracy (Thomas and Associated Press 2000).
- The Urban Institute, in a report prepared for Housing and Urban Development (Turner, Skidmore 1999), concluded: "There is no question that minorities are less likely than whites to obtain mortgage financing and that, if successful, they receive less generous loan amounts and terms." These findings hold true at all levels of the mortgage loan process, even when controlling for income and education.
- In June 2000, American General Life and Accidental Insurance Company agreed to pay $206 million to settle charges of racial discrimination in insurance prices (Samuelson 2000). Blacks had been charged higher prices, even though race-based insurance policies were outlawed in the 1960s.

These are just a few of the more recent cases. The admissions have confirmed the existence of racism plaguing minorities throughout U.S. history.

The government has proven to its citizens its ability to discriminate nationally. Discrimination has been embedded in the basic structures of our society. Combining such evidence with the realities of inaccessible health care systems that disenfranchised people experience clarifies why people believe that society is composed of people with power and those without; individuals with power are capable of performing and hiding actions that may be incomprehensible to others. The case study participants viewed the world in terms of actors and subjects, and most viewed themselves as the subjects.

Early HIV research focusing on Africa as the source and cause of the spread of HIV, even while other theories existed, only enhanced the African American community's belief that racist plots existed to blame them for AIDS while killing them with other minorities. African Americans maintained their beliefs that HIV was part of a genocidal plot, another attempt to wipe out the African American community (Guinan 1993). Therefore, it is not then surprising when African Americans or other minorities mistrust their health and social service providers (Thomas, Quinn 1991; Corbie-Smith et al. 1999), who, in their views, represent only people in power.

Our small sample of case study participants did not display differences in beliefs by race; perhaps being poor and disenfranchised equalizes races and genders in terms of the belief in conspiracy theories. Being disenfranchised means having one's sense of power taken away; it is the sense that others are in control of the world and you can do nothing to influence them. The life histories also did not display racial differences in amount of abuse, neglect, and difficulty with structures meant to help people, such as families, schools, and social services. The hypothesis that poverty is an equalizer in levels of system trust should be further tested.

Discussion

CONFIDENTIALITY

More than half of case study participants and two-thirds of focus group participants had perceived breaches in confidentiality. Although most participants' experiences of breaches were with friends and family members, providers were largely responsible for others. Case study and focus group participants were unwilling to consider legal actions when breaches occurred because such actions would only have heightened their visibility and social discrimination at home. Some participants, like Dean, left his apartment building without a word after being evicted owing to his HIV status. One focus group mom preferred to move her family to a different county rather than make a formal complaint against the health department. Our participants felt completely vulnerable and without realistic recourse.

In rural areas, where patients' families interact with providers' families, an HIV diagnosis becomes a much larger secret to keep. When patients perceive a confidentiality breach, their distrust of the provider system is confirmed. Breaches caused physical, emotional, mental, and financial suffering and loss. Participants reported that they sought care based partly on how well medical staff maintained confidentiality or whether the providers had nonprofessional ties to the patients. Patients avoided institutions where they had either experienced or heard about both breaches in confidentiality and poor medical care. Rural patients, already limited in their health care options, have been compelled to seek health care in even more distant cities; thus, it becomes more difficult for them to attend all their appointments. Increasing geographic barriers to care can lead to a chain of detrimental health effects, which include missing medications and evaluations and lead ultimately to more costly forms of care (Aday et al. 1993).

Because their lives are already so fragile and at times very lonely, people's decisions to keep their HIV status confidential from certain people must be protected; this confidentiality may be the one component of their lives over which HIV patients feel they should have control. To have acquaintances or coworkers recklessly reveal a person's HIV status, while difficult, did not seem as agonizing to the participants as having family or friends do the same thing. When friends and family told others about a person's HIV status, the HIV-positive person had to work through not only the stigma but also the breach of trust by members of the support system. Participants' decisions to share their HIV status with loved ones often revealed the desire for support and acceptance and required a willingness to trust. When that trust was broken, participants felt even more alone than before. Sometimes seen as supporters of last resort, providers likewise disappointed their patients by not being more careful with the knowledge of their patients' HIV status.

Some HIV-positive persons living in rural areas have been willing to forego medical attention in order to protect their privacy (Whetten-Goldstein et al. 2001c). Patients were more willing to risk their health than their jobs, health insurance, anonymity, family honor, or friends. In a system tolerant of breaches in confidentiality, patients may also lie about their personal information and medical condition (Woodward 1995).

From the perspective of patients, a confidentiality policy should require providers to: (1) explain to patients their procedures of sharing information, (2) request patients' consent for sharing of medical records or information, and (3) punish those who breach confidentiality and explain this penalty process to the patients (Whetten-Goldstein et al. 2001c). Patients do not fully understand the current practice of sharing information among health care providers. Accordingly, efforts should focus on enhancing patients' understanding of how sharing medical information can facilitate optimal care. It is unfortunate that such a call for increased patient involvement comes in an era of exploring means to decrease the duration of physician-patient contact as a means of minimizing health care costs (Schwartz 1996; Hellinger 1996). However, patients cannot financially or physically afford to avoid appropriate medical care.

Patient privacy can be further ensured if all persons with access to medical records—including physicians, nurses, secretaries, mental health professionals, and case managers—are trained about the importance of maintaining confidentiality and the consequences if they do not adhere to their institution's confidentiality policy. A true commitment to the privacy interests of patients would be demonstrated by an explicit enforcement system.

Education among all levels of communities (e.g., church groups, schools, health and social service providers of all types, clubs) would benefit people living with HIV. Such education might deter the negative reactions people and providers have had in discovering and disclosing a person's HIV status. A widespread rural HIV education program that would aim to reduce the stigma of the disease could decrease fears of breaches in confidentiality to a more manageable level. If HIV were not such a stigmatized condition, patients would not be as fearful when family, friends, and community members learn of their HIV status. Patients would be able to: widen their support networks; receive care closer to home; forget hiding medicine bottles, physician notes, and educational materials; and feel more comfort about an HIV case manager visiting their homes. Each of these improvements could likewise increase adherence to medications and medical appointments.

CONSPIRACY

With the advent of protease inhibitors and triple-drug therapy, many patients view current prescription medications as an opportunity to live a full life. People living with HIV are living longer than they had ever imagined when diagnosed. But as helpful as these medications have proven to be for numerous patients, many poor and minority individuals still believe that medications are part of the overall conspiracy against them due to their behavior, race, or financial burden on the "system."

Disentangling the participants' fears about, and hopes for, the HIV-related medications is difficult, perhaps because the participants themselves have not reconciled their alternating beliefs and concerns. Of the case study participants, all had been prescribed and taken HIV-related medications at some time since their diagnosis. Nearly all also took medication holidays without informing their providers, and some, like Joni, stopped taking medications altogether because she was concerned about the side effects. As powerful as the medications are, the side effects are also often powerful, frequently causing exhaustion, nausea, and weakness. The medications are seen as harmful, while some believe that the FDA-approved medications are still under clinical study and that impoverished people are being used as guinea pigs. Other patients say that, if they take the drugs, then their HIV will progress to AIDS faster; they believe the drugs are part of a conspiracy effort to cause faster decline in minority HIV patients.

Many believe that persons in the government and/or other persons of authority in this country know "the facts" regarding HIV (e.g., that humans created the virus) but are hiding these facts from citizens (Herek, Capitanio 1994). Understanding the widespread nature of such beliefs is important for policymakers and providers because these beliefs indicate a low level of trust in the care system. Belief in a health care system designed to help and medications designed to improve one's health is important in motivating a person to adhere to difficult treatment protocols and overcome barriers to care.

Conspiracy beliefs do not stand alone; rather, they exert tremendous influence on people's decisions to seek care, adhere to their medication regimens, and talk with others about the need for appropriate health care. Providers and policymakers must understand the depth of such beliefs and the underlying reasoning. Without such an understanding, providers and policymakers have difficulty influencing services significantly and reaching the populations who now avoid care. Proactive interventions may be needed to increase trust and facilitate conversations regarding conspiracy theories. Work can be done with patients individually, in groups, or through community education and discussion facilitation programs.

Chapter 10

Providers, Benefits, and Medications

[My case manager], he's my guardian angel, honey.

Sometimes I just lay in [my bedroom] like my bones aching. Skin is changing. I got this constant cough. . . . I always got a sinus infection. It is affecting my vision. Seems like my ears hurt. My whole body hurts. I just don't feel well ever, and I told you I stopped taking the pills, right? The pills don't make me feel no better.

ACCORDING TO ONE PROVIDER, we have a benefit system in place designed to "equitably distribute drug-resistant HIV." Physicians. Case managers. Mental health and substance abuse counselors. Social service providers. These are just a few providers with whom persons with HIV may need to interact to receive health care and social services. Some programs designed to provide assistance to people include Medicaid, Medicare, Ryan White CARE Act, AIDS Drugs Assistance Programs (ADAPs), Social Security programs, and food stamps. Each program has its own set of eligibility and re-eligibility criteria, with eligibility lasting for differing amounts of time. (See chapter 2 for details regarding benefits programs.) In addition, poor persons are negotiating and purchasing basic necessities such as food, housing, electricity, telephone, water, transportation, clothing, and child care. These are stressful and time-consuming tasks when there is no routine source of income or support. Obtaining and maintaining these sources of financial and subsistence support are complex issues, even for well-educated persons with experience and trust in systems.

The persons presented in this book are not only living with a stigmatized, chronic condition that will kill them, but they are also negotiating complex systems. Their past histories interplay with current living environments and comorbidities, including substance abuse and mental health disorders. These individuals' internal and external characteristics are part of who they are and enter with them into the care system, at which time the systems begin to influence the patients' lives. Patients weigh their own perceived need for care against the barriers to each system. For example, patients consider system-level characteristics such as distance to and cost of care, availability and cost of transportation, availability of child care, and waiting time. People with HIV may also judge more subtle attributes such as trustworthiness of the care system (see chapter 9), whether the providers give quality care, and interpersonal relations between the patient and providers (O'Malley et al. 2000). Therefore, the decision to seek care involves an internal decision-making process that is circular in nature: the person continuously takes in new information, assesses the situation, and makes a new decision based on past events and attributes.

From the viewpoint of the infectious diseases clinic providers, little is known about the patient who first walks through the clinic door. Over time, the clinic providers learn primarily what the patient chooses to share or show through overt behavior. Without tools and experience to assess their patients' relevant life situations, mental health status, and substance abuse history, providers could miss comorbidities such as mental health and substance abuse diagnoses and inaccurately assess readiness for antiretroviral therapies. Physicians are not routinely trained to conduct such detailed nonmedical assessments, nor are they trained to work with people who distrust the system and act guardedly.

In this chapter we discuss participant interaction with health care and social services and treatment adherence. We focus on both barriers to and facilitators of care, inherent in the care system. Participants speak of subsistence-level needs and their interactions with HIV case managers, clinicians, and mental health providers. Participants also speak of their experiences with HIV-related medications. We present literature from the field and data from the Southeast HIV Patient Survey. And we also include in this chapter data from the North Carolina HIV Provider Survey, a survey of random HIV providers.

Voices

BARRIERS AND FACILITATORS TO CARE

All but three case study participants spoke, without being prompted, of their subsistence-level needs. They spoke of worrying about obtaining food for themselves, their children, and, for some, the grandchildren whom they were raising. Participants spoke of their concerns about housing, electrical bills, clothing, and basic necessities such as toilet paper.

The systems that must be navigated to meet subsistence-level needs are at times difficult. Amy spoke of her difficulty in obtaining food from a local agency:

> I'm on all this medication. And I just say, when I call [my case manager] when I'm out of food and stuff and I have to take my medication, I call [my case manager] for a referral, to go to the Salvation Army and get me some food. She'll give me a referral. She says, "Come on. Come on, get you a referral, Amy, because you know you have to eat, so take your medication." You know, and stuff. . . . Last time I went, the lady at the Salvation Army told me, "Don't come back." [cries] . . . They know all about my situation, Social Services, they know all about my situation, Mental Health, and Salvation Army, and when I need food and the lady wouldn't give no food and stuff, I said, "I don't get but fourteen dollars in food stamps."

Amy was a frequent user of social services in a small community, and the service providers may have been tired of serving her. Regardless of the reason for their behavior, according to Amy, the system seemed arbitrary and unkind.

Confidentiality concerns extended beyond medical personnel. Most case study participants received services such as transportation and food stamps through their local Department of Social Services (DSS). In some instances, the DSS personnel, by arranging transportation to clinics or in providing some other help, learn of a person's HIV status while the person is using their services. When she goes for services, Wendy felt that DSS workers, who are also community members, are informed.

Brad discussed the web of services that had to be negotiated to receive his medications. He was determined to live, and, to do so, he wanted to take his medications. He was chronically frustrated by a system that was not arranged in a way that allowed him to meet his goal easily:

> Well, if I can't get Medicaid to pay for [my medications, my case manager] goes through a program through Ryan White, some kind of program they have for state funding, and [my case manager] pays for [the medications] that way. But most of the time, the money is unavailable, and the way that I am put on prescription, that's what I was saying about this deductible—I'm not supposed to miss the dosage. That's why I wish I could really set up with a social worker, wish they could really reconsider, instead of me meet a deductible, just keep [the funding] going, 'cause the medication, I'm not supposed

to miss the dosage, and that mess me up. . . . So that's one of the reasons why I wish honest to God that their resources was a lot better than what they doing now. . . . If it wasn't for [my case manager] trying to get some of my medicine and the money together to pay for the medicine, I think I would be a lot worse off. Because I can't afford it. Some of my medicine is 300 to 500 dollars per bottle, and you know that's a lot of money, and I don't have it. Hopefully, soon, try to make an appointment to see this lady and talk to her about this. And again maybe they reconsider and just knock off this deductible so this way when I am out of my medicine, I will have a way of paying for it. 'Cause right now I'm low, and if I get run out, I don't have no way of getting it. . . . That's why I said the sources down here they stink. They put you through a lot just to get help, and I don't like that. Because, like I said, I need to keep take my medicine, and I guess, like I said, they don't realize the situation.

Brad was speaking of the fact that during the period of time that he had to meet a Medicaid deductible, which can happen every six months, he was not able to purchase his medications.

People under age sixty-five who have been receiving Social Security Disability Income for two years are Medicare-eligible. With Medicare, recipients no longer need to apply every six months and meet deductibles, but prescription medications and dental care are not covered. Case study participants, such as Christine, worried about the high cost of the items not covered by Medicare.

Some persons with HIV find that the system-level barriers to care are too great. Even determined patients such as Brad find themselves thwarted by a system of care that is neither cohesive nor continuous. The benefits structure is a patchwork with large gaps that are particularly dangerous to persons with HIV. Those who represent the new face of the epidemic have limited emotional, financial, or time resources to handle the struggle of applying and reapplying for benefits.

CASE MANAGERS

All the case study clients were identified through their case managers and chosen by the investigators based on demographic characteristics. Thus, the participants had, at a minimum, one person in their lives who knew of their HIV status and who provided them with some assistance. Most participants held their case managers in high esteem. Case managers assisted in making medical appointments, arranging transportation services, and applying for benefits. It is common for applicants to have their applications rejected.

Christine had applied for disability on her own, but it was denied; her case manager helped her reapply, and the application was then accepted. Christine's experience was not unusual, and without case managers, many people would give up. Bill's case manager helped Bill get his credit rating back and did Bill's income taxes one year. The case manager brought Bill glasses, knives, and forks when he moved into subsidized housing. Gary's case manager brought him toilet paper and even went to his wife's funeral. Brad's case manager was helping Brad arrange to take night courses at a community college. Christine's case manager, whom she called her "guardian angel," brought her kerosene for her furnace when she had none in the winter.

Case managers supplied emotional support, as well. In several cases, the participants considered their case managers to be their friends. Some, like Joy, actually named their case managers as their best friends: "So when I have my pity party and get to crying, and say that I'm sick of it, I wish it would end and this and that. And she'd like, you know, she'd tell me something and make me laugh or tell me something, you know. I thank God for her." Rhonda reports that her case manager is on call day and night and that, if there were ever an emergency, the case manager would be the first to be contacted. Rhonda viewed her case manager as someone who "would break her back to help you." Betty said, "Everything I got going for me, [my case manager] did."

Some respondents commented on the high turnover in HIV case management and their frustrations with the paperwork. Lori, ostracized by her family and community, found her providers to be her sole source of support. During the course of the interviews, Lori's HIV case manager resigned from her position, a common phenomenon in areas where salaries are low and resources, training, and support are inadequate. Lori was given some information on getting case management in another city, but "I'm afraid of change, so I don't want to move. I know if I go . . . I'll be closer to my doctor, but I don't know nothing about social services or anything like that, you know."

Although participants may have worried about the confidentiality of their HIV status when they received HIV services from case managers, these participants received immense support from their case managers. Note also that the sample selection procedure may have biased our sample toward those who had good relations with case managers.

PHYSICIANS

For an illness in which proper treatments, counseling, and education are so important, medical providers play crucial roles in the clients' lives. Oftentimes infectious diseases clinicians are heavily relied upon and trusted by clients. Perhaps for the first time in clients' lives, they are given attention and health care by professional medical providers. Our participants did not have family doctors when growing up and, for the most part, experienced only emergency care prior to their HIV diagnosis.

Amy spoke only with her doctors about her HIV status; she refused to talk to anyone else, such as family members, because the burden of the knowledge was too great to place on family members and Amy feared their potential negative reactions. Joey said of his physician: "He's a straight-up guy. That's what I like about him; he's straight-up. He'll tell you, he'll tell you if your medication ain't working. A whole lot of doctors will keep throwing stuff at you. . . . When I leave there, I feel real good when I leave his office." Many participants felt a similar fondness toward their physicians.

At the same time, though, some participants felt that the clinicians did not always have enough time to give them. Gary wanted his physicians to spend more time educating him about HIV and the medications. "But they don't sit down and talk about side effects or none of that shit. I want to know if I'm the only fuckin' person sitting there dealing with fuckin' shakes. I can't even hold a pencil, I can't write a letter because I can't keep my hands still."

A difficulty for physicians and other clinicians is that persons with HIV who have been disenfranchised do not usually raise their questions and concerns unless asked directly and repeatedly. With increasing pressures for clinicians to see more and more patients each day, it becomes increasingly difficult to meet the patients' communication needs.

The quality of the interaction between patient and physician is important for the physician to adequately assess the readiness of the patient to adhere to complicated medical regimens and for continued patient adherence to appointments and medications. Participants complained that they did not regularly see the same physicians at the infectious diseases clinics. Joni was certain that if she had had one doctor who consistently followed her care, she would have adhered to her medications: "See, that [hospital], it is so huge, you know, it is so huge. I'm intimidated by it, you know. You know, you want something a little bit more personable. You know. I don't know, it just sucks; that's all I can tell you. It just sucks."

In chapter 9 we discussed distrust of the medical system, including the results of North Carolina focus groups who demonstrated high levels of distrust among HIV-positive persons living in rural areas and high sensitivity to perceived breaches in confidentiality, even if the breach involved only medical personnel. Some participants waffled between expressing distrust (such as Gina saying that she did not believe her doctor for telling her a cure for HIV does not exist) and great fondness for their infectious diseases physician. It was not possible to disentangle these two opposing views.

LOCAL CLINICIANS

Reactions to local generalist physicians were different from reactions to infectious diseases clinicians. Female participants were more likely than males to have a local clinician because they were seen locally for prenatal care. Although some participants liked their local primary care physicians, others reported very negative experiences with clinicians in the local county health departments. For example, when Lisa decided to have another child, she stopped going to the local health department because she feared their disapproval. As demonstrated in the HIV Cost and Services Utilization Study (HCSUS) and SHIPS data, this decision is not uncommon for HIV-positive women.

MENTAL HEALTH PROVIDERS

The high rate of HIV-positive persons having mental health and/or substance abuse diagnoses is just beginning to be recognized in rural areas. When Joni was asked if she had ever tried to seek mental health counseling, she replied: "I went through some agencies, but it's to me, it's a fucking joke, so I don't talk about it, I don't deal with it, block it out."

Teri, who was struggling to keep free of drugs, refused to seek mental health services because of negative experiences in the past:

Most of the time, I just hold in, I hold in. Because I don't trust nobody. I remember the last time I tried to talk to somebody about myself, I got locked up in the crazy house. . . . And I was so angry one day, and I couldn't hold it in no more, so I tried to talk to them, and all I know, I got locked up in the crazy home, and I refused to talk or tell anybody. Ever since that happened, like I want to kill myself or something, I stay to myself now. If I want to do it, I do it regardless of whatever. I just keep it to myself, if it gets too bad off, I hope that I can come out and tell somebody. I doubt it right now, because since they locked me up that time . . . .

Lori had been seeking mental health counseling for years but stopped because of turnover among mental health providers. Lori, comfortable with her initial counselor, built a trust and willingness to talk with this woman. Lori's new counselor was male, which she said made the transition even more difficult. At one point during her interview, Lori's thoughts sidetracked to a past traumatic event, which signaled the need she had to talk with someone about her feelings. When asked if going to mental health services helped her deal with her issues, Lori responded:

Not really. Because they really don't tell me how to handle it, because sometimes I will have dreams about [the foster mother] and stuff. I will see her beating me. One time, she had made us go out and get our own switches, but we had to get switches with briars in them, and she would plait them up and strip us naked and beat us with them. One time, we were putting plastic up, she put plastic up, and the wind was blowing, and I was holding the plastic while she was cutting, and she took the scissors and gashed my hand with the scissors, but nobody would believe me.

In a seemingly fragile situation, providers did not take significant steps to aid this particular client in her transition to a new counselor, which caused her to dislike the sessions and stop seeking care. In addition, rural areas have a limited choice of providers; for example, Lori had only one choice.

For Amy, however, whenever she confided in someone, it was always a mental health counselor or HIV case manager. Amy often sat alone in her apartment, watching television or even staring at the walls. When she received a telephone call from a counselor at the mental health center, she was pleased to know that someone was watching over her:

[The mental health counselor] would call me every now and then, checking on me. She ain't gonna forget me. She said, "I don't even see you. You're living by yourself? Are you enjoying the place, and is everything all right?" She said, "If anything comes up, just let us know; we will talk about it. We ain't gonna forget you; you're still in our computer." They make me feel good about myself.

Knowing that someone was thinking of her, even if she was just a name in their computer, made Amy feel good.

County mental health providers in the Southeast are often not trained in the provision of mental health services that address the unique concerns of HIV-positive persons. Additionally, services are not structured in a way to provide combined mental health and substance abuse services as a package.

CURRENT MEDICATIONS

On average, participants who were interviewed took eighteen pills per day. Some participants, viewing HIV medications as a means to prolong their life, hoped to live until the day a cure is discovered or shared with them. All twenty-five participants had been or currently were taking HIV medications; almost all of them viewed medications as helpful. But everyone who viewed their regimens as improving their health in terms of their viral loads and CD4 counts also complained of side effects. One participant blamed his impotence on his medications, even though his physicians said the medications were not to blame. Many people living with HIV are forced to choose the better of two evils: taking medications to improve their HIV status or staying off of medicine to avoid the terrible side effects.

Brad made a decision that many others with HIV have made:

> Some of the medicine that I have are giving me side effects like this: my fingernails have never been this dark, never. That's one of the prescriptions. . . . And I stopped taking it. I don't want nothing that's going to make me look worse. And right now, as far as my appearance, if I didn't tell you I was sick, you wouldn't know. So that's why. . . . They want me to continue taking it because it's bringing my viral load down, but with the side effect, making me sick, I don't want to go that way. And that's the choice I make.

When asked why he thinks he's still alive, Brad replied it was because he did not rush into taking medications that were offered to him. Several of his friends had passed away from AIDS, and he blamed their early deaths on medications taken before proper research had been conducted; therefore, doctors did not yet know to tell their patients about possible side effects. Brad agreed that medications had been and could continue to keep him alive (and so did many other participants), but the side effects were too great to ignore. Brad expressed what many people living with HIV feel: they want to avoid physical indications of the virus for as long as possible. If a medication were to take away any lesions Brad might have had, then perhaps he would have stayed on his medications. But at the time of the interviews, medications were only reminding him of his HIV by worsening his appearance.

Lori felt frustrated by having to take medications and regularly go to the doctor: "It's like rubbing it into me . . . to have to take them all the time. Have to take medicine, live off medicine. I don't like going to the doctors. . . . I feel like every time I go, I hear something bad."

On the other hand, several participants felt good about their medications. Dean stated: "I was so happy about taking my medication; it's kind of helping me out, because I have a whole lot more energy than I had before." Christine also faced poor physical appearance in taking her medicines, with her hair falling out, but she said, "I ain't gonna worry about no hair as long as I can get up and clean my house up, cook, eat, and do what I need to do. Go pay bills and have fun if I want to, then I ain't gonna worry about no hair. I say I can glue it in."

When Lisa's physician first approached her to take medications, she responded, "I'm not your rat"—a comment reflecting a common fear that HIV medications are still experimental among minority populations (Erwin, Peters 1999). But she now says that her medications are helping her, even after her gall bladder was removed from medication reactions. For the most part, the participants understood that there could be benefits from taking HIV medications.

Because the participants were identified through their case managers, they were already involved in a care system that was educating them about HIV, medications, and side effects. The relationships they had built with their medical and social service providers enabled them to trust the prescriptions they were given and understand that taking medications lowered their viral load and increased their CD4 count. With the help of their providers this information made sense to them. Even with these beliefs, however, participants such as Joni still participated in drug holidays—times when they would decide that they could not take their medications: "Sometimes I just lay in there like my bones aching. Skin is changing. I got this constant cough. . . . I always got a sinus infection. It is affecting my vision. Seems like my ears hurt. My whole body hurts. I just don't feel well, ever, and I told you I stopped taking the pills right? The pills don't make me feel no better." Drug holidays were taken without informing the physician. The only provider who might have the knowledge that clients were taking drug holidays were the case managers, who are not trained in adherence counseling.

Literature

Many persons currently living with HIV disease have basic subsistence-level needs for such items as food, clothing, and housing (Bonuck et al. 1996; Marx et al. 1997; Piette et al. 1993). Persons with subsistence needs often face a choice of either receiving medical care, which may seem to benefit them only in the distant future, or meeting their immediate daily needs. Therefore, the need for medical care competes with the need for basic subsistence, which becomes an actual barrier to receiving timely care and an invitation to receiving emergency care (Cunningham et al. 1999).

Analysis of data from the national HCSUS indicated that more than one-third of the persons surveyed went without or postponed care because they needed money for food, clothing, or housing; lacked transportation; were unable to get out of work; or were simply too sick (Cunningham et al. 1999). The researchers found that a person with any one or more of these four competing needs was associated with significantly greater odds of requiring an emergency room visit without hospitalization, never receiving antiretroviral agents, and reporting low access to care. Visiting an emergency room without a hospital stay was used as a proxy measure for inappropriate use of care. The odds of reporting low access to care were approximately three times higher among those having one or more competing needs.

Support services such as benefits advocacy, housing, home health care, emotional counseling, and substance abuse treatment are designed to decrease institutional service use such as hospitalization, increase access and adherence to medical care and medications, and improve the quality of life of the HIV-infected individual (Mor et al. 1994; Hughes et al. 1997; Tramarin et al. 1992; Celentano et al. 1998; Strathdee et al. 1998). These supportive services help meet the basic needs of persons with HIV and thereby facilitate their use of medical care and medications. HCSUS inquired about the need for five supportive services in the six months preceding the interview. Respondents were found to be in need of: income assistance or health care benefits (benefits advocacy) (43 percent); a place to live (19 percent); home health care (17 percent); mental health or emotional counseling (33 percent); and drug or alcohol treatment (10 percent) (Katz et al. 2000). In all, 67 percent of the respondents were in need of at least one of the five services.

The decision to prescribe medications is difficult. The clinician must ultimately decide what he or she feels is best for the patient based on whether the clinician thinks (1) the person will benefit from medications and (2) the person can adhere. As described in chapter 1, nonadherence can result in a virus resistant to medications for not only that individual but also those whom the individual might infect (Boden et al. 1999; Wainberg, Friedland 1998).

Being African American, Latino, uninsured and Medicaid-insured, and female and having a nonhomosexual route of exposure to HIV are traits that have all been associated with inferior patterns of HIV care in the United States (Sharpiro et al. 1999). Inferior care refers to both poor health services utilization (e.g., less than two ambulatory visits in a six-month period, at least one emergency department visit that did not lead to hospitalization, or at least one hospitalization) and inadequate medication utilization. The reasons for the inferior care are not entirely clear, but the same groups of people have also been found to have greater subsistence and unmet needs (Cunningham et al. 1999).

Researchers are just beginning to try to understand the patient-doctor interaction and its influence on satisfaction with care, resultant health-related knowledge on the part of the patient, and adherence. Roberts and Volberding (1999) found that HIV/AIDS care physicians engage in pre- and postprescription phases of adherence communication with their patients and that during the preprescription phase, physicians make decisions about the patients' likelihood of adhering to therapy. The researchers noted that physicians have diverse ways of communicating with patients regarding adherence to therapy, that the effect of these techniques has not been assessed, and that there is no common training curriculum. Curtis and colleagues (1999) asked AIDS patients to report on communication with their physicians regarding end-of-life care. Higher-quality communication was associated with higher satisfaction with care. African Americans, Hispanics, females with high-risk sexual partners, and injecting drug users were less likely to report positive communication with their physicians.

SOUTHEAST HIV PATIENT SURVEY (SHIPS)

SHIPS collected information regarding the need for and receipt of different types of services (table 10.1). In the twelve months preceding the interview, survey respondents: needed help paying for prescription medications (39 percent); experienced difficulty applying for benefit programs (28 percent); experienced difficulty with transportation to appointments (18 percent); needed spiritual counseling (38 percent); needed an HIV support group (28 percent); needed emergency housing assistance (28 percent); needed emergency food (26 percent); and needed assistance in obtaining nutritional supplements (25 percent). Nearly three-quarters (71 percent, not shown) did not know where to obtain services or resources for people with HIV/AIDS. Some respondents (12 percent) reported being turned away from health care providers specifically because of their HIV status.

SHIPS asked respondents to rate how often they adhered to their HIV

Table 10.1
Barriers to Care

Barrier to Care	Number	Percentage
Needed help with paying for prescriptions[a]	210	39.4
Applied for benefit programs[a]	265	49.7
Had difficulty if applied for benefit programs	73	27.6
Had difficulty with transportation[a]	98	18.4
Needed spiritual help/pastoral counseling[a]	201	37.7
Needed HIV support group[a]	151	28.3
Needed emergency housing assistance[a]	148	27.8
Needed emergency food[a]	140	26.3
Needed help getting nutritional supplements[a]	131	24.6
Ever turned away by doctor due to HIV	66	12.4
Needed dental care[a]	302	56.7
Did not receive needed dental care	106	35.1
Turned away by dentist due to HIV in past five years	47	8.8

NOTE: Total possible N = 555.

[a]In past year.

medications as prescribed on a five-point Likert scale from "always" to "never" (see appendix A for survey instrument description). We assume self-reporting bias: only those who reported "always" adhering to their medications as prescribed were coded as adherent. Of the respondents 61 percent reported always adhering to medications. This rate is in line with other studies that have reported adherence rates (Gordillo et al. 1999). Multiple logistic regression analysis of SHIPS data examined relationships between adherence and barriers and facilitators of care, including social supports, controlling for other demographic, support, health status, and risk behavior characteristics. An increased likelihood of adherence was associated with: increased distance to their ID clinic (for each additional ten miles of travel the odds of adherence increased by nine); placing importance on AIDS; applying for benefits; and having experienced side effects from medications. Patient characteristics associated with decreased adherence were: ever using illicit drugs; experiencing difficulty with the law in the twelve months preceding the interview; having children under eighteen living at home; a CD4+ cell count between 200 and 500 relative to those with higher CD4+ levels; and having someone to help take the medications. It is likely that respondents who had someone to remind them to take their medications had that person because they were not able to adhere to their medications on their own (see table 10.2). Also HIV case management is associated with greater reception of subsistence-level needs.

Similarly, we examined the number of physician visits in the past year (table 10.3). Respondents who were older, lived further away from the ID clinic, and had children under age eighteen living in the home had fewer physician visits. However, individuals who had a caregiver and were in need of support services had greater physician visits.

NORTH CAROLINA HIV PROVIDER SURVEY AND DISCUSSION
The need to integrate services of medical clinicians and case managers, mental health and substance abuse providers, and departments of social services seems obvious to an outside observer. How else could one cover such large geographical expanses without a continuum of services? Therefore, we conducted the North Carolina HIV Provider Survey in 1997 to assess the degree of services integration in eastern North Carolina. Data from the NC HIV Provider Survey are presented as means of the five-point Likert scale response, with 1 being "none" or "nothing." Categorized by the region in which they were located, providers' knowledge of HIV services in their region indicated a mean response of 1.93 (where 1 is "know nothing") for the other providers listed on their survey (see table 10.4). Generally, the providers made no referrals (1.34) to other agencies and received no referrals (1.20) from other

Table 10.2
Adherent to Medications: Logistic Regression Results from the SHIPS
Database

Adherent	OR	95% CI	P-value
Internal Support			
Have someone to remind respondent to take medications	0.46[a]	0.28, 0.75	0.002
Has caregiver	1.64	0.67, 3.98	0.279
Marital status	1.20	0.60, 2.41	0.600
Children < 18 years old living with respondent	0.70[a]	0.55, 0.90	0.004
Barriers to support services	0.84	0.69, 1.03	0.090
Applied for benefits	1.31[b]	1.05, 1.64	0.018
Had difficulty applying for benefits	1.09	0.53, 2.22	0.824
Attitudes			
Importance of AIDS	1.77[b]	1.02, 3.07	0.043
Experienced medication side-effects	1.20[a]	1.06, 1.36	0.005
Risk Behaviors			
Drug use (6 months)	0.58[b]	0.34, 0.98	0.043
Difficulty with the law (year)	0.43[b]	0.20, 0.94	0.034
Demographics			
Nonwhite	0.83	0.47, 1.47	0.523
Nonmale	0.89	0.48, 1.63	0.694
Gay, lesbian, or bisexual	0.63	0.36, 1.09	0.095
Age	1.03[c]	1.00, 1.06	0.048
Less than high school education	1.11	0.63, 1.95	0.73
Unstable housing	1.32	0.80, 2.18	0.278
Distance to clinic per mile	1.09[b]	1.02, 1.17	0.017
Rural-living[d]	0.61	0.35, 1.08	0.091
Health Status			
CD4 <200	0.45	0.19, 1.03	0.059
CD4 200–500	0.38[b]	0.17, 0.88	0.024

Note: Total N = 430.

[a]Indicates statistical significance at or below the 0.01 level.

[b]Indicates statistical significance between 0.01 and 0.05.

[c]Indicates statistical significance at the 0.05 level.

[d]As defined by zip code and 1990 Census Bureau definition.

agencies. With a mean response of 2.74, rating the satisfaction with the agency was reported to be a nonapplicable question in approximately two-thirds of the cases (65 percent).

These results indicate that there is little to no communication from one provider to the next. Respondents to SHIPS had many nonmedical needs: help with prescription payments, transportation, child care, a support group for people with HIV, emergency housing assistance, emergency food, nutritional supplements, and legal documents. Several of these needs can be addressed by the integration of services: creating a network of HIV providers that serves as a

Table 10.3
Number of Doctor Visits in Past Twelve Months (ordinary least squares)

Independent Variables	Parameter Estimate	Standard Error	P-value
Receive help taking meds	0.02962	0.08467	0.7267
Has caregiver	0.28500	0.13517	0.0355
Marital status	0.15883	0.11435	0.1655
Number of children < 18 living with	−0.04233	0.03420	0.2165
Need support services	0.05723	0.01534	0.0002
Barriers to support services	−0.02968	0.02893	0.3054
Number of benefits programs applied for	−0.0046	0.03522	0.8949
Had difficulty applying for benefits	−0.03767	0.11759	0.7488
People will learn about my HIV	−0.17342	0.16745	0.3009
Local docs unwilling to treat HIV	0.13120	0.18430	0.4769
Self-efficacy scale	−0.00325	0.00311	0.2975
Self-esteem scale	0.00687	0.00416	0.1000
Nonwhite	−0.09817	0.09283	0.2908
Nonmale	0.04069	0.09920	0.6819
Gay, lesbian, or bisexual	0.12187	0.09304	0.1909
Age	−0.01121	0.00502	0.0260
Less than high school education	−0.11800	0.09328	0.2065
Unstable housing	−0.16330	0.08548	0.0567
Distance to clinic rounded off	−0.00211	0.00104	0.0424
Rural-living[a]	0.08543	0.09517	0.3698

NOTE: Total N = 479.
[a]As defined by zip code and 1990 Census Bureau definition.

resource and referral system for persons with HIV. Although patients have many social service and health care needs, the NC HIV Provider Survey illustrates that providers of services for persons who are HIV-positive are not familiar with one another. This lack of knowledge and coordination may further inhibit HIV-positive patients from learning about helpful services that would help stabilize their lives in ways to promote self-care.

THE INCREASES IN THE number and proportion of persons with HIV living in rural areas who abuse illicit substances, have mental health problems, are of low economic status (with associated instability in living conditions), and have primary responsibility for children have brought a host of long-term issues to providers. When compounded by chronic HIV and apparent weak provider knowledge of care sources, these patient characteristics may hinder the ability of rural HIV providers to care for a disease that is no longer acute. The ability of persons to adhere to complex therapies over long periods of time is greatly affected by the changing face of the virus. If all social needs are not met concurrently with clinical therapy, then HIV treatment may be not

Table 10.4
Provider Survey Responses

Question	Mean Actual Responses
Knowledge of named agency[a]	1.93
Referrals to named agency[a]	1.34
Referrals from named agency[a]	1.20
Satisfaction with Relationship with Named Agency[b]	2.74

NOTE: Total N=101 from North Carolina HIV Provider Survey.
[a]Scale: 1–5: 1=None.
[b]Scale: 1–4: 1=Not at all satisfied.

as effective and even dangerous by creating strains of drug resistant virus through nonadherence.

Case management is funded for HIV-positive persons by the Ryan White CARE Act and by state Medicaid programs with the intention of providing persons with HIV or AIDS greater access to support services (Fleishman et al. 1991; Jellinek 1988; Mor et al. 1989; Riley 1992; Sonsel 1989). Studies have demonstrated that persons with case managers are more likely to receive benefits advocacy, housing, home health care, substance abuse services, psychological services, and emotional and practical support (Fleishman et al. 1991; Katz et al. 2000; London et al. 1998; Wight et al. 1995) and even increased HIV medication use (Katz et al. 2001). HCSUS data indicate that approximately 60 percent of HIV-positive persons who seek care nationally have case managers (Katz et al. 2000). Having patients with such diverse and complicated needs, clinicians should want to be in close contact with the case managers who both help the client negotiate systems and work with the client regularly in their home environment.

Models of care that combine health and social services are being tested in urban areas (Master et al. 1996). Such models often involve the formal collaboration of a small number of provider agencies. In rural areas, models of integrated care might need to be expanded by incorporating greater numbers of agencies over greater distances. For example, it is not feasible to contract with one or two HIV case management agencies to serve a large region. In North Carolina, where one infectious diseases clinic treats patients from more than fifty counties, to create an integrated system of care each infectious diseases clinic would need to communicate with fifty or more case management agencies that serve individuals with multiple chronic diseases. This need is true even as outreach infectious diseases clinics are being funded and arranged because, as seen in the case studies, clients still choose to travel longer distances to major centers to better protect their confidentiality. Each case management agency needs to be in contact with a host of local service providers and multiple infectious diseases clinics to meet clients' needs. Such integration of care and communication networks may seem daunting, but with ingenuity and modern communication techniques we may be able to create integrated systems of care in the face of large obstacles.

North Carolina is attempting to integrate services through a computer network that links infectious diseases clinics with each case management agency through a program called the North Carolina Services Integration Program (NC SIP; originally a Special Projects of National Significance [SPNS] Program sponsored by the Ryan White CARE Act). The computer network also maintains resource directories that include local resources for HIV-positive persons, eligibility requirements for benefits programs, and connections to national HIV information databases. The North Carolina AIDS Care Unit collaborates with NC SIP to offer substantive trainings to case managers. Trainings include such issues as recognizing mental health and substance abuse needs, self-care, vicarious traumatization, and working with a difficult client. NC SIP provided a sounding board for isolated case managers and attempted to link case managers with each other. NC SIP has incorporated another Ryan White Title V funded program, the North Carolina HIV Training and Information Center, which focuses on the provision of HIV-related training to clinicians. NC SIP is testing models of integrated substance abuse, mental health, and HIV services with funding from the Substance Abuse and Mental Health Services Administration, the Health Resources and Services Administration, and the National Institutes of Health (HIV/AIDS Treatment Adherence, Health Outcomes and Cost Study Group 2001).

The integration of care services is extremely difficult in the rural South when working with such a vast number of agencies, each with its own provider cultures, rules and regulations, bureaucracies, and providers. Integration, requiring tenacity and patience, is made more difficult by the constant turnover in care providers.

In states such as Alabama, Louisiana, and North Carolina, HIV case managers are not responsible for providing adherence counseling of any type for fear that they might tell patients how to take specific medications. As a result of such policies, case managers cannot be trained on simple adherence skills such as ways to organize one's life around taking medications (see chapter 11).

Standards must be developed for educating providers and screening for issues to influence an individual's willingness and ability to adhere to clinic visits and medications. Gerbert and colleagues (1999) found that the health outcomes and experiences were improved among HIV-positive persons when their clinicians used a "relationship-centered approach" to their care. They found that three life circumstances served as teachable moments or, as psychological theorists would describe, times of readiness for change. These moments were at the time of the HIV/AIDS diagnosis, at the onset of symptoms, and at the beginning of medication treatment. At these times, HIV-positive persons became more involved with their health care. Therefore, instruction on communication methods is important for clinicians and should be added to the growing list of things physicians must learn to provide care that requires highly active patient involvement.

Brad hoped that by participating in the case study, someone in a decision-making position would hear his voice and realize that the systems in place were causing him improper medication utilization, which would hasten his death. Because the benefits are difficult to maintain, it is easy for a person to go for periods of time without coverage. Clearly the lack of medication coverage most concerned the case study participants. Maine recently received a Medicaid waiver to expand coverage to people with HIV who are poor but not yet disabled; thus, patients could benefit from early treatment (Levi, Kates 2000).

Case managers informed us that they instruct their clients first to run up medical bills to meet their deductible and then ignore the letters from medical centers requesting payment that the clients have no means of paying. Physicians have told us that they have ordered unnecessary procedures and overnight stays so that patients can meet their deductible quicker and remain on Medicaid to maintain continuous prescription medication coverage. Providers are engaging in these practices in an attempt to provide the best medical care for their patients and clients in a system that is not structured to allow for best, or even adequate, medical care for poor chronically ill persons who require continuous expensive medications.

Instead of forcing providers and patients to try to find ways to work around the system, policymakers should work with them to improve the system to fit the real day-to-day needs of the chronically ill patient. Within states and within federal agencies, policymakers must realize that the paperwork, application, and reapplication processes that they implement are far from beneficial to the patients' care needs. These bureaucracies frustrate not only the most appreciated providers, who sometimes leave the field because of exhaustion, but also the patients, who lack energy or time when their own health and their family's well-being are at stake. In spite of all the trauma and victimization that the case study participants experienced in their childhood and adulthood lives, they want to live and are trying to survive. As they struggle with decisions either to feed themselves and their children in the short term or to pay for medicines that may help them in the long term, should not we reorganize our systems of care to support them so they can eliminate the struggle and meet both needs?

Part V

Theory and Policy

Chapter 11

Theoretical Framework and Policy Recommendations

Central to this book is the belief that individuals make logical behavioral decisions given the context of their lives, including comorbidities. If we do not understand the way in which people are behaving, then we are not sufficiently understanding the context of their lives. If providers, policymakers, and researchers begin their work with a deeper knowledge of the many forces influencing an individual's and population's behavior, then practical service and policy changes can be made given societal will. An holistic understanding of the context into which HIV enters a person's life allows us to better understand behaviors and therefore leads to more appropriate policies and interventions. Such an understanding must also lead us to the conclusion that the underlying causes—perhaps the most powerful and fundamental causes—of behavior, treatment, and health outcomes are deeply ingrained in our societal structures, beliefs, and political ideologies in ways that cannot be altered by simple changes in health policy (see Tesh 1988 for similar arguments).

In the first section of this chapter we focus on theories of health-related behavior by combining other researchers' work with the participants' contributions. Theories or frameworks allow one to enmesh new knowledge into the perspective of past work and thereby pinpoint areas for potential change. The second section draws policy implications from the theories, the voices, and current system structures.

Theoretical Framework

The framework presented below combines important elements from both the health services and psychological literature. While the framework is presented in a linear fashion, all relationships (with the exception of immutable

Health Services Utilization and Treatment Adherence

- Utilization of Medical Services (appropriate or inappropriate)
- Regular Clinic Visits
- Medication Adherence
- Decrease Risky Behavior
- Increase Health Promotion Behavior
- Use of Ancillary Services

Figure 11.1. Health Services Utilization and Treatment Adherence

characteristics) are reciprocal and presented as such in the final figure. The model is not meant to be exclusive for our understanding of HIV, but it should be more broadly considered for all chronically ill populations and particularly for poor, disenfranchised, and disengaged individuals. Likewise, the review of literature is not entirely specific to HIV, nor is it exhaustive of HIV research. The primary outcomes of interest are behaviors related to health promotion (including social and health services utilization), treatment adherence (including adherence to medication recommendations), risk reduction, and ancillary services (see fig. 11.1).

Health services researchers and those from the field of psychology present different and complementary explanations for how people make decisions about health services utilization. Health services researchers such as Aday and colleagues (1974, 1993) explain variation in service utilization through a combination of personal characteristics, health status, environmental characteristics, availability and accessibility of services, and satisfaction (see fig. 11.2). Psychological theory focuses in part on internal cognitive processes that lead to decisions regarding behaviors such as service utilization or adherence to treatment plans (Myers, Midence 1998) (fig. 11.3). This decision-making process is a black box for health services researchers.

Utilization of health services, medication adherence, risk behaviors, and health promotion are usually studied separately. Although these behaviors occur in different locations (e.g., in the home, on the streets, or traveling to clinics) and with differing degrees of frequency, they are each human behaviors that could be predicted by the environment, personal characteristics, health status, and internal decision-making processes. Depending on a given outcome the magnitude of the effects and even the direction of the effects may differ.

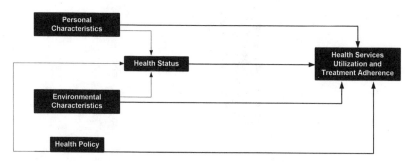

Figure 11.2. Simplified Health Services Research Model of Determinants of Health Services Utilization and Medication Adherence

HEALTH SERVICES UTILIZATION AND TREATMENT ADHERENCE: INTERNAL DECISION-MAKING PROCESS

People often stop taking their medications before they should; some actively decide not to take their medications either because they believe the medications are not needed when they feel healthy or because the medications have negative side effects (Weidle et al. 1999). Others simply forget to take their medications. Recent studies indicate that even under the best of circumstances, only 67 percent of patients appropriately adhere to their medication regimens, even for short-term medications, such as a ten-day course of antibiotics (Lee et al. 1999).

The way in which a person who needs services decides how, when, and where to seek services is a complex internal cognitive process (see fig. 11.4). An understanding of this process delves into the very nature of human actions, feelings, and interactions, where the individual consciously and subconsciously accounts for innumerable factors. The public health and health services literature has focused primarily on the cognitive process, consisting of one's knowledge, attitudes, and beliefs that translate into action. Knowledge includes knowing about the symptoms of a disease or need for services, recognizing the seriousness of that disease, and understanding that services are available. Defined in this way, knowledge has been shown to be associated with increased utilization of services given the same level of need (Delorme et al. 1999; Cole et al. 1997). When symptoms of a disease are not present, a person's attitudes toward the health care system and the disease are important in determining utilization of services. Finally, beliefs about a disease's curability and the usefulness of services also influence when care is sought.

Utilization of health care services and medication adherence have been found to be associated with the individual's perception of the seriousness of

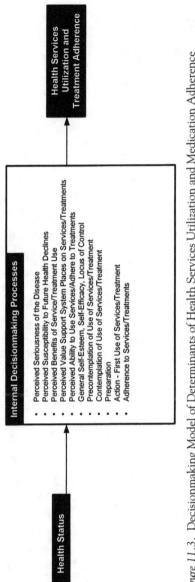

Figure 11.3. Decisionmaking Model of Determinants of Health Services Utilization and Medication Adherence

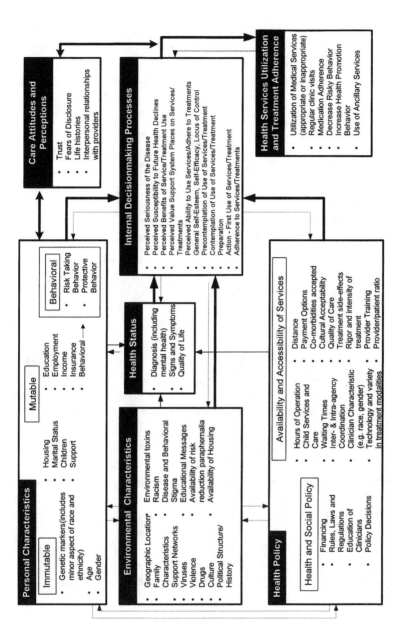

Personal Characteristics

Immutable
- Genetic markers (includes minor aspect of race and ethnicity)
- Age
- Gender

Mutable
- Housing
- Marital Status
- Children
- Support
- Education
- Employment
- Income
- Insurance
- Behavioral →

Behavioral
- Risk Taking Behavior
- Protective Behavior

Environmental Characteristics
- Geographic Location*
- Family Characteristics
- Support Networks
- Viruses
- Violence
- Drugs
- Culture
- Political Structure/ History
- Environmental toxins
- Racism
- Disease and Behavioral Stigma
- Educational Messages
- Availability of risk reduction paraphernalia
- Availability of Housing

Health Policy

Health and Social Policy
- Financing
- Rules, Laws and Regulations
- Education of Clinicians
- Policy Decisions

Health Status
- Diagnosis (including mental health)
- Signs and Symptoms
- Quality of Life

Availability and Accessibility of Services
- Hours of Operation
- Child Services and Care
- Waiting Times
- Inter- & Intra-agency Coordination
- Clinician Characteristic (e.g. race, gender)
- Technology and variety in treatment modalities
- Distance
- Payment Options
- Co-morbidities accepted
- Cultural Acceptability
- Quality of Care
- Treatment side-effects
- Rigor and intensity of treatment
- Provider Training
- Provider/patient ratio

Care Attitudes and Perceptions
- Trust
- Fears of Disclosure
- Life histories
- Interpersonal relationships with providers

Internal Decisionmaking Processes
- Perceived Seriousness of the Disease
- Perceived Susceptibility to Future Health Declines
- Perceived Benefits of Service/Treatment Use
- Perceived Value Support System Places on Services/ Treatments
- Perceived Ability to Use Services/Adhere to Treatments
- General Self-Esteem, Self-Efficacy, Locus of Control
- Precontemplation of Use of Services/Treatment
- Contemplation of Use of Services/Treatment
- Preparation
- Action - First Use of Services/Treatment
- Adherence to Services/Treatments

Health Services Utilization and Treatment Adherence
- Utilization of Medical Services (appropriate or inappropriate)
- Regular clinic visits
- Medication Adherence
- Increase Health Promotion Behavior
- Decrease Risky Behavior
- Use of Ancillary Services

Figure 11.4. Detailed Determinants of Health Services Utilization and Treatment Adherence (Bi-Directional)

the disease, the perceived susceptibility to the disease or disease progression, and an assessment of the benefits from the recommended course of action. The patient weighs these benefits against perceived barriers to the action (Horne, Weinman 1998; Kelley, Scott 1990) (see fig 11.4). For example, adherence to zidovudine monotherapy has been found to be associated with patient belief that zidovudine prolongs life (Samet et al. 1992).

Various psychological theories provide an even richer explanation of human behavior (Fishbein, Guinan 1996). Psychological theories have further developed the link between the apparent need for service or treatment and its utilization. The most widely tested theoretical models of care-seeking behavior are Social Cognition Models, which emphasize the individual's perceptions regarding the disease and the best treatment for its perceived condition, and Stage Models, which emphasize the individual's readiness to engage in treatment (Conner, Norman 1996). Both models are explained more fully below and are correlated with adherence to medication in chronic and acute diseases (Cochran, Gitlin 1988; Horne 1997; Miller et al. 1992; Ried, Christensen 1988; Ried et al. 1985), practicing safer sex (Abraham et al. 1996; Chan, Fishbein 1993), smoking cessation (DiClemente et al. 1991; Godin et al. 1992; Velicer et al. 1992), dietary changes (Curry et al. 1992; McCann et al. 1996), and exercise changes (Godin et al. 1989; Godin et al. 1991; Marcus et al. 1992; Norman, Smith 1995).

Perceptions about disease form the base of the Health Belief Model (our model integrates the Health Belief Model and the Theory of Reasoned Action extended by Perceived Behavioral Control, which are the primary Social Cognition Models), one of the Social Cognition Models (Rosenstock 1974) involving a "cue to action" as an important trigger to initiating treatment (Becker, Maiman 1975). Such a cue might be an HIV diagnosis or a friend's death from HIV. Results from one meta-analysis indicate that the combined components of the Health Belief Model explain nearly one-fourth of the variation in health promotion behavior (Zimmerman, Vernberg 1994).

Equally important in the decision-making process is the value that patients place on a treatment's potential outcome (Ajzen, Fishbein 1980). A patient who believes a treatment is effective and attainable may still not place a high value on its outcome, such as improved health or changed behavior. For example, a patient may first need to believe that adhering to clinic visits will stop the decline in health status *and* must also believe that a decline in health status is a negative outcome. A patient's assessment of how the support network (e.g., family and friends) views the treatment and its outcome is another important motivator to engage the patient in treatment. Believing that others want the individual to go to the doctor *and* wanting to please others may further influence patient intentions.

Self-esteem, self-efficacy, and locus of control (see fig. 11.4) are also important in determining a patient's perception of ability to engage in treatment (Pearlin, Schooler 1978; Rosenberg 1965). Self-esteem is a measure of how worthy a person feels. Self-efficacy is the degree to which the patient feels control over life and environment. Similarly, locus of control is where a patient feels control lies for personal behaviors and the events that occur (Rotter 1966). Individuals differ in perceptions of their control over their environments and their own behaviors; these differences are important in predicting treatment-related behavior (Ajzen 1985). In analyses of behavior, using questions regarding perceived behavioral control improves predictions of patients' intentions and behavior (Ajzen 1991; Conner, Sparks 1996).

Even understanding the above relationships does not explain the behavior of all patients. For example, a patient who would appear to have everything in place to appropriately engage in treatment may still not utilize services. This patient may recognize the importance of clinic visits, have a support system composed of individuals encouraging use of services, and may appear to have the self-esteem and sense of self-efficacy needed for the necessary behavioral change. Why would this individual still not engage in care? The answer can be partially answered by examining the patient's readiness for the required change in behavior.

The Stages of Change Model suggests that improving and maintaining health behavior occurs in five progressive stages: precontemplation, contemplation, preparation, action, and maintenance (Prochaska, DiClemente 1983) (see fig. 11.4). Precontemplation is characterized by not even thinking of change as a possibility. In the contemplative stage, the person is considering, but not committed to, a behavioral change. Preparation is defined as having a plan for change in the near future. Action involves attempts to change or to engage in the planned behavior. Maintenance, or adherence, occurs when the person attempts to prevent returning to previous undesired behaviors. Individuals pass through these phases in a cyclical manner. At the same time, past and current experiences in utilization of services and treatment adherence influence the internal decision-making process regarding future behavior. (This bi-directionality between the internal decision-making process and health services utilization and treatment adherence is not indicated in figure 11.3 but is in figure 11.4.)

While an individual who needs treatment is undergoing a complex internal decision-making process, external or noncognitive circumstances simultaneously contribute to whether the individual finally receives treatment. These noncognitive influences include health status, personal characteristics (e.g., age, education), environmental factors (e.g., support network encouragement or discouragement), and the availability of care. Past research has emphasized the importance of health status in determining a person's utilization of services and adherence to medications. Even nationally important published documents as recent as *Healthy People 2010* (Office of Disease Prevention and Health Promotion 2000), listing the health objectives for the next decade, included noncognitive factors but not the integral psychological factors in health services/health outcome models. Our work supports the equally important roles that both noncognitive influences and the internal decision-making process have in determining utilization and adherence; we state that both can be understood and modified with appropriate intervention.

DETERMINANTS OF UTILIZATION AND ADHERENCE:
HEALTH STATUS

Health status determines need for health services. An individual's health status is defined objectively by medical diagnoses, signs, and symptoms of disease(s) and quality of life (fig. 11.4). A diagnosis includes conditions such as HIV, a mental health or substance abuse disorder, and other comorbidities including diabetes and heart disease, all of which have high prevalence rates in the South (Zheng et al. 1997) and particularly among African Americans (National Center for Health Statistics 1994). Signs and symptoms of the diagnosis, or medical condition, might include night sweats and weight loss associated with HIV or anxiety associated with a mental health disorder. They may also include more general effects such as ability to function (e.g., dress, eat, use the toilet) or experiences of pain and fatigue (Ware et al. 1993). Quality of life includes all aspects of how patients feel about their lives, including the functional limitations just described (Ware et al. 1993).

Health status is influenced by genetic endowment, prosperity, the social and physical environment, a feeling of well-being, the individual's response to personal and environmental influences, existent and accessible health care services, and the manner in which individuals are treated within health care systems (Evans, Stoddard 1990; Evans et al. 1994; Andersen et al. 2000). Individuals vary in their need for health care services and therapies at any given time. As explained below, many characteristics and behaviors that influence health status also independently and directly influence service utilization and adherence patterns.

INFLUENCE OF PERSONAL CHARACTERISTICS AND ENVIRONMENTAL FACTORS DIRECTLY ON HEALTH STATUS AND INDEPENDENTLY ON UTILIZATION AND ADHERENCE

The realization that both personal characteristics and the environment affect health status dates as far back as the fifth century B.C.E. Hippocrates, in his exploration of population differences in health status, noted the importance of "the seasons, the winds, the rising of the sun, the waters (marshy and soft or hard and running from above), the ground (naked or wooded and well watered), whether inhabitants are fond of drinking and eating in excess or are fond of labor and exercise." While having no knowledge of the direct biological causes of disease, Hippocrates demonstrated a preliminary understanding of the importance of behavior and environment on health.

PERSONAL CHARACTERISTICS AFFECTING HEALTH STATUS. Personal characteristics consist of those traits that most obviously and objectively describe a person to an observer. These include demographic factors that are immutable (cannot be changed), sociodemographic factors that are mutable (can be altered), and behaviors in which a person engages (Aday et al. 1993) (fig. 11.4). Immutable characteristics include age, gender (recognizing that gender can be defined in different ways and can be altered), skin color, genetic makeup, and sexual orientation. Mutable personal characteristics can include: marital status, geographic living location, housing status, number of children, years of education, occupation, income, and health insurance.

GENDER. Some diseases differ in occurrence by gender: multiple sclerosis is more common in women (Franklin, Nelson 1993), while men are more likely to experience heart disease (Smith, Pratt 1993). Women's mortality rate from HIV is higher than men's, possibly owing to less access to health care (Cohen 1996; Shapiro et al. 1999), poorer utilization of available services, and/or worse adherence to treatment protocols. Differences between men and women exist in the relationship between virus replication, CD4+ decline, and responses to drug therapy (Currier et al. 2000), as well as in HIV progression overall (Anastos et al. 2000).

POVERTY. Social class and income inequalities influence how long and how well people live (Lochner et al. 2001; Shi et al. 1999; Kawachi, Kennedy 1999) and affect the trade-offs made between quantity and quality of life (Patrick, Erickson 1993). People with lower levels of education, lower income, manual and low-paying jobs and without insurance and stable housing have higher rates of morbidity and mortality (Evans et al. 1994). The influence of poverty on health has been documented since the mid-1800s (Susser, Susser 1996). Lower income level is often used as a proxy for lower educational level, and vice versa; both have been shown to be associated with poorer health habits, higher rates of high-risk behaviors, higher maternal mortality rates, lack of prenatal care, misuse of treatment, higher barriers to care, and higher morbidity and mortality. These problems affect health care for individuals and their children, related to all illnesses including cancer, heart disease, diabetes, and HIV (Guendelman et al. 2000; Potvin et al. 2000; Hardy et al. 2000; Cook et al. 1999; Lee 1999; Luginaah et al. 1999; Eachus et al. 1999; Mandelblatt et al. 1999; Anglin, White 1999; Evans et al. 1994). Socioeconomic status also negatively affects the way in which patients are treated in medical settings (Magnus, Mick 2000; Rathore et al. 2000) and their quantity and quality of life (van Ryn, Burke 2000; Patrick, Erickson 1993). Poverty can be viewed as a Catch-22, whereby the person does not have sufficient funds to access appropriate care and services, which leads to poorer health and decreased opportunities to find well-paying jobs. There is an interrelationship between poverty and HIV whereby factors associated with poverty predispose one to HIV; for example, subsistence living can lead one to exchange sex for money or housing or simply allow greater exposure to high-risk activities and greater need for escape.

RACE AND SEXUAL ORIENTATION. There is little genetic evidence that individuals of any race or ethnicity are more or less susceptible to HIV, yet rates differ dramatically by race. Often, race and ethnicity are included as immutable characteristics. However, there is no scientifically accepted definition of race or ethnicity, and there is little consistency in the use of these terms in health care research (Schulman et al. 1995). Measures of skin color do not capture culture, biology, values, or behavior (LaVeist 1994). Research has found few genetic differences by race, and even these are dwarfed by differences among population groups defined by all other characteristics previously listed. People with different skin colors experience different levels of racism that then influences health status (LaVeist 1996; LaVeist 2000; Williams 1997; Williams et al. 1994). For example, social discrimination directly influences health status as measured by such indicators as self-rated health status (Schulz et al. 2000), blood pressure (Krieger, Sidney 1996; Krieger 1990), and general morbidity and mortality (Ren et al. 1999; Williams 1999). Researchers are only just beginning to develop sophisticated measures of discrimination (Krieger 1999; Krieger 2000).

Races in the United States differ in their common history, be it one of slavery and oppression or one of coming to the United States with a vision of opportunity (Wilkinson, King 1987). The interaction of social forces on groups defined by skin color and ethnicity has resulted in differences in income, housing, education, employment, use of drugs, violence, family characteristics, and health status (Wilkinson, King 1987). Although socioeconomic status is a powerful predictor of health (Kawachi, Kennedy 1999; Krieger et al. 1997; Lochner et al. 2001; Shi et al. 1999), studies indicate that even when controlling for income and other measures of socioeconomic status, racial disparities continue (Lillie-Blanton, LaVeist 1996). In addition, cultural differences may influence eating and exercise habits, marital status, and childbearing (Corin 1994). HIV is ecologically associated with the personal and environmental poverty frequently found in minority communities.

Similar arguments regarding discrimination can be made for sexual orientation, possibly defined by genetic markers (Pillard, Bailey 1998; Bailey et al. 1999). Sexual orientation influences such mutable characteristics as marital status, number of children, and education. A person's sexual orientation may also lead to different environmental experiences of discrimination and related stress.

RURAL LIVING. The rural nature of the surrounding environment influences the type of care networks that can be created and the limitations people face in trying to access services. People living in rural areas are provided less aggressive care, have higher age-specific mortality and morbidity rates, and are most costly to the system (Nickens 1995; General Accounting Office 1991; Ford, Cooper 1995; Ricketts et al. 1994). Specifically with HIV, studies have shown that better care is given by providers with higher volumes of HIV-positive patients because treatment regimens, being so complex, require extensive experience (Brosgart et al. 1999; Willard et al. 1999). Yet many rural doctors have little or no experience treating HIV/AIDS (Voelker 1998).

The nature of small communities, where confidentiality is difficult to protect and reliable transportation is hard to find, can further decrease care accessibility. Although basic care may be offered by the local health department, the fear of encountering a relative's neighbor who works there may hinder the person from seeking care locally (Whetten-Goldstein et al. 2001c). Rural-living, HIV-positive persons travel long distances for care because they are concerned about confidentiality and believe that local physicians are not knowledgeable in HIV care (Mainous, Matheny 1996). Furthermore, to access the next-closest available care source may require traveling for hours. If such transportation is even available, it can be very tiring and costly.

Relative to urban-living HIV-positive persons, rural-living HIV-positive patients have lower satisfaction with life, lower perceptions of social support from family and friends, reduced access to medical and mental health care, higher levels of loneliness, more perceived stigma, greater fear that their HIV serostatus would be learned by others, and more maladaptive coping strategies (Heckman et al. 1998a). There is a common perception that persons living in rural areas may be protected from the risk behaviors and violence that occur more frequently in urban areas. While incidence rates of homicides and crack use are lower in rural areas, these high-risk behaviors still occur (Gilliland et al. 2000; McCoy, H. et al. 1999; McCoy, C. et al. 1999), and for the population of interest, the rates are not entirely known. One study of female crack-cocaine users that compared crack use, sexual practices, and potential for HIV infection and transmission between rural and urban women found few differences (Forney et al. 1992).

BEHAVIORAL CHARACTERISTICS. A subcategory of mutable characteristics is behavioral characteristics (see fig 11.4), which can vary by immutable characteristics. For example, general population studies clearly indicate that females generally engage in less risk-taking behavior than males (e.g., substance abuse, smoking, number of sexual partners) (Brady, Randall 1999; Moon et al. 1999), but a study of crack users, many of whom were HIV-infected, revealed that women reported more sexual partners than men, particularly in exchange for drugs or money (Tortu et al. 1998). McGinnis and Foege (1993) found that human behavior was responsible for approximately half of the 2,148,000 deaths of United States citizens in 1990. The researchers examined studies conducted from 1977 to 1993 to use best evidence in estimating predictors of death. The most prominent contributors to the deaths in a single year were: tobacco (400,000 deaths); diet and activity patterns (300,000 deaths); sexual behavior (30,000 deaths); motor vehicles (25,000 deaths); and illicit drug use (20,000 deaths).

Risk-taking and protective behaviors are mutable and interact bidirectionally with health status and internal decision-making processes. It is possible to help someone stop taking extreme risks to self and others and engage in protective behaviors. In our model, such protective behaviors are also part of the outcome behaviors. Some interventions designed to reduce high-risk sexual and needle-sharing behavior among HIV-positive persons have been successful (Lurie, Drucker 1997; Lurie et al. 1998). Likewise, one's risk-taking behavior is influenced by the environment (e.g., prevalence of guns in the community) and also influences the environment of others.

PERSONAL CHARACTERISTICS AFFECTING UTILIZATION AND ADHERENCE INDEPENDENT OF HEALTH STATUS

GENDER. Among the general population, studies indicate that chronically ill women tend to utilize services more frequently than men. Women with HIV were more likely than men to use the emergency room, which is considered inappropriate care because it is neither prevention nor maintenance but rather emergency (last-minute) care (Kissinger et al. 1995). Although some studies indicate no difference in adherence to HIV medications between men and women (Haubrich et al. 1999; Kaplan et al. 1999; Holzemer et al. 1999), SHIPS data indicate that women are less likely to report adherence to HIV medication regimens if they have children under age eighteen living at home. Women with early HIV infection also report lower quality of life than men (Lenderking et al. 1997). And in a study of AIDS patients, women reported greater pain intensity and poorer functional status (Breitbart et al. 1996).

RACE. Nonwhite, HIV-infected persons experience more pain, functional impairment, HIV-related medical symptoms, and lower CD4+ lymphocyte counts compared to white, HIV-infected persons (Lenderking et al. 1997; Breitbart et al. 1996). Additionally, African Americans and Hispanics have shorter survival expectancies with more opportunistic infections than Caucasians (Bright et al. 1996; Murrain 1996; Easterbrook et al. 1991; Del Amo et al. 1998). In spite of the high HIV infection rate among nonwhite groups, some studies focusing on high-risk populations (e.g., homosexuals, injecting drug users) have shown that African Americans report less sexual risk-taking (e.g., receptive anal intercourse, anonymous partners, unprotected sex) (Easterbrook et al. 1993; Koblin et al. 1990), although they report more past sexually transmitted diseases (Easterbrook et al. 1993; Heckman et al. 1999).

African Americans also have increasing rates of HIV infection and troubling utilization of services and treatment adherence. African Americans and Hispanics have proportionately more HIV infection than Caucasians (Easterbrook et al. 1993; Koblin et al. 1990; Centers for Disease Control and Prevention 1999c) and enter HIV treatment at later disease stages than Caucasians (Easterbrook et al. 1993), which result in higher mortality rates (Bright et al. 1996; Murrain 1996). Studies indicate that minority populations are less likely to receive a protease inhibitor, non-nucleoside analog, or other antiretroviral therapy, controlling for disease stage (Kaplan et al. 1999; Moore et al. 1994). African American, HIV-positive persons report higher rates of hospital admissions and longer lengths of inpatient stays than white persons; perhaps this indicates delayed health care (Moore et al. 1994; Fleishman et al. 1994).

One hypothesis used to explain differences in health care utilization is that African Americans are less likely to have insurance. However, in a study of gay, HIV-positive men, where African Americans and whites were equally likely to have health insurance, whites were still more likely than African Americans to use outpatient and dental services (Kass 1999). In a separate study of HIV-positive patients who had access to free or low-cost treatment, African Americans were more likely to miss outpatient appointments and have emergency room visits (Kissinger et al. 1995). Some of these utilization and treatment differences may be owing to inequalities in a health care system that treats African Americans differently from Caucasians, racial differences in beliefs about the health care system (e.g., distrust, fear of stigma), and efficacy of treatments.

POVERTY. Consistent with research in other populations, poor, HIV-infected persons have fewer outpatient visits and more emergency room visits (Fleishman et al. 1994; Tramarin et al. 1997). Those without health insurance have fewer visits of any kind (Fleishman et al. 1994). Better quality of life among HIV-infected patients is associated with higher income and employment (Swindells et al. 1999). Higher levels of education are positively associated with treatment adherence (Kalichman et al. 1999).

Among HIV-negative, gay men, lower educational levels are associated with more unprotected sex with casual partners (Strathdee et al. 1997). Additionally, a national probability sample of men and women showed that less education was associated with less condom use in casual relationships (Anderson et al. 1999).

ENVIRONMENTAL FACTORS AFFECTING HEALTH STATUS

The environment plays a large role in the health of both a community and an individual. Investigators routinely observe differences in mortality, disease prevalence, and other measures of health status between and within nations, countries, states, regions, metropolitan or rural areas, cities, and neighborhoods (Patrick, Wickizer 1995).

The twentieth century led to a tremendous expansion in our understanding of the associations among environment, personal characteristics, risk-taking or protective behavior, and health status (fig. 11.4). Studies demonstrated the correlations between health status and environmental influences:

- Environmental toxins directly influence the health status of individuals. Such toxins are most often stored near the poorest neighborhoods (Farer, Schieffelbein 1987; McGinnis, Foege 1993).

- Violence in a community has a direct effect on the health status of individuals who are injured in violent events. Violence witnessed in the home or on the street also alters people's perceptions of their permanency in the world, their willingness to take risks, and their locus of control. Post-traumatic stress disorder can make it difficult for a person to engage in beneficial activities (e.g., seeking health services for a deadly disease) (Whitmire et al. 1999).

- Support networks for children, beginning with family structural characteristics (e.g., the number of adults available to care for a child and the quality of their relationships), influence the risk-taking behavior of children and the future mutable personal characteristics of the child such as marital status, education, and income (Schor, Menaghan 1995).

- Infectious diseases continue to emerge and reemerge in communities (Satcher 1995), and they pose a direct health threat to those who come into contact with them. Likewise, from a clinical perspective, different strands of drug-resistant viruses are prevalent in different regions of the country.

- The availability of illicit drugs in a community often leads to lower educational attainment, lower aggregate incomes, more violence, and weak family support networks (Schor, Menaghan 1995).

- Culture is an environmental factor associated with personal characteristics such as nutritional habits, marital status, and the importance of education. Culture can be described as a shared, learned, or intergenerationally transmitted pattern of customs, beliefs, values, and behaviors (Corin 1995).

- Educational messages and mass media influence a person's mutable personal characteristics, knowledge, attitudes, beliefs, and therefore behaviors (Patterson et al. 1996).

- Availability of risk reduction paraphernalia is associated with its use. For example, the availability of condoms is associated with condom use (Cohen et al. 1999; Kirby et al. 1999) and the availability of clean needles is associated with the use of those needles (Lurie, Drucker 1997).

- Racism and other forms of sustained discrimination influence self-esteem, which, in turn, influences a person's ability to seek care. In addition, there is evidence that the stress of living in environments that do not accept a person's personal characteristics—such as race or sexual orientation—can, in itself, take a toll on the body and lead to lower immune system functioning (Patrick, Erickson 1993).

Chronic stress weakens the immune system and increases the likelihood of heart disease and cancer (Stefanski, Engler 1998; Lawrence, Kim 2000).

- Support networks have been found to strongly influence personal behavior (Ell 1996).
- Family characteristics such as marital status of parents and degree of severe discipline and violence can predict mental health disorders and unwanted pregnancies among teenagers (Schor, Menaghan 1995).
- Disease stigma such as the stigma related to being HIV-positive affects health status by reducing a person's willingness to discuss disease prevention measures or disclose one's HIV status, thereby putting others at risk of being infected (Demas et al. 1995).
- Social capital describes an individual in terms of social relationships. These include levels of trust (see below) and expectations of help from and to others. Social capital in itself is predictive of health status because of its role in the functioning of community life (Kawachi 1999; Kawachi et al. 1999). McLeroy and colleagues (1998) suggest that we examine health, health care, and promotion from an ecological perspective that includes focusing attention on both the individual and social environmental factors. Changes in the social environment produce changes in individuals, and, given the bidirectional nature of this relationship, support of individuals leads to implementation of needed change in the environment.

Not only does the environment influence personal characteristics, behavior, and health status, but personal characteristics and behavior also influence the environment of others because many environmental influences stem from others' actions.

Clearly, the environment plays an important role in health status. Environmental factors are important contributors to the risk of having HIV. First, the virus must be present in the environment. Second, environmental factors influence mutable and behavioral characteristics as well as internal decision making (see below), which then influences behavioral characteristics that could lead to HIV infection. As exemplified in the case studies presented in this book, family characteristics, such as the amount of parental fighting or love and attention offered to the children, influence the children's development of their own sense of self-esteem and self-efficacy in the world, thereby later influencing their life decisions and their risk for HIV. Further important factors are the availability of illicit drugs, clean needles, educational messages indicating the need to use clean needles (Lurie, Drucker 1997), and condoms.

Finally, the lack of support networks in one's environment increases a person's willingness to engage in HIV-related risk-taking behavior (Montoya 1998).

ENVIRONMENTAL FACTORS AFFECTING UTILIZATION AND ADHERENCE INDEPENDENT OF HEALTH STATUS

Many of the same environmental characteristics that take a toll on health also influence health service utilization (see fig. 11.4). For example, health education messages may increase a person's knowledge about self care and where to go for particular services, thereby increasing service use directly. Likewise, a chaotic environment may make seeking routine services difficult because of lack of support by family and friends and difficulties in accessing transportation. A community culture in which health care services are not highly valued may decrease service utilization. Below are a few specific examples of the environment's impact on service utilization.

VIOLENCE AND TRAUMA. Chapter 4 examined the lives of our case study participants in light of the growing body of research demonstrating that past and chronic experiences of trauma, abuse, and neglect influence health status, health care utilization, and health promotion activities. Past chronic trauma may be highly prevalent among the new generation of HIV-positive persons. Cohen and colleagues (2000) found a 66 percent lifetime prevalence of domestic violence and a 31 percent chance of experiencing sexual abuse during childhood among women with HIV or at high risk for HIV. Childhood sexual abuse was strongly associated with a lifetime history of domestic violence and high-risk behaviors. The prevalence of trauma in our very small sample of case study participants was 100 percent. The life histories presented in this book indicate that similar rates of abuse may be found among women and both homosexual and heterosexual HIV-positive men. If this abuse experience is characteristic of the new face of HIV, integration of trauma therapy with HIV care may be an effective means of increasing health service utilization and treatment adherence for a significant proportion of patients.

SOCIAL SUPPORT. Social support is defined as having people one can confide in and/or having people whom one can depend on to help when in need. Chapter 6 provided literature demonstrating the importance of social supports for care utilization and health promotion. The case study participants did not generally have strong support networks, as either children or adults.

STIGMA IN THE ENVIRONMENT. The participants identified a factor missing in past theoretical models: the importance of stigma around HIV, issues of sexuality, sexual behavior, and illicit drug use—all of which are factors in HIV transmission. In rural areas, where confidentiality is difficult to maintain, HIV stigma is rampant, and concerns about discrimination and ostracism for being seropositive are high (Lundberg 1998; McKinney 1998; Rumley, Esinhart 1993). Therefore, disease stigma is an environmental characteristic to consider when examining potentially stigmatizing conditions. The case study and focus group participants expressed high levels of concern around issues of confidentiality, fear of discrimination, and stigma within the community. Chapter 9 further explored past research regarding stigma.

The stigma of HIV, homosexuality, and engaging in unaccepted behaviors in a rural community deters both utilization of health services and treatment adherence. As examples, the already difficult task of arranging transportation to and from an infectious diseases clinic becomes even more daunting when one cannot tell others why one is going for care. Brochures given to patients in the clinics are thrown out at the door to prevent others seeing them at home. Case managers report that rural HIV patients occasionally mix all their medications into one bottle to avoid identifiable labels. Patients also decline to take home medication instructions. Clinicians report that patients often do not want case managers, who can help in getting transportation and medications, to come to their houses because the community links the case manager to HIV-related work.

POLITICAL STRUCTURE AND HISTORY. The political structure of the environment and past policies influence the general trust that disenfranchised populations have in systems, including systems of care. Examples of past discrimination provided in chapter 9 show the continued presence of racism and discrimination in our society. Discrimination results in distrust of systems and lower perceived control over the environment. Persons with less perceived environmental control are less likely to engage in health promotion activities.

HEALTH POLICY AFFECTING HEALTH STATUS

Health policy directly influences the availability and accessibility of services. Health policies include laws, rules, regulations, and decisions regarding how and whether disease prevention and health promotion activities, including curative care, are financed and organized at all levels. They include the amount of staffing and resources allocated to an area or problem and decisions to adopt certain standards of care or practice (Spasoff 1999). Health policies influence health status and create environments that allow for availability and accessibility of disease prevention and health promotion activities (fig.

11.4). For, example, laws that allow needle exchange programs can reduce HIV transmission without increasing drug use (Doherty et al. 2000; Lurie, Drucker 1997) while policies to provide condoms in high schools do not increase rates of sexual activity (Kirby et al. 1999) but do increase rates of safe sexual practices among teens (Wolk, Rosenbaum 1995; Schuster et al. 1998; Guttmacher et al. 1997). The availability and accessibility of health education messages that are appropriate and understandable to the target population are also determined by health policy decisions. Laws, regulations, and taxes can cause people to behave more cautiously than they would otherwise. For example, laws and regulations regarding alcohol consumption (Whetten-Goldstein et al. 2000b; Sloan et al. 2000) and cigarette smoking (Siegel, Biener 2000; Smith et al. 2000) have been instrumental in changing risk-taking behavior. Decisions to increase taxes on items such as alcohol and tobacco may reduce consumption of these goods among the poor, thereby positively affecting their health status (Cook, Moore 1999).

Policy decisions influence the availability and accessibility of treatment (Spasoff 1999). For example, closing down proximal health care centers can adversely affect the health of those with limited resources by decreasing their use of routine care and thereby causing decreased health status. Decisions about the size of copayments may overdeter poorer individuals and families from seeking care and also result in lower health status. Decisions at the federal and state levels to fund particular areas of research and care also influence the availability of information and treatment and, therefore, health status. In the case of HIV, the decision to fund AIDS Drugs Assistance Programs (ADAP) created an environment of available HIV medications for HIV-positive patients who would otherwise not have been able to afford them. Individual decisions regarding HIV testing are influenced, in part, by state confidentiality policies (Paringer et al. 1991).

HEALTH POLICY AFFECTING UTILIZATION AND ADHERENCE INDEPENDENT OF HEALTH STATUS

The availability of services can be measured in terms of the geographic distance to the closest services needed, a ratio of the number of service providers to the population in need, the service provider's acceptance of the patient's condition, and/or the service provider's acceptance of the payment the individual can offer. The distance a patient must travel to see a clinician familiar with HIV complications and treatments is an indicator of the availability of care.

Services or medications might be available but not accessible to the patient. Although a service may be located a block from the client, it may not be offered at a time when the individual needs to receive or is able to seek services. Hours of operation are less of a problem for those with acute service needs than for those with chronic needs. For example, studies have shown that hours of operation influence the ability of women receiving Medicaid to attend prenatal care appointments. Many employers of low-income earners do not allow their employees to repeatedly take leave for appointments. Likewise, if HIV-positive patients must depend on transportation provided by the county Department of Social Services to get to medical care, and transportation is offered only on the one day per week that clinic care is not offered, then the care is not accessible. Low perceived access through long distances, high costs, or poor clinic hours is associated with poor health–related quality of life (Cunningham et al. 1995).

Long waiting times to see a clinician (Aday et al. 1993) can deter utilization of services because of other life needs such as employment and child care. In addition, cultural appropriateness of the way in which a service is delivered can influence the service's accessibility (Goicoechea-Balbona 1997). For example, when services are provided in English to a migrant farm worker population that speaks Spanish, clients may be hesitant to seek services and may not follow protocols because they either do not understand them or have not developed a trusting relationship with a provider.

Accessibility is also determined by the payments available to and accepted by providers. For poor, HIV-positive patients dependent on Medicaid, if a needed service is not covered or sufficiently reimbursed by Medicaid, then a provider may decide not to make that service accessible to such patients. Therefore, lack of insurance results in negative service use (Fleishman et al.1994). In rural areas, services such as mental health counseling for persons with HIV may not be accessible because the magnitude of the problem has not yet been recognized (Aruffo et al. 1995; Heckman et al. 1996); thus, no policies have been put in place to appropriately train and fund mental health counselors.

The rigorousness of the desired or prescribed treatment influences patient desire and ability to adhere to appointment and treatment protocols (McElnay, McCallion 1998) and should be included as service characteristics. Adherence to treatments involving more frequent health care appointments is more difficult. The characteristics of the medication regimen, such as its complexity (e.g., multiple medications and dosage intervals) and the extent to which medications have perceived beneficial effects or deleterious side effects (determined as part of the internal decision-making process) all likely bear on treatment adherence (Blackwell 1996; Cramer, Rosenheck 1998; Kelley et al. 1987).

HIV poses a unique set of circumstances that may further reduce health service utilization. In the case of rural HIV, testing often occurs at health departments where the staff are members of the same community as the clients. Patients are embarrassed to let staff know that they engaged in behaviors that put them at risk for HIV; they are even more embarrassed for the staff to confirm that they have HIV. They are sometimes equally embarrassed that their partners might have engaged in such behaviors (e.g., having a promiscuous spouse might suggest that one cannot keep one's partner satisfied). Therefore, familiarity with health department staff reduces the accessibility of local care providers for stigmatizing conditions. The same is true for substance abuse and mental health services that clients need. Decreased accessibility of services diminishes the effects of preventive measures and HIV testing for the individual and others in their network of friends and associates.

ATTITUDES AND PERCEPTIONS

Adding to previous theoretical frameworks, case study and focus group participants maintained attitudes and perceptions that influenced their propensity to seek medical care. Many case study participants believed that the government created HIV to kill off populations, and some considered taking medication to be allowing oneself to be treated as a guinea pig. It was not clear how case study participants reconciled these beliefs with the role of their medications or trust of their physicians or other providers. Literature previously cited indicates that low trust of the health care system is one reason for lower rates of appropriate health services use. In addition, perceptions of how well providers at a particular clinic were able to maintain confidentiality influenced where care was sought. However, some clinic characteristics were beyond the providers' control, such as proximity of the clinic to the patient's home.

The perception that providers cared for them was important to the participants. In speaking about their physicians and case managers, participants spoke of the length of time that the provider spent with them. Any words of praise or encouragement from providers were welcomed. When case study participants were asked to draw a "family tree" in any form that they wanted, several participants included their case managers because the case manager was there for them to call on and available to listen. In the focus groups, when participants were asked if they would trust having their information put into a computer system, the participants replied that if they trusted the health or social service professional entering the data, then they would also trust the system.

Policy and Future Research Recommendations

The new wave of the HIV epidemic is characterized by persons who have been disenfranchised as members of minority groups and as low-income persons. As individuals, they have been disenfranchised as persons whose parents were far from upstanding members of the community, who had few to no social supports, and whose problems were not handled by "systems" such as family, education, or social service. The new wave of the epidemic is both disenfranchised and disengaged from care structures. Addressing these fundamental issues requires national debate and reform that occurs at community, county, state, and federal levels. The recommendations below focus on serving patients such as the case study participants today, but they do not address all the societal issues that lead to the patients being in their current position.

MENTAL HEALTH AND SUBSTANCE ABUSE SERVICES

Life histories provided by the case study participants and SHIPS data indicate high levels of need for mental health and substance abuse services among individuals representing the new wave of the HIV epidemic. Integration of mental health and substance abuse services could enable a person to better care for HIV disease.

A survey conducted by the North Carolina Division of Medical Assistance (2001) of HIV-case managers revealed that 54 percent of agencies represented reported that mental health services were not "reasonably accessible" for Medicaid-eligible clients. The reasons for lack of access were varied and not all HIV-specific: long waiting lists for services; high mental health provider turnover; lack of transportation; therapists uncomfortable seeing HIV-positive clients; lack of provider empathy; and poor quality of services. The case study participants illustrated examples of inaccessibility of services by citing staff turnover and perceived poor quality services. Our survey of case managers in Alabama, Georgia, Louisiana, Mississippi, and South Carolina revealed similar information regarding the inaccessibility of mental health services.

The cultural competence of counseling staff is important given that such a high proportion of newly infected people are minorities. For example, since the early 1990s, racial differences have been recognized in the length of time it takes for the client to feel comfortable with the counselor (Priest 1991; Midgette, Meggert 1991). These differences correspond to differences both in client expectations of the counseling process and its outcome and in communication styles (e.g., verbal and nonverbal cues). Effective treatment of African American clients may take longer than for European Americans.

Dually and triply diagnosed clients are affected by the stigma associated with not only HIV disease but also mental illness. Research continues to show that many people, particularly those in rural areas, do not view mental illness equally with a physical illness (Johnsen et al. 1997). In rural areas of North Carolina, interviews indicated that mental health care is for "crazy people." Thus, stigmatizing attitudes about mental health and substance disorders may influence the availability and accessibility of services in rural areas (Johnsen et al. 1997).

Ideally, appropriate services provided by competent staff could be offered in every state, with staffing in each county. Such services would require training for service providers in issues unique to persons with HIV: for example, dealing with disease stigma with family and community, addressing sexual risk-taking behavior, discussing stigma related to homosexuality and bisexuality, and recommending and offering harm reduction models of substance abuse treatment that take relapse into account rather than offering only abstinence models. Policymakers could require that such training be offered and taken by mental health and substance abuse treatment centers that accept state and federal funds; this mandate, however, would require extra expenditures to train agencies and to serve new clients.

Contrary to popular belief, rural mental illness rates are as high or higher than those of urban areas (American Psychological Association 2001; Blank et al. 1995). However, the lack of specialized mental health services generally is a problem in such areas (Fox et al. 1995; Blank et al. 1995; Merwin et al. 1995). Rural counties do not have a critical mass of clients to make financially feasible the provision of specialized mental health or substance abuse services. Yet, the needs presented by the case study participants were complex; HIV is just one more complexity.

If the county mental health systems are not able or willing to provide care, then states could allow private mental health counselors, neither affiliated with the county mental health system nor licensed physicians, to bill Medicaid or Ryan White for services. A recent court case forced North Carolina's Division of Medical Assistance to make such a change in provider billing eligibility for HIV-positive persons under age twenty-one. Extending this type of policy to adults is one way to increase accessibility. Other states have tried other initiatives including carve-outs (funds specifically set aside) for mental health services.

Substance abuse services are reported to be even less available and accessible than mental health services outside of urban areas. Respondents to the informal Five States Survey of Case Managers noted a problem: a high proportion of the few substance abuse services available are abstinence-based models of treatment where clients must discontinue services if they abuse drugs or alcohol. (The Five States Survey consisted of interviews with at least ten geographically dispersed HIV case managers in Alabama, Georgia, Louisiana, Michigan, and South Carolina and was conducted at Duke University by Whetten-Goldstein.) The alternative is a more realistic harm-reduction model of treatment that moves clients toward abstinence by allowing for occasional relapses. Harm reduction models have been found highly effective in treating substance abuse. With sexually transmitted diseases the added public health defense favors harm-reduction models: any amount of time that a client is kept off drugs is a positive outcome because the risk of disease transmission is reduced during that time period. Harm-reduction models are now accepted and promoted by researchers and the federal government, but they are not widely used (U.S. Department of Health and Human Services 1999).

Another NC SIP initiative is examining the costs and effectiveness of providing integrated HIV, substance abuse, and mental health services. People receive care for their HIV disease at one of five infectious diseases clinics in a seventeen-county region and travel to one of two outpatient mental health and substance abuse clinics for care one to three times per week. One of the most time-consuming components of the initiative is addressing issues of transportation, which, for some clients, costs more than $350 per month. Although the project appears successful for those who engage in services, it remains to be seen if there are cost offsets, such as reduced emergency room visits, that would make the funding of such programs more feasible.

Slightly different is a model providing counseling and substance abuse services within the infectious diseases clinics for a one-stop-shopping model; this can be effective for persons who live near the clinics but difficult for those who do not. Such a model of care is currently being tested in Chicago (HIV/AIDS Treatment Adherence, Health Outcomes and Cost Study Group 2001). With sufficient outreach and transportation resources, such a model could be effective for a wider rural area. However, previous research has indicated that people are willing to travel greater distances for clinical care than for other health-related services that are needed more frequently (Graduate Medical Education National Advisory Committee 1980; Ricketts et al. 1994). Ideally, because of the necessarily high frequency of mental health and substance abuse services, they should be located more closely to the client.

HIV CASE MANAGEMENT

Studies have demonstrated that HIV case management has positive effects on appropriate service utilization and health outcomes of poor, HIV-positive persons (Katz et al. 2000). The job of an HIV case manager is difficult. To integrate job duties—applying for benefits and meeting subsistence-level needs such as obtaining food, clothing, housing, electricity, and even toilet paper—a case manager must not only have detailed knowledge of multiple service systems and benefits programs but also be able to work with and understand clients who can be very difficult because their lives are often in crisis. Yet HIV-case managers are often not provided the training required to perform these tasks, and their salaries are not commensurate with their responsibilities.

ADHERENCE COUNSELING. The HIV case managers are often more familiar with the day-to-day lives of the patients than are providers in medical settings. HIV case managers often visit patients' homes and work with patients on many issues within their own environment. The opportunity to provide adherence counseling and basic information is great. Yet case managers in Alabama, Georgia, Louisiana, and North Carolina report restrictions on billing Medicaid for adherence counseling; South Carolina and Mississippi do not have any Medicaid-reimbursed HIV case management. One survey confirmed that respondents provided adherence counseling but were not billing for their services. Almost all the case managers who participated in this survey (95 percent) expressed a strong desire for training in adherence-related case management activities (Reif et al. 2001).

The North Carolina Division of Medical Assistance has some concerns: if case managers provide adherence counseling, then they will encounter situations where patients will ask them to give information about specific medications, which would violate regulations. However, models of adherence counseling, such as those distributed by the Health Resources and Services Administration-funded AIDS Education and Training Networks, can be used to train case managers to help patients organize their lives in ways that incorporate medication-taking at regular intervals. Case managers could also inquire as to whether the client is adhering to medications and, with the client's permission, talk with the clinician about potential concerns. Case managers report that they are now providing adherence counseling because clients want them to do so; case managers feel that counseling is important, but, because the policy regulations are unclear, formal trainings regarding best methods for providing adherence counseling cannot be conducted. Alternatively, states could look to specifically support medical case management, which orients case managers toward prioritizing medical issues. (Medical case managers must have a clinical background and therefore can provide adherence counseling.)

PROVIDER RELATIONSHIPS WITH THE PATIENTS

Systems need to recognize that we are working with populations demonstrating a high level of system distrust. Building trust should become an accepted component of care. Little research has been done on appropriate and effective methods to enhance patient trust, but such efforts should be undertaken. As noted previously, the therapeutic alliance between client and counselor can take longer for African Americans than for European Americans, and providers must be aware of potential differences in communication styles and client expectations (Priest 1991; Midgette, Meggert 1991). Solid research on methods of trust building is needed. Providers should be reimbursed for their time in building stronger relationships with patients. Providing care in ways that account for the many factors that influence behavior may improve accessibility of care (Stokols 2000).

EDUCATION AND RISK-REDUCTION COUNSELING

RELATIONSHIP AND PARENTING EDUCATION. Many of the case study participants discussed the emotionally complex issues of engaging in safe sex with a partner with whom a participant wants to have a lasting relationship. Most of the participants' partners were HIV-negative. Some male partners refused to engage in safe sex, which caused anger and guilt among the female participants. Gary expressed disbelief that his wife could stay with him and sometimes wished that she would become HIV-positive so that he would not have to worry about infecting her any more. Participants expressed the fear of disclosing their status to potential sexual partners, knew the importance of safe sex, and, for the most part, knew how to engage in safe sex (although one participant mistakenly used two condoms at a time as a safer method). The missing education that the participants needed was how to negotiate safe sex with their partners. Educational techniques such as role-playing and hearing from others with the same problems might have helped these individuals. Behavioral education that incorporates both basic safe sex and needle use practices and relationship negotiation strategies could reduce HIV infection and reinfection rates.

Many women spoke of wanting to stop the cycle of abuse with their children and grandchildren. They wanted something better for their children, and yet they did not always succeed in containing their anger. Parenting education is viewed as a type of luxury counseling not often provided to poor, HIV-positive persons. Yet, in the long run, helping future generations to live more positive lives may be one of the best preventive measures policymakers and providers should consider.

CONFIDENTIALITY. Confidentiality, of great concern to many case study participants, has been shown through work previously cited to be of greater concern to rural-living patients than to urban-living patients. The focus group participants suggested specific ways that confidentiality concerns could be addressed (see chapter 9 for more detail). Providers should attend training sessions that address confidentiality issues for HIV-positive persons, including concerns about serostatus information being passed from one provider to another. Training must to be particularly intensive for providers serving patients whom they and/or their families know personally.

GENDER. With increasing rates of HIV among women and specific needs associated with them (i.e., socioeconomic dependence on men, role as family caregiver), providers and policymakers are recognizing the need to address women's needs through the structure of care offered (Fullilove et al., Policy Brief Number 1; Aranda-Naranjo, Policy Brief Number 1). Women were concerned about not only their children's care when they sought services but also issues related to becoming pregnant again and negotiating safe sex with long-term partners who controlled sexual relations. Clinicians may need training on both gaining the trust of and treating women who have been sexually abused.

HIV STIGMA. HIV stigma results in increased stress for patients as they try to hide their diagnosis from family and friends. Parents worry that their children will be ostracized at home and in school. HIV stigma could be reduced by having community organizations, leaders, and churches regularly discuss HIV and invite HIV-positive persons to speak and interact with them. Modes of HIV-transmission and treatment should be explained. Plays could be written and performed in schools and churches.

CONSPIRACY AND HIV MEDICATIONS. Community education should address not only HIV transmission and treatment but also HIV conspiracy theories. As with HIV stigma, attitudes will not immediately change, but the dialogue must begin. Conspiracy theories are imbedded in notions of unjust and arbitrary treatment delivered by those in power to those without power. It is hard to argue against these theories as we continue to experience and learn of minority mistreatment such as those discussed in chapter 9. Clinicians who are also good community educators should be invited to speak at local schools, churches, and clubs. Community leaders should also open discussions about past racially related treatment and potential future actions.

SPIRITUAL COMMUNITY

Many case study participants spoke of spiritual beliefs. While participants, for the most part, were not attending church when they became infected with HIV, some were turning to these communities for spiritual support once they discovered their HIV status. The spiritual community is a powerful force in rural southern communities for norm setting. Churches can help deliver health and HIV-related messages to the community (Hatch, Derthick 1992) and thereby reduce the stigma of HIV. Churches with primarily black congregations have served their communities' health and human service needs throughout U.S. history. Thomas and colleagues (1994) found that among northern African American churches, community health outreach programs could be predicted by church size and the minister's educational level. Health promotion messages have been successfully distributed through churches. For example, nutritional habits of churchgoers were successfully changed over the course of an intensive program through the churches (Campbell et al. 2000). In some regions, such as areas in Mississippi, churches have put together funds that are used to pay for emergency HIV-medications. In regions where religious organizations play an important role in the culture, working with churches could be a powerful instrument for change.

SCHOOLS

Education regarding HIV transmission and protection is difficult in some states with regulations that allow only abstinence-based sexual education. Such regulations have made schools hesitant to allow any discussion of HIV. In some areas, local health departments have gained permission to bus "high-risk" children from school to the health department to receive more detailed information. Such models create problems of their own such as the definition of "high-risk" by excluding a number of "low-risk" children who could still benefit from education; being bused from school also attaches a stigma to the high-risk children. Models of HIV education that promote abstinence do exist and are also being utilized in schools.

BENEFIT PROGRAMS

MEDICAID. State Medicaid programs each have their own eligibility rules. Although some people qualify categorically, others must pay copayments, deductibles, or spend a percentage of their income on medical expenses. As has been discussed, Georgia and North Carolina have Medicaid spend-down requirements for those who are not categorically eligible for Medicaid (see chapter 2). Such regulations put providers in a difficult situation of helping people receive optimal care while trying to negotiate a bureaucratic system that is not designed to adequately provide continuous insurance coverage (see chapter 10); therefore, clinical care and medications cannot be regularly obtained. Thus, the current system is apparently creating health care that is negatively driven by administrative policy; as a result, patients and providers suffer great stress as they worry about how their medications will be paid for as they move from one source of payment to another.

States have applied for waivers to be able to cover more HIV-positive people under Medicaid; the waivers expand coverage to more people, but the system remains cumbersome. Maine has applied for a waiver that would expand coverage to people earlier in the HIV disease progression, but it includes six-month eligibility reviews and copayments, which for some are as high as $80 per month (Anonymous 2000).

Researchers and policymakers need to conduct thorough investigations of the number of people who are not able to negotiate current systems before expanding the same system. Because each state has its own set of eligibility criteria, it is difficult to make generalizable recommendations.

INTEGRATED CARE

The case study participants and SHIPS respondents had multiple services needs. If we examine the needs expressed, we see that respondents needed care that included: HIV clinical care; mental heath treatment; substance abuse treatment; care for other comorbidities such as diabetes and hypertension; housing services; food services; income support benefits; support groups; legal services; and HIV-specific educational information and resource knowledge. Our informal Five State HIV Case Manager Survey indicated that the level of needed services is not unique to North Carolina.

In states that are largely urban, care networks specific to the needs of HIV positive people have been developed that are made possible by the urban nature of the state, such as New York (84 percent urban), Maryland (81 percent), and Michigan (71 percent). Reliable and inexpensive transportation is available to bring people into a network of proximal providers offering primary care, case management, substance abuse and mental health treatment, and employment rehabilitation. With research documenting the importance and power of integrated care and supportive services (Piro, Doctor 1998; Katz et al. 2000; Ricketts et al. 1994; Chandler et al. 1996; Porter et al. 1996; Hampson et al. 1996; Ulmer et al. 1997; Racine et al. 1998), providers and policymakers working in primarily rural regions must learn how to develop the means to offer such coordinated care across vast distances to improve the health of their patient population.

Models of care that combine health and social services are being tested in urban areas (Master et al. 1996). Furthermore, demonstration projects in St. Louis, Detroit, Chicago, Boston, Seattle, New York City, Philadelphia, and North Carolina are testing the effectiveness and costs of treating persons with HIV, substance abuse, and mental health diagnoses in more integrated ways (Department of Health and Human Services 1998). Such models often involve the formal collaboration of a small number of provider agencies.

In rural areas, models of integrated care might need to be expanded by incorporating greater numbers of agencies because of distance. For example, it is not feasible to contract with one or two HIV-case management agencies to serve a large region. In North Carolina, where one infectious diseases clinic treats patients from more than fifty counties, in order to create an integrated system of care, it would be necessary for each infectious diseases clinic to communicate with fifty or more case management agencies that serve individuals with multiple chronic diseases. This need is true even as outreach infectious diseases clinics are being funded and arranged because, as seen in the case studies, clients still choose to travel longer distances to major centers to better protect their confidentiality. Such integration of care and communication networks may seem daunting to create, but with ingenuity and modern communication techniques, we may be able to create integrated systems of care in the face of large obstacles.

Clinical care could be provided through shared care models where infectious diseases clinics communicate and collaborate with local primary care physicians. Alternatively, as has been done in parts of Georgia and is being tested in North Carolina, the more urban clinics can create satellite clinics. These satellite clinics can either have their own full-time staff linked to the urban centers or the ID clinics can send clinicians to satellite sites on a weekly or bimonthly basis, depending on the need. Finally, urban-based clinics can train interested local providers in HIV-related care so they can meet the needs of the local client population. These alternatives should be tested while keeping in mind that some individuals will still seek care farther from home because distance helps protect confidentiality. Satellite clinics could incorporate mental health and substance abuse treatment, as well as HIV case managers who can assist in negotiating the other needed support services (e.g., housing, food, income supports, electricity, legal supports).

Rural HIV in the South and Other Chronic Diseases

The setting of this book is the South. Throughout the book, there has been an undertone of barriers and situations that are unique or more prevalent in rural and/or southern areas. Similarly, a report of the unique mental health needs of rural-living women released by the American Psychological Association (2001) addressed many of the same issues in comparing rural and urban individuals. Rural-living women experienced higher poverty rates, lower educational levels, higher rates of single-headed households, higher rates of depression and anxiety (41 percent of rural women, compared to 13 to 20 percent of urban women), higher rates of suicide, much higher rates of teen pregnancy (30 to 40 percent higher than their urban counterparts), higher rates of comorbidities that include higher increases in AIDS rates, and more stigma for lesbians. Barriers to rural treatment included lack of access, awareness of services, and services themselves, higher cost than urban care, and cultural misunderstanding. Thus, we see providers must face the same issues in treating rural-living individuals, whether they are male or female or whether the treatment is for mental illness, HIV, or another chronic condition.

The stereotypes of rural communities being supportive and close were not borne out by the participants. Participants usually lacked close community supports. Participants often relied on family members who at times further isolated the participant through their fear of "catching" HIV and through telling community members of the diagnosis. The fear of HIV status disclosure led participants to behave in ways that they would not have otherwise behaved, including not following clinical recommendations. Studies indicate that this fear is higher in rural than in urban areas. Issues of isolation and fears of disclosure must be addressed if we are to provide good care to rural-living, HIV-positive persons.

Many participants held strong religious beliefs, but most had been outside the church when they became HIV-positive. Participants struggled to reconcile their disease with their spiritual beliefs; some believed that God had given them the disease to help them live better and with more respect. The church is a place where caring and support could be provided for some HIV-positive individuals. Working with religious leaders could reduce community stigma and increase personal support for clients.

Rural areas have lower population densities, which translate to fewer people within a geographic radius with any particular disease. This small patient population makes it difficult for specialty clinicians to provide services in rural areas because they cannot care for sufficient numbers of patients to make their practice financially feasible. As a result, poor rural-living patients must travel long distances to obtain HIV-related care, but transportation to clinics located outside a county is often not readily available. New models of care organization and integration, as described above, must be tested and developed.

Generally, as was shown in the American Psychological Association report (2001), rural residents face all the problems of their urban counterparts, but they can muster fewer resources and wear a different cultural veil. The cultural veil extends not only to populations considered minority (e.g., African American, Hispanic, Native American), but also to poor European Americans who might live outside the community mores. As indicated in research conducted by Thomas and colleagues (1999), we find that sociophysical factors related to not only race but also poverty (e.g., race relations, employment opportunities, interagency coordination, intercommunity dynamics), which plays a role in the spread of sexually transmitted diseases in the South. Such research should be further conducted beyond the diseases of syphilis and HIV so that we can better understand cultural effects on disease, care access, and service utilization. If we can create comprehensive and sensitive models of care that increase access to care for HIV-positive persons, similar models could be used for other diseases that affect people in the South.

Resources

Many of the suggested changes require financial resources and political will to alter the status quo. However, once changes are implemented, accompanying good research may find that cost offsets would make society willing to pay potential marginal increases for the resultant decreases in new HIV infections and the improved quality of life and health status of individuals infected with HIV. Efforts by the Special Projects of National Significance division of the Health Resources and Services Administration, by the Substance Abuse and Mental Health Services Administration, by the National Institutes of Health, by state agencies, and by private funding to test new and improved models of care and education should be applauded. The importance of rigorous evaluation of these initiatives should be strongly encouraged so that policymakers can make decisions with as much information as possible regarding potential risks. In addition, it should be noted that not all the proposed changes require complete restructuring of systems; some are merely incremental steps.

This section focused on areas of investigation for change within the health policy realm of the determinant of health services utilization and treatment adherence. As indicated in the bidirectional figure 11.4, health and social policy influences individuals and environments in multiple ways. Through policy, social and service environments are altered, possibly reducing barriers to care and improving its quality.

The voices and numbers presented in this book help us understand the lives of persons who are within the new wave of the HIV epidemic in the South. Understanding should lead to reevaluation of what providers, policymakers, and researchers know about providing services and arranging care structures in ways that are most appropriate and accessible. Large-scale studies of southerners with HIV and other chronic diseases and how persons cope with their disease must be conducted to further inform providers and policy-makers. Hypotheses from these case studies should be further tested; consider, for instance, the prevalence rates of past and current trauma, substance abuse, and unstable housing. Unique care needs should be investigated, and models should be tested that are appropriate for care across geographic distances and across diseases.

The policy recommendations are tempered with the knowledge that reduced HIV transmission stems from reduced levels of risk behavior, which are often the result of past life events grounded in injustice and inequalities. Although an underlying focus of this discussion is on changing current patient behavior through an enriched understanding of patients' lives and meeting patients where they are today, we could alternatively focus our enriched understanding on altering our societal fabric so that individuals in our society no longer experience many of the negative forces that our partici-pants experienced in their homes, communities, and educational, social serv-ice, and care systems.

Appendix A   *Data Collection Methods*

This appendix introduces the five data collection sources used in this book. The primary sources of information are the twenty-five life histories. To complement this data, we added data from the Southeast HIV Patient Survey, the North Carolina HIV Provider Survey, and focus groups.

Selecting the Participants

Throughout the spring and summer of 1998, we worked with HIV case managers and Ryan White Title II CARE Act consortia administrators in eastern North Carolina to identify potential case study participants. The consortium administrators recommended case managers with whom we should work. The only requirements were that the clients be from North Carolina and be willing to meet with interviewers multiple times to talk about their entire lives. The interviews would be audiorecorded and used in nonidentifying ways in a book. Participants would also receive $15 grocery store vouchers for each interview. The case managers were asked to provide a list of candidates, identifying them only by their gender, race, mode of transmission, and age.

Participant selection was based only on the demographic characteristics of the potential participants in order to represent different geographical areas, modes of transmission, and genders. Because we had to identify interviewees through their case managers, one bias of our sample is that they are all of low-income status and receive any number of benefits such as Medicaid, Medicare, or Ryan White CARE Act funding.

The project director developed a research protocol, and we obtained IRB approval. We developed a five-page, open-ended survey instrument (see Appendix B), which Duke's Institutional Review Board approved. Evaluators of SPNS in other rural sites (including Alabama, Arkansas, Navajo Nation, Alaska, and Latino border communities in Texas) critiqued and approved the instrument.

We pretested the instrument with three respondents who completed three interviews each. Two students, who were hired on the basis of their interpersonal skills, abilities, past experiences, and interest in the interviewing effort, conducted the remainder of the interviews during the summer of 1998. Students were hired because they were removed from all health care and social service systems. This separation from what may be perceived as The Authorities or The System sought to promote a connection and honest conversation with the participants that a social worker or case manager may not have been able to have because clients rely on them for benefits and aid. The hiring process for the interviewers was very selective because they had to be able to put participants at ease, think quickly, and be empathetic to human suffering but not be swallowed by emotion. The project director had more than thirteen years of experience in counseling and interviewing disenfranchised populations as well as training interviewers. We used gender matching in an effort to provide a comfortable and safe environment for the case study participants. The female interviewer was black, while the male interviewer was white. The decision to choose a white interviewer was difficult because of the predominately minority status of participants, but the interviewer possessed other characteristics that enabled him to bond quickly with the male respondents.

When our interviewers first spoke with each client via telephone, they confirmed that the clients wanted to be interviewed three times for two hours per interview, would permit audiotaping, understood that they would never be identified by name, and would receive compensation for each interview. All the selected clients agreed to be interviewed, although one dropped out after the first interview and one woman did not complete the entire interview process. Participants chose where to conduct the interviews, most often choosing their own homes, but some participants asked to meet at their case manager's office or somewhere else. Although the interviewers had with them a list of topics and questions, they did not use them during the meeting, so as to elicit a conversation rather than an interview. During the final interview, each participant was asked to draw a timeline that listed the important events in his or her life, to draw a family tree that listed people who she or he considered family (blood-related or not), and to complete two standardized questionnaires about traumatic events and self-esteem and self-efficacy (see appendix C for a list of the trauma questions).

The authors listened to the taped interviews between each interview session. The authors then met with the interviewers to discuss new topics of discussion and areas on which to focus and to clarify issues when the interviewer and the authors understood the respondent in different ways. In addition, using a standard approach to case series studies, the authors added questions to the list for all respondents as themes emerged from the respondents.

The Records: Tapes and Transcripts

The nearly two hundred hours of tapes were then transcribed verbatim and checked for accuracy. The authors read the transcripts, separately coding each line according to themes and topics. Two research assistants compiled the two sets of codes onto one transcript, allowing for the complete set of codes to be entered into QSR NUD*IST 4, a software package designed to facilitate qualitative analysis by compiling the data into categories specified by the authors (Qualitative Solutions and Research Pty Ltd, 1997). Upon completion of the data entry, the interviews were presented according to theme, allowing for tabulation of clients' quotes and stories according to topic.

Southeast HIV Patient Survey (SHIPS)

Throughout the book, we provide results from a unique source of data from three of our target states (Alabama, North Carolina, South Carolina). The results provide additional quantitative data regarding HIV in the South. During the summer of 1997, consecutive patients who were HIV-positive and Medicaid-eligible (based on their medical records as identified by the front-desk clerk) and attended one of seven infectious diseases clinics were asked if they would participate in a periodic telephone survey and have their medical records examined annually for four years. The recruitment techniques were rigorous; Duke-trained staff conducted the recruitment at the sites to ensure that both the study was not forgotten and the sample did not become one of convenience rather than consecutive patients.

The ID clinics were selected based on their similarity to one another in their provider and patient population. The clinics were located in academic medical centers in North Carolina (Bowman Gray School of Medicine, Duke University Medical Center, East Carolina University School of Medicine, and the University of North Carolina at Chapel Hill Hospital), South Carolina (Medical University of South Carolina), Alabama (the University of Alabama at Birmingham), and Florida (University of Florida, Gainesville). The Florida sample was subsequently dropped from analyses because the population was demographically dissimilar and the enrollment technique was not sequential.

Based on power calculations and budgetary constraints, we set a target of eight hundred study participants enabling small subanalyses of groups consisting of ten percent of the total sample. Of the 909 patients approached to participate in the survey, 858 consented, for an acceptance rate of 94.4 percent. Patients were asked to provide three contact telephone numbers to facilitate tracking. Those who refused participation reported that they did so because they were not interested or did not have the time.

Clinicians conducted medical record abstractions for each person who had consented to participate in the study and who had not passed away at the time of chart review (N=834). The chart data was used to collect more clinical information (e.g., CD4 counts over time, viral loads, and medications prescribed). From this sample, the survey firm Louis Harris and Associates conducted 555 patient surveys from October 1997 until July 1998. There were 804 potential survey respondents after accounting for those who were deceased (N=4), HIV-negative (N=3), or not interviewable due to communication barriers (N=15), imprisonment (N=6), or hospitalization (N=2). Of those 804 remaining, 23 refused to participate and 226 either had moved (N=41), provided pager or cellular telephone numbers no longer in service (N=5), did not answer (N=57), had telephone numbers that were not in service or were disconnected (N=69), or had provided incorrect telephone numbers (N=54). The final survey response rate was 70 percent.

The SHIPS was patterned after validated national and chronic disease surveys in collaboration with the Evaluation and Technical Assistance Center (ETAC) at the Columbia University School of Public Health and with investigators from more than thirty HIV research sites nationally who were funded in the 1996 round of SPNS under HRSA. The specific instruments of the survey chosen by this national team have been used in other studies of the chronically ill, including those with HIV. Reported physical and mental health functioning were indices of questions from the Medical Outcomes Study Short-Form 21 (MOS SF-21), a standard health status rating instrument created from the original MOS SF-36 specifically to measure health-related quality of life of HIV-positive persons. The physical and mental health subscales are the most highly predictive subscales of the summary scales and stand on their own. With the subscales, the health ratings can be compared to ratings from the SF-36 that have been normed nationally for different types of populations defined by demographics and disease type. The survey obtained information on: the respondent's current general health functioning (Bozzette et al. 1995; Wu et al. 1991); limitations in activities of daily living (Ware 1993); HIV/AIDS specific signs and symptoms (Bozzette et al. 1995; Wu et al. 1991); self-esteem (Rosenberg 1965) and self-efficacy (Pearlin and Schooler

1978); medication use (Chesney et al. 2000); the amount and sources of care received in the recent past because of disability (Whetten-Goldstein et al. 1997, 1999); use of a hospital or a nursing home during the previous year; visits to physicians and mental health professionals; expenditures on prescription drugs during the past month (previous year if no visits/expenditures during the past month); domestic help other than to assist in personal care of the respondent; access to care; health insurance; housing; detailed demographic information; mode of HIV transmission allowing for multiple responses; and illicit substance use.

The consecutive sampling technique is as strong as random selection over a period of time. Therefore, the survey participants represent Medicaid-eligible, HIV-positive patients who attend academic medical centers for care in at least the three states studied in the South. While individuals receiving Medicaid represent the majority of patients in infectious diseases clinics in the South, the eligibility criteria of the study limit the generalizability of the findings from this population. In addition, participants were selected from infectious diseases clinics, thereby creating a selection bias toward those who engage in the health care system at academic medical centers. The sample was likely biased in the direction of those who were more engaged in the health care system and in more stable living conditions because interviewers were able to contact the sample to conduct the survey. Therefore, the results obtained concerning barriers to care are conservative and should be viewed as such.

North Carolina HIV Provider Survey

The NC HIV Provider Survey was based on the Infrastructure Grid developed by a group of investigators from sites around the nation involved in testing the effectiveness of various interventions designed to alter HIV provider communication and integration of services. This initiative was funded under Title V of the Ryan White CARE Act (Measurement Group 1999). The instrument sought to ascertain the level of knowledge, interaction, and satisfaction among HIV service providers within eastern North Carolina based on regions defined by Ryan White CARE Act Consortium. The eastern half of North Carolina, a land mass larger than West Virginia or South Carolina (U.S. Census Bureau 1995), contains ten of the state's fourteen North Carolina Ryan White CARE Act Consortia. The state divided itself into these fourteen regions so that Ryan White CARE Act funding could be appropriately distributed throughout the state.

In June 1997, each of the ten consortia directors was asked to provide a list of providers who serviced HIV clients in their region. The directors identified 462 providers; these providers' services included case management, medical care, legal aid, and HIV testing. We divided the providers into regions defined as areas in which an individual would seek various services, that is, in which providers would be expected to have knowledge of each other so as to provide referrals for their clients. In most cases, the area was the region defined by the consortia, but more densely populated consortia were subdivided by county or by county and surrounding counties. In an effort to survey at least 100 providers for adequate power, we randomly sampled 120 providers. The sample was weighted by region to oversample less densely populated areas based on standard statistical techniques.

Included in the sample were case management agencies, AIDS service organizations, primary medical care providers, mental health providers, community-based organizations, hospitals, HIV testing organizations, home health or hospice, specialty care providers, task forces, public benefits offices, dental care, legal services, transportation services, and long-term care facilities that serve HIV-positive persons. Agencies were asked to write in organizations with which they worked that the survey did not capture. The mail-back survey consisted of four questions relative to the listed HIV providers (Lin et al. 1998): (1) How much do you know about the HIV/AIDS services at this agency? (2) What percent of your HIV/AIDS clients-patients does your agency refer to this agency? (3) What percent of the incoming HIV/AIDS clients-patients in your agency comes from referrals from this agency? and (4) How satisfied are you with your working relationship with this agency? Answers were on a five-point scale, with an additional category for "information unavailable." We requested that one of the personnel who worked most closely with the organization's HIV/AIDS patients complete the survey. The response rate to the survey was 85 percent, for a total sample of 101.

Focus Groups

Three separate focus groups were conducted in 1997 with IRB approval. Participants were asked to discuss their experiences with breaches in confidentiality, positive and negative aspects of computers, how computer systems can affect confidentiality, and under what conditions they would trust a computer system to store medical information (Whetten-Goldstein et al. 2001c). The focus groups, conducted in three different regions of eastern North Carolina, were led by a trained facilitator and a research assistant, who taped the session and took notes (Krueger 1994). Knowing beforehand the topic that would be discussed during the focus group meeting, a total of fifteen HIV-positive patients participated in the three focus groups: nine participants were African American, and seven were female. This participation represented a high turnout given that, on average, the three support groups attracted a combined total of sixteen participants. Pizza and soft drinks were available during two focus groups, and participants in the third group received grocery store gift certificates. A focus group guide was used to trigger conversation and ensure that domains of interest were discussed. Audiotapes of the focus groups were transcribed verbatim and checked for accuracy. The authors separately, and then together, coded each transcript, inductively developing codes to account for themes that emerged from the discussions. (See Whetten-Goldstein et al. 2001c for a list of themes.) Data were entered into QSR NUD-IST 4, the same software package used in analyzing the case study interviews (QSR Pty Ltd. 1997).

Appendix B: Case Study Interview Protocol

Interviewers did not follow an exact script. Not all respondents answered every area of questioning.

I. Childhood

Let's start by talking about your childhood.

When and where were you born?

How many brothers and sisters did you have?

How would you describe the place you lived in as a child?

How would you describe the community in which you grew up?

Can you tell me about your parents and/or other adults who cared for you?

INTERVIEWER: PROBE FOR MARITAL STATUS AND EMPLOYMENT OF PARENT OR CARETAKER.

How would you describe your childhood?

What was your home life like?

Can you share with me some memories that you have of your childhood that are really good, or make you feel happy?

Can you share with me some childhood memories that are not good?

II. Growing up:

Did you move around much when you were growing up?

For how many years did you go to school, and what was school like for you?

Are there one or two people who you would say really shaped who you are today, either negatively or positively?

> IF YES: Could you please describe these people and how they influenced you?

Was there anything you wanted to do when you grew up; aspirations for a career, lifestyle, etc.?

III. Spiritual beliefs

Do you have any spiritual or religious beliefs?

> IF YES: How would you describe those beliefs?

> IF NO: Is there anything that you would say that you believe in?

IV. Source of illnesses

Where do you think HIV came from, how did it get started?

How do you think people become infected with HIV?

How do you think that you became infected with HIV?

When did you find out that you were HIV-positive?

What does being HIV-positive mean to you?

How does being HIV-positive affect your daily life?

What does HIV do to your body?

How did you find out that you were HIV-positive?

Who else knows that you are HIV-positive?

V. Care-seeking behavior

Where do you go for help when you are sick? [PROBE FOR MEDICAL CARE, ALTERNATIVE (SPIRITUAL) SOURCES OF CARE, HELP FROM FRIENDS, RELATIVES, ETC.]

When do you seek medical care in a doctor's office, clinic, or hospital?

What problems do you face when you are sick and want medical attention?

IF USES ALTERNATIVE OR SPIRITUAL SOURCES OF CARE: When do you use alternative or spiritual sources of care?

Have you ever changed doctors, hospitals, or other care providers due to feelings of discrimination? If so, why?

> IF YES: Have you ever wanted to change care providers due to feelings of discrimination, but were unable to do so for any reason?

VI. Treatment drugs, health providers, social workers and case managers

Are you taking medications for your HIV?

Do you think that medications prescribed by your health care provider help you, hurt you, or do nothing for you?

> IF HELP OR HURT: How do they [HELP, HURT]?

> IF DO NOTHING: Why do you think that the medications do nothing?

Do you think that there is a cure for HIV/AIDS?

How would you describe your relationship with your doctor?

What would you like your relationship with your doctor to be like?

Is there someone who talks with you about difficulties that you are having?

> IF YES: REPEAT THE FOLLOWING SET OF QUESTIONS FOR EACH PERSON

> Who is this person?

> What do they do for you?

> What would you like them to do for you?

Do doctors and other health care workers maintain confidentiality?

Have you had experiences where people have found out about your HIV status without your wanting them to?

> IF YES: Could you tell me about these experiences?

Have you heard of others who have had their HIV status told to people that they did not want to know?

> IF YES: Could you tell me about these experiences?

VII. Demographics

We are almost done. I am just going to ask you a few more questions about your educational background, race/ethnicity, work history, marital status, and children.

How would you describe your racial and/or ethnic background?

How much school education have you completed?

Are you currently married or live with a partner?

IF MARRIED: Where does your spouse live?

How many children have you given birth to, adopted, or cared for?

IF ONE OR MORE: Could you please tell me about your children?

Are you working for money?

IF YES: What do you do? [PROBE FOR HOURS PER WEEK]

IF NO: Did you ever work for money?

IF YES: What did you do?

When did you stop working?

Why did you stop working?

Do you have goals or aspirations for the future?

IF YES: Do you intend to pursue them?

VIII. Additional Questions dependent on demographics of case study interviewee:

What was it like growing up black in North Carolina?

Are any providers racist?

What experiences have you had with racism?

Describe your community.

How are rural areas different from urban areas?

Why did you and why do others come back to rural areas such as North Carolina?

Appendix C: List of Traumatic Events Read by Interviewer to Respondent

People often have traumatic experiences. I mean terrible, frightening events. I am going to read a list of some possible events that sometimes happen to people. Please tell me if you ever experienced:

1. A serious accident/fire at home or at your job?
2. A natural disaster such as a hurricane, major earthquake, flood, or other similar disaster?
3. Direct combat experience in a war?
4. Physical assault or abuse by your partner?
5. Physical assault or abuse in your adult life by someone other than your partner?
6. Physical assault or abuse as a child?
7. Seeing people hitting or harming one another in your family when you were growing up?
8. Sexual assault or rape in your adult life?
9. Sexual assault or rape as a child?
10. Seeing someone physically assaulted or abused?
11. Seeing someone seriously injured or violently killed?
12. Losing a child through death?
13. Death or permanent separation from parent or someone who was like a parent to you before you were age eighteen?
14. Death of a spouse, partner, or loved one when you were an adult?

References

Abraham, C., P. Sheeran, D. Abrams, R. Speers. 1996. Health Beliefs and Teenage Condom Use: A Prospective Study. *Psychology and Health* 11:641–655.

Adam, B.D., A. Sears. 1994(a). Negotiating Sexual Relationships After Testing HIV-Positive. *Medical Anthropology* 16:63–77.

———. 1994(b). *People with HIV/AIDS Talk . . . About Life, Love, Work, and Family.* Windsor, Ontario: AIDS Committee of Windsor.

———. 1996. *Experiencing HIV: Personal, Family, and Work Relationships.* New York: Columbia University Press.

Adams, J.A., P.L. East. 1999. Past Physical Abuse is Significantly Correlated with Pregnancy as an Adolescent. *Journal of Pediatric and Adolescent Gynecology* 12: 133–138.

Adams, M., C. Hanssens, T. Lazarus. 1998. Battling HIV on Many Fronts [letter]. *New England Journal of Medicine* 338(3):198.

Aday, L.A., R. Andersen. 1974. A Framework for the Study of Access to Medical Care. *Health Services Research* 9(3):208–220.

Aday, L.A., C.E. Begley, D.R. Lairson, C.H. Slater. 1993. *Evaluating the Medical Care System: Effectiveness, Efficiency, and Equity.* Ann Arbor, Mich.: Health Administration Press.

Ajzen, I. 1985. From Intentions to Actions: A Theory of Planned Behavior. In *Action-Control from Cognition to Behaviour,* ed. J. Kuhl, J. Beckmann. Heidelberg: Springer-Verlag.

———. 1991. The Theory of Planned Behavior. *Organizational Behavior and Human Decision Processes* 50:179–211.

Ajzen, I., M. Fishbein. 1980. *Understanding Attitudes and Predicting Social Behavior.* Englewood Cliffs, N. J.: Prentice Hall.

Alexander, P.C., S.J. Lupfer. 1987. Connections between Childhood Abuse and HIV Infection. *Archives of Sexual Behavior* 16:235–245.

Allen, J.D., G. Sorensen, A.M. Stoddard, G. Colditz, K. Peterson. 1998. Intention to Have a Mammogram in the Future Among Women Who Have Underused Mammography in the Past. *Health Education and Behavior* 25:474–488.

Allers, C.T., K.J. Benjack, N.T. Allers. 1992. Unresolved Childhood Sexual Abuse: Are Older Adults Impacted? *Journal of Counseling and Development* 71:14–27.

American Psychiatric Association. 1994. *Diagnostic and Statistical Manual of Mental*

Disorders Fourth Edition: DSM-IV. Washington, D. C.: American Psychiatric Association.

American Psychological Association. May 2001. An APA Report: The Behavioral Health Care Needs of Rural Women: The Report of the Rural Women's Work Group and the Committee on Rural Health.

Anastos K., S.J. Gange, B. Lau et al. 2000. Association of Race and Gender with HIV-1 RNA Levels and Immunologic Progression. *Journal of Acquired Immune Deficiency Syndromes* 24:218–226.

Andersen R., S. Bozzette, M. Shapiro, P. St Clair, S. Morton, S. Crystal et al. 2000. Access in Vulnerable Groups to Antiretroviral Therapy among Persons in Care for HIV Disease in the United States. HCSUS Consortium. HIV Cost and Services Utilization Study. *Health Services Review* 35:389–416.

Andersen, J.E., R.W. Wilson, P. Barker, L. Doll, T.S. Jones, D. Holtgrave. 1999. Prevalence of Sexual and Drug-Related HIV Risk Behaviors in the U.S. Adult Population: Results of the 1996 National Household Survey on Drug Abuse. *Journal of Acquired Immune Deficiency Syndromes* 21:148–156.

Andrews, G., C. Tennant, D. Hewson, M. Schonell. 1978. The Relation of Social Factors to Physical and Psychiatric Illness. *American Journal of Epidemiology* 108: 27–35.

Anglin, M.K., J.C. White. 1999. Poverty, Health Care, and Problems of Prescription Medication: A Case Study. *Substance Use and Misuse* 34:2073–2093.

Anonymous. 2000. Maine HIV/AIDS 115 Demonstration: Operational Protocol.

Antoni, M.H., L. Baggett, G. Ironson, A. LaPerriere, S. August, N. Klimas, N. Schneiderman, M.A. Fletcher. 1991. Cognitive-Behavioral Stress Management Intervention Buffers Distress Responses and Immunologic Changes Following Notification of HIV-1 Seropositivity. *Journal of Consulting and Clinical Psychology* 59:906–915.

Antoni, M.H., D. Goldstein, G. Ironson, A. LaPerriere, M.A. Fletcher, N. Schneiderman. 1995. Coping Responses to HIV-1 Serostatus Notification Predict Concurrent and Prospective Immunologic Status. *Clinical Psychology and Psychotherapy* 2:234–248.

Aranda-Naranjo, B., C. Portillo, H. Schietinger, G. Norgan. Policy Brief Number 1. Impact of the Ryan White CARE Act on Services Provided to Women, Children, and Families. *Directions in HIV Service Delivery and Care: Vulnerable Populations.* HIV/AIDS Bureau: Health Resources and Services Administration.

Aruffo, J.F., R.G. Thompson, A.A. Gottlieb, W.N. Dobbins. 1995. An AIDS Training Program for Rural Mental Health Providers. *Psychiatric Services* 46:79–81.

Associated Press. December 8, 1999. Jury: Martin Luther King's Death a Conspiracy.

Bailey, J.M., R.C. Pillard, K. Dawood, M.B. Miller, L.A. Farrer, S. Trivedi, R.L. Murphy. 1999. A Family History Study of Male Sexual Orientation Using Three Independent Samples. *Behavior Genetics* 29:79–86.

Barnhoorn F., H. Adriaanse 1992. In Search of Factors Responsible for Noncompliance among Tuberculosis Patients in Wardha District, India. *Social Science and Medicine.* 34:291–306.

Bartholow, B.N., L.S. Doll, D. Joy, J.M. Douglas, Jr., G. Bolan, J.S. Harrison, P.M. Moss, D. McKirnan. 1994. Emotional, Behavioral, and HIV Risks Associated with Sexual Abuse among Adult Homosexual and Bisexual Men. *Child Abuse and Neglect* 18:747–761.

Bartlett, J.G., J.E. Gallant. 2000–2001. *Medical Management of HIV Infection.* Baltimore, Md.: Johns Hopkins University, Department of Infectious Diseases.

Bates, K.G. 1990. Is it Genocide? *Essence* September, 76–118.

Becker, M.H., L.A. Maiman. 1975. Sociobehavioral Determinants of Compliance with Health and Medical Care Recommendations. *Medical Care* 13:10–24.

Berry, D.E., M.M. McKinney, K.M. Marconi. 1997. A Typological Approach to the Study of Rural HIV Service Delivery Networks. *Journal of Rural Health* 13:216–225.

Black, M.M., H. Dubowitz, R.H. Starr, Jr. 1999. African American Fathers in Low Income, Urban Families: Development, Behavior and Home Environment of Their Three-Year-Old Children. *Child Development* 70:967–978.

Blackwell, B. 1996. From Compliance to Alliance: A Quarter Century of Research. *Netherlands Journal of Medicine* 48:140–149.

Blank, M.B., J.C. Fox, D.S. Hargrove, J.T. Turner. 1995. Critical Issues in Reforming Rural Mental Health Service Delivery. *Community Mental Health Journal* 31:511–524.

Blank, M.B., F.L. Tetrick III, D.F. Brinkley, H.O. Smith, V. Doheny. 1994. Racial Matching and Service Utilization among Seriously Mentally Ill Consumers in the Rural South. *Community Mental Health Journal* 30:271–281.

Blume, A.W., K.B. Schmaling. 1996. Loss and Readiness to Change Substance Abuse. *Addictive Behaviors* 21:527–530.

———. 1998. Regret, Substance Abuse, and Readiness to Change in a Dually Diagnosed Sample. *Addictive Behaviors* 23:693–697.

Boden, D., A. Hurley, L. Zhang, Y. Cao, Y. Guo, E. Jones, J. Tsay, J. Ip, C. Farthing, K. Limoli, N. Parkin, M. Markowitz. 1999. HIV-1 Drug Resistance in Newly Infected Individuals. *Journal of the American Medical Association* 282:1135–1141.

Bonuck, K.A., P.S. Arno, J. Green, J. Fleisham, C.L. Bennett, M.C. Fahs, C. Maffeo. 1996. Self-Perceived Unmet Health Care Needs of Persons Enrolled in HIV Care. *Journal of Community Health* 21:183–198.

Boyce, P., M. Harris, D. Silove, A. Morgan, K. Wilheim, D. Hadzi-Pavlovic. 1998. Psychosocial Factors Associated with Depression: A Study of Socially Disadvantaged Women and Young Children. *Journal of Nervous and Mental Disease* 186:3–11.

Bozzette, S.A., R.D. Hays, S.H. Berry, D.E. Kanouse, A.W. Wu. 1995. Derivation and Properties of a Brief Health Status Assessment for Use in HIV Disease. *Journal of Acquired Immune Deficiency Syndromes* 8:253–265.

Brady, K.T., C.L. Randall. 1999. Gender Differences in Substance Use Disorders. *Psychiatric Clinics of North America* 22:241–252.

Brashers, D.E., J.L. Neidig, L.W. Cardillo, L.K. Dobbs, J.A. Russell, S.M. Haas. 1999. "In an Important Way, I Did Die": Uncertainty and Revival in Persons Living with HIV or AIDS. *AIDS Care* 11:201–219.

Breitbart, W., M.V. McDonald, B. Rosenfeld, S.D. Passik, D. Hewitt, H. Thaler, R.K. Portenoy. 1996. Pain in Ambulatory AIDS Patients. I: Pain Characteristics and Medical Correlates. *Pain* 68:315–321.

Bremner, J.D. 1999. Does Stress Damage the Brain? *Biological Psychiatry* 45:797–805.

Bremner, J.D., M. Narayan. 1998. The Effects of Stress on Memory and the Hippocampus throughout the Life Cycle: Implications for Childhood Development and Aging. *Development and Psychopathology* 10:871–885.

Bremner, J.D., M. Narayan, L. Staib, S. Southwick, T. McGlashan, D. Charney. 1999. Neural Correlates of Memories of Childhood Sexual Abuse in Women with and without Posttraumatic Stress Disorder. *American Journal of Psychiatry* 156:1787–1795.

Briere, J., M. Runtz. 1988. Symptomatology Associated with Childhood Sexual Victimization in a Nonclinical Adult Sample. *Child Abuse and Neglect* 12:51–59.

Bright, P.E., D.K. Arnett, C. Blair, M. Bayona. 1996. Gender and Ethnic Differences in Survival in a Cohort of HIV Positive Clients. *Ethnicity and Health* 1:77–85.

Brody, G.H., D.L. Flor, N.M. Gibson. 1999. Linking Maternal Efficacy Beliefs, Developmental Goals, Parenting Practices, and Child Competence in Rural Single-Parent African American Families. *Child Development* 70:1197–1208.

Brook, J.S., D.W. Brook, P.T. Win, M. Whiteman, J.R. Masci, J. de Catalogne, J. Roberto, F. Amundsen. 1997. Coping with AIDS: A Longitudinal Study. *American Journal on Addictions* 6:11–20.

Brosgart, C.L., T.F. Mitchell, R.F. Coleman, T. Dyner, K.E. Stephenson, and D.I. Abrams. 1999. Clinical Experience and Choice of Drug Therapy for Human Immunodeficiency Virus Disease. *Clinical Infectious Diseases* 28:14–22.

Broun, S.N. 1998. Understanding Post-AIDS Survivor Syndrome: A Record of Personal Experiences. *AIDS Patient Care* 12:481–488.

Browne, A., D. Finkelhor. 1986. Initial and Long-Term Effects: A Review of the Research. In *A Sourcebook of Child Sexual Abuse*, 1 ed., ed. D. Finkelhor. Beverly Hills, Calif.: Sage Publications.

Campbell, M.K., B.M. Motsinger, A. Ingram, D. Jewell, C. Makarushka, B. Beatty, J. Dodds, J. McClelland, S. Demissie, W. Demark-Wahnefried. 2000. The North Carolina Black Churches United for Better Health Project: Intervention and Process Evaluation. *Health Education and Behavior* 27:241–253.

Caplan, R.D., E.A.R. Robinson, J.R.P. French Jr., J.R. Caldwell, M. Shinn. 1976. *Adhering to Medical Regimens: Pilot Experiments in Patient Education and Social Support.* Ann Arbor: University of Michigan Press.

Carosella, A.M., E.J. Ossip-Klein, C.A. Owens. 1999. Smoking Attitudes, Beliefs, and Readiness to Change among Acute and Long Term Care Inpatients with Psychiatric Diagnoses. *Addictive Behaviors* 24: 331–344.

Carver, C.S., M.F. Scheier, J.K. Weintraub. 1989. Assessing Coping Strategies: A Theoretically Based Approach. *Journal of Personality and Social Psychology* 56:267–283.

Caspi, A., B. Henry, R.O. McGee, T.E. Moffitt, P.A. Silva. 1995. Temperamental Origins of Child and Adolescent Behavior Problems: From Age 3 to Age 15. *Child Development* 66:55–68.

Catalan, J., A. Beevor, L. Cassidy, A.P. Burgess, J. Meadows, A. Pergami, B. Gazzard, S. Barton. 1996. Women and HIV Infection: Investigation of Its Psychosocial Consequences. *Journal of Psychosomatic Research* 41:39–47.

Celentano, D.D., D. Vlahov, S. Cohn, V.M. Shadle, O. Obasanjo, R.D. Moore. 1998. Self-Reported Antiretroviral Therapy in Injection Drug Users. *Journal of the American Medical Association* 280:544–546.

Center for Disease Control (CDC). Summary of Notifiable Diseases, United States [1989–1999] *Morbidity and Mortality Weekly Report* 1990(38(53)); 1991(39(53)); 1992(40(53)); 1993(41(53)); 1994(42(53)); 1995(43(53)); 1996(44(53)); 1997(45(53)); 1998(46(54)); 1999(47(53)); 2001(48(53)).

———. 1997; 1998a; 1998b; 1999a; 1999b. *HIV/AIDS Surveillance Report.* Atlanta, Ga.: CDC. (9)1; 10(1); 10(2); 11(1); 11(2).

———. 1999c. Emerging Infectious Diseases: A Public Health Response. Atlanta, Ga.: CDC.

———. 2000a. HIV/AIDS among Racial/Ethnic Minority Men Who Have Sex with Men. United States, 1989-1998. *Morbidity and Mortality Weekly Report* 49:4–11.

———. 2000b. Preventing Emerging Infections: Addressing the Problem of Antimicrobial Resistance. Atlanta, Ga.: Centers for Disease Control and Prevention. 2000.

Center for Medicaid and State Operations. 2000. Fact Sheet: Medicaid and Acquired Immune Deficiency Syndrome (AIDS) And Human Immunodeficiency Virus (HIV) Infection. Department of Health and Human Services.

Chaix, C., C. Grenier-Sennelier, P. Clevenbergh, J. Durant, J.M. Schapiro, P. Dellamonica, I. Durand-Zaleski. 2000. Economic Evaluation of Drug Resistance Genotyping for the Adaptation of Treatment in HIV-Infected Patients in the VIRADAPT Study. *Journal of Acquired Immune Deficiency Syndromes* 24:227–231.

Chan, D.K., M. Fishbein. 1993. Determinants of College Women's Intentions to Tell Their Partners to Use Condoms. *Journal of Applied Social Psychology* 23:1455–1470.

Chandler, D., J. Meisel, M. McGowen, J. Mintz, K. Madison. 1996. Client Outcomes in Two Model Capitated Integrated Service Agencies. *Psychiatric Services.* 47:175–180.

Chesney, M., S. Folkman. 1994. Psychological Impact of HIV Disease and Implications for Intervention. *Psychiatric Clinics of North America* 17:163–182.

Chesney, M.A., J.R. Ickovics, D.B. Chambers, A.L. Gifford, J. Neidig, B. Zwickl, A.W. Wu. 2000. Self-Reported Adherence to Antiretroviral Medications among Participants in HIV Clinical Trials: The AACTG Adherence Instruments. Patient Care Committee and Adherence Working Group of the Outcomes Committee of the Adult AIDS Clinical Trials Group (AACTG). *AIDS Care* 2:255–266.

Chesson, A.L., Jr., P.W. Murphy, C.L. Arnold, T.C. Davis. 1998. Presentation and Reading Level of Sleep Brochures: Are They Appropriate for Sleep Disorders Patients? *Sleep* 21:406–412.

Clarke, J., M.D. Stein, M. Sobota, M. Marisi, L. Hanna. 1999. Victims as Victimizers: Physical Aggression by Persons with a History of Childhood Abuse. *Archives of Internal Medicine* 159:1920–1924.

Cochran, S.D., M.J. Gitlin. 1988. Attitudinal Correlates of Lithium Compliance in Bipolar Affective Disorders. *Journal of Nervous and Mental Disease* 176:457–464.

Cohen, D.A., T.A. Farley, J.R. Bedimo-Etame, R. Scribner, W. Ward, C. Kendall, J. Rice. 1999. Implementation of Condom Social Marketing in Louisiana, 1993 to 1996. *American Journal of Public Health* 89:204–208.

Cohen, M. 1996. Natural History of HIV Infection in Women. *Obstetrics and Gynecology Clinics of North America* 24:743–758.

Cohen, M., C. Deamant, S. Barkan, J. Richardson, M. Young, S. Holman, K. Anastos, J. Choen, S. Melnick. 2000. Domestic Violence and Children Sexual Abuse in HIV-Infected Women and Women at Risk for HIV. *American Journal of Public Health* 90:560–565.

Cohen, S., T.A. Wills. 1985. Stress, Social Support, and the Buffering Hypothesis. *Psychological Bulletin* 98:310–357.

Cohn, S.E., J.D. Klein, J.E. Mohr, C.M. Van der Horst, D.J. Weber. 1994. The Geography of AIDS: Patterns of Urban and Rural Migration. *Southern Medical Journal* 87:599–606.

Cole, S.R., C.A. Bryant, R.J. McDermott, C. Sorrell, M. Flynn. 1997. Beliefs and Mammography Screening. *American Journal of Preventive Medicine* 13:439–443.

Coleman, C.L., W.L. Holzemer. 1999. Spirituality, Psychological Well-Being, and HIV Symptoms for African Americans Living with HIV Disease. *Journal of the Association of Nurses in AIDS Care* 10:42–50.

Conduct Problem Prevention Research Group. 1999. Initial Impact of the Fast Track Prevention Trial for Conduct Problems: I. The High-Risk Sample. *Journal of Consulting and Clinical Psychology* 67:631–647.

Conner, M., P. Norman. 1996. *Predicting Health Behaviour.* Buckingham, U.K.: Open University Press.

Conner, M., P. Sparks. 1996. The Theory of Planned Behaviour and Health Behaviours. In *Predicting Health Behaviour*, ed. M. Conner, P. Norman. Buckingham, U.K.: Open University Press.

Cook, C.A., K.L. Selig, B.J. Wedge, E.A. Gohn-Baube. 1999. Access Barriers and the Use of Prenatal Care by Low-Income, Inner-City Women. *Social Work* 44: 129–139.

Cook, P.J., M.J. Moore. 1999. Alcohol. In *Handbook of Health Economics*, ed. A. Cuyler and J. Newhouse. Amsterdam: Elsevier.

Cooper-Patrick, L., J.J. Gallo, J.J. Gonzales, H.T. Vu, N.R. Powe, C. Nelsen, D.E. Ford. 1999. Race, Gender, and Partnership in the Physician-Patient Relationship. *Journal of the American Medical Association* 282:583–589.

Corbie-Smith, G., S.B. Thomas, M.V. Williams, S. Moody-Ayers. 1999. Attitudes and Beliefs of African Americans toward Participation in Medical Research. *Journal of General Internal Medicine* 14:537–546.

Corin, E. 1994. The Social and Cultural Matrix of Health and Disease. In *Why Some People are Healthy and Others are Not? The Determinants of Health of Populations*, eds. R.G. Evans, M.L. Barer, T.R. Marmor. Hawthorne, N.Y.: Aldine De Gruyer.

———. 1995. The Cultural Frame: Context and Meaning in the Construction of Health. In *Society and Health*, eds. B.C. Amick, S. Levine, A.R. Tarlov, D.C. Walsh. New York: Oxford University Press.

Cramer, J., A. Rosenheck. 1998. Compliance with Medication Regimens for Mental and Physical Disorders. *Psychiatric Services* 49:196–201.

Crimp, D., A. Rolston. 1990. *AIDS Demographics*. Seattle, Wash.: Bay Press.

Cunningham, R.M., A.R. Stiffman, P. Dore, F. Earls. 1994. The Association of Physical and Sexual Abuse with HIV Risk Behaviors in Adolescence and Young Adulthood: Implications for Public Health. *Child Abuse and Neglect* 18:233–245.

Cunningham, W.E., R.M. Andersen, M.H. Katz, M.D. Stein, B.J. Turner, S. Crystal, S. Zierler, K. Kuromiya, S.C. Morton, P. St. Clair, S.A. Bozzette, M.F. Shapiro. 1999. The Impact of Competing Subsistence Needs and Barriers on Access to Medical Care for Persons with Human Immunodeficiency Virus Receiving Care in the United States. *Medical Care* 37:1270–1281.

Cunningham, W.E., R. Hays, K. Williams, K. Beck, W. Dixon, M. Shapiro. 1995. Access to Medical Care and Health-Related Quality of Life for Low-Income Persons with Symptomatic Human Immunodeficiency Virus. *Medical Care* 33: 739–754.

Currier, J.S., C. Spino, J. Grimes et al. 2000. Differences between Women and Men in Adverse Events and CD4+ Responses to Nucleoside Analogue Therapy for HIV Infection. The AIDS Clinical Trials Group 175 Team. *Journal of Acquired Immune Deficiency Syndromes* 24:316–324.

Curry, S.J., A.R. Kristal, D.J. Bowen. 1992. An Application of the Stage Model of Behavior Change to Dietary Fat. *Health Education Research* 7:97–105.

Curtis, J.R., D.L. Patrick, E. Caldwell, H. Greenlee, A.C. Collier. 1999. The Quality of Patient-Doctor Communication about End-of-Life Care: A Study of Patients with Advanced AIDS and Their Primary Care Clinicians. *AIDS* 13:1123–1131.

Dalaker, J., U.S. Census Bureau. 1999. Current Population Reports, Series P60-207, Poverty in the United States: 1998. Washington, D.C.: U.S. Government Printing Office.

Damasio, H., T. Grabowski, R. Frank, A.M. Galaburda, A.R. Damasio. 1994. The Return of Phineas Gage: Clues about the Brain from the Skull of a Famous Patient. *Science* 264:1102–1105.

Dancy, B.L., R. Marcantonio, K. Norr. 2000. The Long-Term Effectiveness of an HIV Prevention Intervention for Low-Income African American Women. *AIDS Education and Prevention* 12:113–125.

Davis, K., J. Stapleton. 1991. Migration to Rural Areas By HIV Patients: Impact on HIV-Related Healthcare Use. *Infection Control and Hospital Epidemiology* 12:540–543.

Davis, S.F., R.H. Byers, Jr., M.L. Lindegren, M.B. Caldwell, J.M. Karon, M. Gwinn. 1995. Prevalence and Incidence of Vertically Acquired HIV Infection in the United States. *Journal of the American Medical Association* 274:952–955.

Deater-Deckard, K., K.A. Dodge, J.E. Bates, G.S. Petit. 1998. Multiple Risk Factors in the Development of Externalizing Behavior Problems: Group and Individual Differences. *Development and Psychopathology* 10:469–493.

Deeks, S.G., M. Smith, M. Holodniy, J.O. Kahn. 1997. HIV-1 Protease Inhibitors: A Review for Clinicians. *Journal of the American Medical Association* 277:145–153.

Del Amo, J., A. Petruckevitch, A. Phillips, A.M. Johnson, J. Stephenson, N. Desmond, T. Hanscheid, N. Low, A. Newell, A. Obasi, K. Paine, A. Pym, C.M. Theodore, K.M. De Cock. 1998. Disease Progression and Survival in HIV-1-Infected Africans in London. *AIDS* 12:1203–1209.

Delorme, D., M. Rotily, N. Escaffre, A. Galinier-Pujol, A. Loundou, J.P. Moatti. 1999. Knowledge, Beliefs, and Attitudes of Inmates towards AIDS and HIV Infection: A Survey in a Marseille Penitentiary Center. *Revue d' Epidemiologie et de Santé Publique* 47:229–238.

DeMarco, R.F., K.H. Miller, C.A. Patsdaughter, M. Chisholm M, C.G. Grindel. 1998. From Silencing the Self to Action: Experiences of Women Living with HIV/AIDS. *Health Care for Women International* 19:539–552.

Demas, P., E. Schoenbaum, T. Wills, L. Doll, R. Klein. 1995. Stress, Coping, and Attitudes toward HIV Treatment in Injecting Drug Users: A Qualitative Study. *AIDS Education and Prevention* 7:429–442.

Department of Health and Human Sciences. 1998. Cooperative Agreements for an HIV/AIDS Treatment Adherence, Health Outcomes, and Cost Study. Guidance for Applicants No. SM 98-007. Catalog of Federal Domestic Assistance No. 93.230. Washington, D.C.

Devinsky, O., M.J. Morrell, B.A. Vogt. 1995. Contributions of Anterior Cingulate to Behavior. *Brain* 118:279–306.

DiClemente, C.C., J.O. Prochaska, S.K. Fairhurst, W.F. Velicer, M.M. Velasquez, J.S. Rossi. 1991. The Process of Smoking Cessation: An Analysis of Precontemplation, Contemplation and Preparation Stages of Change. *Journal of Consulting and Clinical Psychology* 59:295–304.

Dietz, P.M., A.M. Spitz, R.F. Anda, D.F. Williamson. P.M. McMahon, J.S. Santelli, D.F. Nordenberg, V.J. Felitti, J.S. Dendrick. 1999. Unintended Pregnancy among Adult Women Exposed to Abuse or Household Dysfunction During their Childhood. *Journal of the American Medical Association* 282:1359–1364.

Dilorio, C., W.N. Dudley, J. Soet, J. Watkins, E. Maibach. 2000. A Social Cognitive-Based Model for Condom Use Among College Students. *Nursing Research* 49:208–214.

Dodge, K.A. 1996. Biopsychosocial Perspectives on the Development of Conduct Disorder. Invited Address to the NIMH Prevention Research Conference. McLean, Va.

Doherty, M.C., B. Junge, P. Rathouz, R.S. Garfein, E. Riley, D. Vlahov. 2000. The Effect of a Needle Exchange Program on Numbers of Discarded Needles: A 2-Year Follow-Up. *American Journal of Public Health* 90:936–939.

Drake, R.E., K.T. Mueser, R.E. Clark, M.A. Wallach. 1996. The Course, Treatment, and Outcome of Substance Disorder in Persons with Severe Mental Illness. *American Journal of Orthopsychiatry* 66:42–51.

Drake, R.E., M.A. Wallach. 1989. Substance Abuse among the Chronic Mentally Ill. *Hospital and Community Psychiatry* 40:1041–1046.

Dressler, W. 1991. Social Class, Skin Color, and Arterial Blood Pressure in Two Societies. *Ethnicity and Disease* 1:60–77.

Drossman, D.A., J. Leserman, G. Nachman, Z.M. Li, H. Gluck, T.C. Toomey, C.M. Mitchell. 1990. Sexual and Physical Abuse in Women with Functional or Organic Gastrointestinal Disorders. *Annals of Internal Medicine* 113:828–833.

Duncan, R.D., B.E. Saunders, D.G. Kilpatrick, R.F. Hanson, H.S. Resnick. 1996.

Childhood Physical Assault as a Risk Factor for PTSD, Depression, and Substance Abuse: Findings from a National Survey. *American Journal of Orthopsychiatry* 66:437–448.

Eachus, J., P. Chan, N. Pearson, C. Propper, G. Davey Smith. 1999. An Additional Dimension to Health Inequalities: Disease Severity and Socioeconomic Position [see comments]. *Journal of Epidemiology and Community Health* 53:603–611.

Easterbrook, P.J., J.S. Chmiel, D.R. Hoover, A.J. Saah, R.A. Kaslow, L.A. Kingsley, R. Detels. 1993. Racial and Ethnic Differences in Human Immunodeficiency Virus Type 1 (HIV-1) Seroprevalence Among Homosexual and Bisexual Men. The Multicenter AIDS Cohort Study. *American Journal of Epidemiology* 138: 415–429.

Easterbrook, P.J., J.C. Keruly, T. Creagh-Kirk, D.D. Richman, R.E. Chaisson, R.D. Moore. 1991. Racial and Ethnic Differences in Outcome in Zidovudine-Treated Patients with Advanced HIV Disease. Zidovudine Epidemiology Study Group. *Journal of the American Medical Association* 266:2713–2718.

El-Bassel, N., L. Gilbert, S. Krishnan, R. Schilling, T. Gaeta, S. Purpura, S.S. Witte. 1998. Partner Violence and Sexual HIV-Risk Behaviors among Women in an Inner-City Emergency Department. *Violence and Victims* 13:377–393.

Ell, K. 1986. Coping with Serious Illness: On Integrating Constructs to Enhance Clinical Research Assessment and Intervention. *International Journal of Psychiatry in Medicine* 15:335–356.

———. 1996. Social Networks, Social Support, and Coping with Serious Illness: The Family Connection. *Social Science and Medicine* 42(2):173–183.

Ensink, K., B.A. Robertson, C. Zissis, P. Leger. 1997. Post-Traumatic Stress Disorder in Children Exposed to Violence. *South African Medical Journal* 87:1526–1530.

Epstein, J.N., B.E. Saunders, D.G. Kilpatrick, H.S. Resnick. 1998. PTSD as a Mediator between Childhood Rape and Alcohol Use in Adult Women. *Child Abuse and Neglect* 22:223–234.

Erwin, J., B. Peters. 1999. Treatment Issues for HIV+ Africans in London. *Social Science and Medicine* 49:1519–1528.

Evans, R.G., M.L. Barer, T.R. Marmor. 1994. *Why Are Some People Healthy and Others Not? The Determinants of Health of Populations*. New York: Aldine de Gruyter.

Evans, R.G., G.L. Stoddard. 1990. Producing Health, Consuming Health Care. *Social Science and Medicine* 31:1347–1363.

Fahs, M.C., D. Waite, M. Sesholtz, C. Muller, E.A. Hintz, C. Maffeo, P. Arno, C. Bennett. 1994. Results of the ACSUS for Pediatric AIDS Patients: Utilization of Services, Functional Status, and Social Severity. *Health Services Research* 29:549–568.

Faithfull, J. 1997. HIV-Positive and AIDS-Infected Women: Challenges and Difficulties of Mothering. *American Journal of Orthopsychiatry* 67:144–151.

Farer, L.S., C.W. Schieffelbein. 1987. Respiratory Diseases. *American Journal of Preventive Medicine* 3 Suppl:115–124.

Fawzy, F.I., S. Namir, D.L. Wolcott. 1989. Structured Group Intervention Model for AIDS Patients. *Psychiatric Medicine* 7:35–45.

Feagin, J. 1991. The Continuing Significance of Race: Antiblack Discrimination in Public Places. *American Sociological Review* 56:101–116.

Federal Medicare Agency. 2000. 2000 Guide to Health Insurance for People with Medicare. Health Care Financing Administration.

Federal Register. February 15, 2000. 65, no. 31: 7555–7557.

Felitti, V.J. 1991. Long-Term Medical Consequences of Incest, Rape, and Molestation. *Southern Medical Journal* 84:328–331.

Felitti, V.J., R.F. Anda, D. Nordenberg, D.F. Williamson, A.M. Spitz, V. Edwards, M.P. Koss, J.S. Marks. 1998. Relationship of Childhood Abuse and Household

Dysfunction to Many of the Leading Causes of Death in Adults. *American Journal of Preventive Medicine* 14:245–258.

Fernando, D. 1993. *AIDS and Intravenous Drug Use: The Influence of Morality, Politics, Social Science, and Race in the Making of a Tragedy.* Westport, Conn.: Praeger.

Fishbein, M., M. Guinan. 1996. Behavioral Science and Public Health: A Necessary Partnership for HIV Prevention. *Public Health Reports* 2 Suppl 3:5–10.

Flaskerud, J.H., E.R. Calvillo. 1991. Beliefs About AIDS, Health, and Illness Among Low-Income Latina Women. *Research in Nursing and Health* 14:431–438.

Fleishman, J.A., D.C. Hsia, F.J. Hellinger. 1994. Correlates of Medical Service Utilization among People with HIV Infection. *Health Services Research* 29:527–548.

Fleishman, J.A., V. Mor, J. Piette. 1991. AIDS Case Management: The Client's Perspective. *Health Services Research* 26:447–470.

Foa, E.B., T.M. Keane, M.J. Friedman, eds. 2000. *Effective Treatments for PTSD: Practice Guidelines from the International Society for Traumatic Stress Studies.* New York: Guilford Press.

Folkman, S., M. Chesney, L. McKusick, G. Ironson, D.S. Johnson, T.J. Coates. 1991. Translating Coping Theory into Intervention. In *The Social Context of Coping,* ed. J. Eckenrode, 239–259. New York: Plenum.

Food and Nutrition Service. 2000. Food Stamp Program: Frequently Asked Questions. U.S. Department of Agriculture.

Ford, E.S., R.S. Cooper. 1995. Racial/Ethnic Differences in Health Care Utilization of Cardiovascular Procedures: A Review of the Evidence. *Health Services Research* 30:237–252.

Forney, M.A., J.A. Inciardi, D. Lockwood. 1992. Exchanging Sex for Crack-Cocaine: A Comparison of Women from Rural and Urban Communities. *Journal of Community Health* 17:73–85.

Fox, J.C., E. Merwin, M.B. Blank. 1995. De Facto Mental Health Services in the Rural South. *Journal of Health Care for the Poor and Underserved* 64:434–468.

Franklin, G.M., L.M. Nelson. 1993. Chronic Neurologic Disorders. In *Chronic Disease Epidemiology and Control,* eds. R.C. Brownson, P.I. Remington, J.R. Davis. Washington, D.C.: American Public Health Association.

Freedberg, K.A., J.A. Scharfstein, G.R. Seage III, E. Losina, M.C. Weinstein, D.E. Craven, A.D. Paltiel. 1998. The Cost-Effectiveness of Preventing AIDS-Related Opportunistic Infections. *Journal of the American Medical Association* 279:130–136.

Friedland, J., R. Renwick, M. McColl. 1996. Coping and Social Support as Determinants of Quality of Life in HIV/AIDS. *AIDS Care* 8:15–31.

Fry, G. 1975. *Night Riders in Black Folk History.* Knoxville: University of Tennessee Press.

Fullilove, M.T., R. Fullilove, J. Stevens, L. Green. 2000. Policy Brief Number 1. Women's Equity in AIDS Resources. Directions in HIV Service Delivery and Care: Vulnerable Populations. HIV/AIDS Bureau: Health Resources and Services Administration. Rockville, Md.

Fullilove, R. 1998. How the Past Haunts Minority Care Today: The Legacy of Tuskegee. *Innovations.* HIV/AIDS Bureau: Health Resources and Services Administration. Rockville, Md.

Gabbard, G.O., S.G. Lazar, J. Hornberger, D. Spiegal. 1997. The Economic Impact of Psychotherapy: A Review. *American Journal of Psychiatry* 154:147–155.

General Accounting Office: Rural Hospitals. 1991. Federal Hospitals Should Target Areas Where Closures Would Threaten Access to Care. February. Report GAO/HRD-91-41. Washington, D.C.

General Accounting Office. March 2000. HIV/AIDS: Use of Ryan White CARE Act and Other Assistance Grant Funds. HEHS-00-54. Washington, D.C.

Gerbert, B., C. Love, N. Caspers, K. Linkins, J.H. Burack. 1999. Making All the Difference in the World: How Physicians Can Help HIV-Seropositive Patients Become More Involved in their Healthcare. AIDS Patient Care and STDS 13: 29–39.

Gilliland, M.G., P.R. Spence, R.L. Spence. 2000. Lethal Domestic Violence in Eastern North Carolina. North Carolina Medical Journal 61:287–290.

Glickman, D. January 5, 1999. Remarks of Secretary of Agriculture Dan Glickman: Black Farmers Class Action Settlement Announcement. Washington, D.C.

Godin, G., P. Valois, J. Jobin, A. Ross. 1991. Prediction of Intention to Exercise in Individuals Who Have Suffered from Coronary Heart Disease. Journal of Clinical Psychology 47:762–772.

Godin, G., P. Valois, L. Lepage, R. Desharnais. 1992. Predictors of Smoking Behaviour—An Application of Ajzen Theory of Planned Behaviour. British Journal of Addiction 87:1335–1343.

Godin, G., L. Vezina, O. LeCerc. 1989. Factors Influencing the Intention of Pregnant Women to Exercise after Giving Birth. Public Health Reports 104:188–195.

Goicoechea-Balbona, A.M. 1997. Culturally Specific Health Care Model for Ensuring Health Care Use by Rural, Ethnically Diverse Families Affected by HIV/AIDS. Health and Social Work 22:172–180.

Golding, J.M. 1994. Sexual Assault History and Physical Health in Randomly Selected Los Angeles Women. Health Psychology 13:130–138.

Goodman, L.A., R.D. Fallot. 1998. HIV Risk-Behavior in Poor Urban Women with Serious Mental Disorders: Association with Childhood Physical and Sexual Abuse. American Journal of Orthopsychiatry 68:73–83.

Goodman, L.A., S.D. Rosenberg, K.T. Mueser, R.E. Drake. 1997. Physical and Sexual Assault History in Women with Serious Mental Illness: Prevalence, Correlates, Treatment, and Future Research Directions. Schizophrenia Bulletin 23:685–696.

Gordillo, V., J. Del Amo, V. Soriano, J. Gonzalez-Lahoz. 1999. Sociodemographic and Psychological Variables Influencing Adherence to Antiretroviral Therapy. AIDS 13:1763–1769.

Gornick, M., P. Eggers, T. Reilley, R. Mentnech, L. Fitterman, L. Kucken, B. Vladeck. 1996. Effects of Race and Income on Mortality and Use of Services Among Medicare Beneficiaries. New England Journal of Medicine 335:791–798.

Graduate Medical Education National Advisory Committee. 1980. Geographic Distribution Report, Vol. III. DHHS Publication No. (HRA) 81–653. Washington, D.C.: U.S. Government Printing Office.

Graham, R.P., M.L. Forrester, J.A. Wysong, T.C. Rosenthal, P.A. James. 1995. HIV/AIDS in the Rural United States: Epidemiology and Health Services Delivery. Medical Care Research and Review 52:435–452.

Guendelman, S., R. Wyn, Y.W. Tsai. 2000. Children of Working Low-Income Families in California: Does Parental Work Benefit Children's Insurance Status, Access, and Utilization of Primary Health Care? Health Services Research 35:417–441.

Guinan, M.E. 1993. Black Communities' Belief in AIDS as Genocide: A Barrier to Overcome for HIV Prevention. Annals of Epidemiology 3:193–195.

Gutman, L.M., J.S. Eccles. 1999. Financial Strain, Parenting Behaviors, and Adolescents' Achievement: Testing Model Equivalence Between African American and European American Single- and Two-Parent Families. Child Development 70:1464–1476.

Guttmacher, S., L. Lieberman, D. Ward, N. Freudenberg, A. Radosh, D. Des Jarlais. 1997. Condom Availability in New York City Public High Schools: Relationships to Condom Use and Sexual Behavior. American Journal of Public Health 87: 1427–1433.

Hackl, K.L., A.M. Somlai, J.A. Kelly, S.C. Kalichman. 1997. Women Living with HIV/AIDS: The Dual Challenge of Being a Patient and Caregiver. *Health and Social Work* 22:53–62.

Hampson, J.P., R.I. Roberts, D.A. Morgan. 1996. Shared Care: A Review of the Literature. *Family Practice* 13:264–279.

Hardy, R.E., N.U. Ahmed, M.K. Hargreaves, K.A. Semenya, L. Wu, Y. Belay, A.J. Cebrun. 2000. Difficulty in Reaching Low-Income Women for Screening Mammography. *Journal of Health Care for the Poor and Underserved* 11:45–57.

Harlow, L.L., J.S. Rose, P.J. Morokoff, K. Quina, K. Mayer, K. Mitchell, R. Schnoll. 1998. Women HIV Sexual Risk Takers: Related Behaviors, Interpersonal Issues, and Attitudes. *Women's Health* 4:407–439.

Harmer, A.L., J. Sanderson, P. Mertin. 1999. Influence of Negative Childhood Experiences on Psychological Functioning, Social Support, and Parenting for Mothers Recovering from Addiction. *Child Abuse and Neglect* 23:421–433.

Hatch J., S. Derthick. 1992. Empowering Black Churches for Health Promotion. *Health Values* 16:3–9.

Haubrich, R.H., S.J. Little, J.S. Currier, D.N. Forthal, C.A. Kemper, G.N. Beall, D. Johnson, M.P. Dube, J.Y. Hwang, J.A. McCutchan. 1999. The Value of Patient-Reported Adherence to Antiretroviral Therapy in Predicting Virologic and Immunologic Response. California Collaborative Treatment Group. *AIDS* 13:1099–1107.

He, H., H.V. McCoy, S.J. Stevens, M.J. Stark. 1998. Violence and HIV Sexual Risk Behaviors among Female Sex Partners of Male Drug Users. *Women and Health* 27:161–175.

Heckman, T.G., J.A. Kelly, L.M. Bogart, S.C. Kalichman, D.J. Rompa. 1999. HIV Risk Differences between African American and White Men Who Have Sex with Men. *Journal of the National Medical Association* 91:92–100.

Heckman, T.G., A.M. Somlai, S.C. Kalichman, S.L. Franzoi, J.A. Kelly. 1998(a). Psychosocial Differences Between Urban and Rural People Living with HIV/AIDS. *Journal of Rural Health* 14:138–145.

Heckman, T.G., A.M. Somlai, J.A. Kelly, L.Y. Stevenson, K. Galdabini. 1996. Reducing Barriers to Care and Improving Quality of Life for Rural Persons with HIV. *AIDS Patient Care and STDS* 10:37–43.

Heckman, T.G., A.M. Somlai, J. Peters, J. Walker, L. Otto-Salaj, C.A. Galdabini, J.A. Kelly. 1998(b). Barriers to Care Among Persons Living with HIV/AIDS in Urban and Rural Areas. *AIDS Care* 10:365–375.

Heckman, T.G., A.M. Somlai, K.J. Sikkema, J.A. Kelly, S.L. Franzoi. 1997. Psychosocial Predictors of Life Satisfaction Among Persons Living with HIV Infection and AIDS. *Journal of the Association of Nurses in AIDS Care* 8:21–30.

Heim, C., D.J. Newport, S. Heit, Y.P. Graham, M. Wicox, R. Bonsall, A.H. Miller, C.B. Nemeroff. 2000. Pituitary-Adrenal and Autonomic Responses to Stress in Women after Sexual and Physical Abuse in Childhood. *Journal of the American Medical Association* 284:592–597.

Hellinger, F.J. 1996. The Impact of Financial Incentives on Physician Behavior in Managed Care Plans: A Review of the Evidence. *Managed Care Research and Review* 53:294–314.

Herek, G.M., J.P. Capitanio. 1994. Conspiracies, Contagion, and Compassion: Trust and Public Reactions to AIDS. *AIDS Education and Prevention* 6:365–375.

Hidalgo, R.B., J.R. Davidson. 2000. Posttraumatic Stress Disorder: Epidemiology and Health-Related Considerations. *Journal of Clinical Psychiatry* 61 Suppl. 7:5–13.

Himelein, M.J., R.E. Vogel, D.G. Wachowiak. 1994. Nonconsensual Sexual Experiences in Precollege Women: Prevalence and Risk Factors. *Journal of Counseling and Development* 72:411–415.

HIV/AIDS Bureau. 2000(a). Fact Sheet: AIDS Drug Assistance Programs (ADAPs) Funding Overview. Health Resources and Services Administration. Rockville, Md.

————. 2000(b). Fact Sheet: AIDS Drug Assistance Programs (ADAPs) Eligibility Criteria. Health Resources and Services Administration. Rockville, Md.

————. 2000(c). CARE Act Programs and Funding. Health Resources and Services Administration. Rockville, Md.

————. 2000(d). Delivering HIV Services to Vulnerable Populations: What Have We Learned? HIV/AIDS Evaluation Monograph Series. #6. Health Resources and Services Administration. Rockville, Md.

HIV/STD Prevention and Care Branch, Epidemiology, and Special Studies Unit. 1999a. 1999 HIV/AIDS Surveillance Report. North Carolina Department of Health and Human Services, Department of Public Health. Raleigh, N.C.

————. 1999b. 1999 STD Surveillance Report. North Carolina Department of Health and Human Services, Department of Public Health. Raleigh, N.C.

Hochman, J.S., J.E. Tamis, T.D. Thompson, W.D. Weaver, H.D. White, F. Van de Werf, P. Aylward, E.J. Topol, R.M. Califf. 1999. Sex, Clinical Presentation, and Outcome in Patients with Acute Coronary Syndromes. *New England Journal of Medicine* 341:226–232.

Hoffman, E.D. Jr., B.S. Klees, C.A. Curtis. 2000. Brief Summaries of Medicare and Medicaid Title XVIII and Title XIX of The Social Security Act. Office of the Actuary, Health Care Financing Administration, Department of Health and Human Services. Washington, D.C.: GPO.

Hoffman, M.A. 1991. Counseling the HIV-Infected Client: A Psycho-Social Model for Assessment and Intervention. *Counseling Psychology* 19:467–542.

Holtgrave, D.R., S.D. Pinkerton. 1997. Updates of Cost of Illness and Quality of Life Estimates for Use in Economic Evaluations of HIV Prevention Programs. *Journal of Acquired Immune Deficiency Syndromes* 16:54–62.

Holzemer, W.L., I.B. Corless, K.M. Nokes, J.G. Turner, M.A. Brown, G.M. Powell-Cope, J. Inouye, S.B. Henry, P.K. Nicholas, C.J. Portillo. 1999. Predictors of Self-Reported Adherence in Persons Living with HIV Disease. *AIDS Patient Care and STD* 13:185–197.

Hooper, E. 1999. *The River: A Journey to the Source of HIV and AIDS.* New York: Little, Brown and Company.

Horberg, M., B. Schatz. 1998. Battling HIV on Many Fronts [letter]. *New England Journal of Medicine* 338:98.

Horne, R. 1997. Representations of Medication and Treatment: Advances in Theory and Measurement. In *Perceptions of Health and Illness: Current Research and Applications*, eds. K.J. Petrie, J. Weinman. London: Harwood Academic Publishers.

Horne, R., J. Weinman. 1998. Predicting Treatment Adherence: An Overview of Theoretical Models. In *Adherence to Treatment in Medical Conditions*, eds. L.B. Myers, K. Midence. Amsterdam: Harwood Academic Publishers.

Howard G., R.T. Anderson, G. Russell, V.J. Howard, G.L. Burke. 2000. Race, Socioeconomic Status, and Cause-Specific Mortality. *Annals of Epidemiology* 10:214–223.

Hughes, S.L., A. Ulasevich, F.M. Weaver, W. Henderson, L. Manheim, J.D. Kubal, F. Bonarigo. 1997. Impact of Home Care on Hospital Days: A Meta Analysis. *Health Services Research* 32:415–429.

Hurst, D.F., D.L. Boswell, S.E. Boogaard, M.W. Watson. 1997. The Relationship of Self-Esteem to the Health-Related Behaviors of the Patients of a Primary Care Clinic. *Archives of Family Medicine* 6:67–70.

Ingram, K.M., D.A. Jones, R.J. Fass, J.L. Neidig, Y.S. Song. 1999. Social Support and

Unsupportive Social Interactions: Their Association with Depression Among People Living with HIV. *AIDS Care* 11:313–329.

Ironson, G., A. Friedman, N. Klimas, 1994. Distress, Denial, and Low Adherence to Behavioral Interventions Predict Faster Disease Progression in Gay Men Infected with Human Immunodeficiency Virus. *International Journal of Behavioral Medicine* 1:90–105.

Ito, Y., M.H. Teicher, C.A. Glod, and E. Ackerman. 1998. Preliminary Evidence for Aberrant Cortical Development in Abused Children: A Quantitative EEG Study. *Journal of Neuropsychiatry and Clinical Neurosciences* 10:298–307.

Jellinek, P.S. 1988. Case-Managing AIDS. *Issues in Science and Technology* 4:59–63.

Johnsen, M.C., J.P. Morrissey, M.O. Calloway, B.J. Fried, M.B. Blank, B.E. Starrett. 1997. Rural Mental Health Leaders' Perceptions of Stigma and Community Issues. *Journal of Rural Health* 13:59–70.

Johnson, J.G., P. Chohen, J. Brown, E.M. Samiles, D.P. Bernstein. 1999. Childhood Maltreatment Increases Risk for Personality Disorders during Early Adulthood. *Archives of General Psychiatry* 56:607–608.

Jones, J. 1993. *Bad Blood: The Tuskegee Syphilis Experiment: Tragedy of Race and Medicine.* New York: Free Press.

Joslin, D., R. Harrison. 1998. The "Hidden Patient." Older Relatives Raising Children Orphaned by AIDS. *Journal of the American Medical Association* 53:65–76.

Kaldjian, L.C., J.F. Jekel, G. Friedland. 1998. End-of-Life Decisions in HIV-Positive Patients: The Role of Spiritual Beliefs. *AIDS* 12:103–107.

Kalichman, S.C., B. Ramachandran, S. Catz. 1999. Adherence to Combination Antiretroviral Therapies in HIV Patients of Low Health Literacy. *Journal of General Internal Medicine* 14:267–273.

Kaplan, J.E., D.L. Parham, L. Soto-Torres, K. Van Dyck, J.A. Greaves, K. Rauch, B. Ellis, H.E. Amandus. 1999. Adherence to Guidelines for Antiretroviral Therapy and for Preventing Opportunistic Infections in HIV-Infected Adults and Adolescents in Ryan White-Funded Facilities in the United States. *Journal of Acquired Immune Deficiency Syndromes* 21:228–235.

Kass, N., C. Flynn, L. Jacobson, J.S. Chmiel, E.G. Bing. 1999. Effect of Race on Insurance Coverage and Health Service Use for HIV-Infected Gay Men. *Journal of Acquired Immune Deficiency Syndrome* 20:85–92.

Katz, M.H., W.E. Cunningham, V. Mor, R.M. Andersen, T. Kellogg, S. Zierler, S.C. Crystal, M.D. Stein, K. Cylar, S.A. Bozzette, M.F. Shapiro. 2000. Prevalence and Predictors of Unmet Need for Supportive Services among HIV-Infected Persons: Impact of Case Management. *Medical Care* 38:58–69.

Katz M.H., W.E. Cunningham, J.A. Fleishman, K.M. Andersen, T. Kellogg, S.A. Bozzette, M.F. Shapiro. 2001. Effect of Case Management on Unmet Needs and Utilization of Medical Care and Medications among HIV-Infected Persons. *Annals of Internal Medicine* 135:557–565.

Kawachi, I. 1999. Social Capital and Community Effects on Population and Individual Health. *Annals of the New York Academy of Science* 896:120–130.

Kawachi, I., B.P. Kennedy. 1999. Income Inequality and Health: Pathways and Mechanisms. *Health Services Research* 34:215–227.

Kawachi, I., B.P. Kennedy, R. Glass. 1999. Social Capital and Self-Rated Health: A Contextual Analysis. *American Journal of Public Health* 89:1187–1193.

Keenan, T. 1998. The Impact of HIV/AIDS Treatment Advance on Community Based AIDS Service Organisations. *International Conference on AIDS* 12:745 (Astract No. 34310).

Kelley, G.R., J.A. Mannon, J.E. Scott. 1987. Utility of the Health Belief Model and

Examining Medication Compliance among Psychiatric Outpatients. *Social Science and Medicine* 25:1205–1211.

Kelley, G.R., J.E. Scott. 1990. Medication Compliance and Health Education among Outpatients with Chronic Mental Disabilities. *Medical Care* 28:1181–1187.

Kelly, B., B. Raphael, D. Statham, M. Ross, H. Eastwood, S. McLean, B. O'Loughlin, K. Brittain. 1996. A Comparison of the Psychosocial Aspects of AIDS and Cancer-Related Bereavement. *International Journal of Psychiatry in Medicine* 26(1): 35–49.

Kelly, J.A., D.A. Murphy, R. Bahr, S.C. Kalichman, M.G. Morgan, L.Y. Stevenson, J.J. Koob, T.L. Brasfield, B.M. Bernstein. 1993. Outcome of Cognitive-Behavioral and Support Group Brief Therapies for Depressed, HIV-Infected Persons. *American Journal of Psychiatry* 150:1679–1686.

Kessler, R.C., A. Sonnega, E. Bromet, M. Hughes, C.B. Nelson. 1995. Posttraumatic Stress Disorder in the National Comorbidity Survey. *Archives of General Psychiatry* 52:1048–1060.

Kilpatrick, K.L., M. Litt, L.M. Williams. 1997. Post-Traumatic Stress Disorder in Child Witnesses to Domestic Violence. *American Journal of Orthopsychiatry* 67(4): 639–644.

Kimerling, R., L. Armistead, R. Forehand. 1999. Victimization Experiences and HIV Infection in Women: Associations with Serostatus, Psychological Symptoms, and Health Status. *Journal of Traumatic Stress* 12:41–58.

Kindig, D.A. 1997. *Purchasing Population Health: Paying for Results*. Ann Arbor: University of Michigan Press.

Kirby, D., N.D. Brener, N.L. Brown, N. Peterfreund, P. Hillard, R. Harrist. 1999. The Impact of Condom Availability in Seattle Schools on Sexual Behavior and Condom Use. *American Journal of Public Health* 89:182–187.

Kissinger, P., D. Cohen, W. Brandon, J. Rice, A. Morse, R. Clark. 1995. Compliance with Public Sector HIV Medical Care. *Journal of the National Medical Association* 87:19–24.

Klonoff, E.A., H. Landrine. 1999. Do Blacks Believe That HIV/AIDS Is a Government Conspiracy against Them? *Preventive Medicine* 28:451–457.

Koblin, B.A., J. McCusker, B.F. Lewis, J.L. Sullivan. 1990. Racial/Ethnic Differences in HIV-1 Seroprevalence and Risky Behaviors Among Intravenous Drug Users in a Multisite Study. *American Journal of Epidemiology* 132:837–846.

Krieger, N. 1990. Racial and Gender Discrimination: Risk Factors for High Blood Pressure? *Social Science and Medicine* 30:1273–1281.

———. 1999. Embodying Inequality: A Review of Concepts, Measures, and Methods for Studying Health Consequences of Discrimination. *International Journal of Health Services* 29:295–352.

———. 2000. Refiguring "Race": Epidemiology, Racialized Biology, and Biological Expressions of Race Relations. *International Journal of Health Services* 30:211–216.

Krieger, N., S. Sidney. 1996. Racial Discrimination and Blood Pressures: The CARDIA Study of Young Black and White Adults. *American Journal of Public Health* 86:1370–1378.

Krieger, N., D.R. Williams, N.E. Moss. 1997. Measuring Social Class in U.S. Public Health Research: Concepts, Methodologies, and Guidelines. *Annual Review of Public Health* 18:341–378.

Krueger, R. A. 1994. *Focus Groups: A Practical Guide for Applied Research*. Thousand Oaks, Calif.: Sage Publications.

Lam, N.S., and K. Liu. 1994. Spread of AIDS in Rural America, 1982–1990. *Journal of Acquired Immune Deficiency Syndrome* 7:485–490.

Lansky A., A.K. Nakahima, T., Diaz, et al. 2000. Human Immunodeficiency Virus

Infection in Rural Areas and Small Cities in the Southeast: Contributions of Migration and Behavior. *Journal of Rural Health* 16:20–30.

LaVeist, T.A. 1994. Beyond Dummy Variables and Sample Selection: What Health Services Researchers Ought to Know About Race as a Variable. *Health Services Research* 29:1–16.

———. 1996. Why We Should Continue To Study Race…But Do a Better Job: An Essay on Race, Racism, and Health. *Ethnicity and Disease* 6:21–29.

———. 2000. On the Study of Race, Racism, and Health: A Shift From Description to Explanation. *International Journal of Health Services* 30:217–219.

Lawrence, D.A., D. Kim. 2000. Central/Peripheral Nervous System and Immune Responses. *Toxicology* 142:189–201.

Lechner, M.E., M.E. Vogel, L.M. Garcia-Shelton, J.L. Leichter, K.R. Steibel. 1993. Self-Reported Medical Problems of Adult Female Survivors of Childhood Sexual Abuse. *Journal of Family Practice* 36:633–638.

LeDoux, J.L. 1993. Emotional Memory: In Search of Systems and Synapses. *Annals of the New York Academy of Science* 702:149–157.

Lee, M., J.A. Kemp, A. Canning, C. Egan, G. Tataronis, F. Farraye. 1999. A Randomized Controlled Trial of an Enhanced Patient Compliance Program for Helicobacter Pylori Therapy. *Archives of Internal Medicine* 159:2312–2316.

Lee, P.R. 1999. Socioeconomic Status and Health. Policy Implications in Research, Public Health, and Medical Care. *Annals of the New York Academy of Science* 896:294–301.

Lenderking, W.R., C. Wold, K.H. Mayer, R. Goldstein, E. Losina, G.R. Seage. 1997. Childhood Sexual Abuse among Homosexual Men: Prevalence and Association with Unsafe Sex. *Journal of General Internal Medicine* 12:250–253.

Leserman, J., D.A. Drossman, Z. Li, T.C. Toomey, G. Nachman, L. Glogau. 1996. Sexual and Physical Abuse History in Gastroenterology Practice: How Types of Abuse Impact Health Status. *Psychosomatic Medicine* 58:4–15.

Leserman, J., E.D. Jackson, J.M. Petitto, R.N. Golden, S.G. Silva, D.O. Perkins, J. Cai, J.D. Folds, D.L. Evans. 1999. Progression to AIDS: The Effects of Stress, Depressive Symptoms, and Social Support. *Psychosomatic Medicine* 61:397–406.

Leserman, J., Z. Li, D.A. Drossman, Y.J.B. Hu. 1998. Selected Symptoms Associated with Sexual and Physical Abuse History among Female Patients with Gastrointestinal Disorders: The Impact on Subsequent Health Care Visits. *Psychological Medicine* 28:417–425.

Leserman, J., D.O. Perkins, D.L. Evans. 1992. Coping with the Threat of AIDS: The Role of Social Support. *American Journal of Psychiatry* 149:1514–1520.

Leserman, J., J.M. Petitto, R.N. Golden, H. Gu, D.O. Perkins, S.G. Silva, J.D. Folds, D.L. Evans. 2000. The Impact of Stress, Depression, Social Support, Coping, and Cortisol on Progression to AIDS. *American Journal of Psychiatry* 157:1221–1228.

Levi, J., J. Hidalgo, S. Wyatt. 2000. The Impact of State Variation in Entitlement Programs on the Ryan White CARE Act and Access to Services for Underserved Populations. *Directions in HIV Service Delivery and Care: A Policy Brief.* Health Resources and Services Administration. Number 2.

Levi, J., J. Kates. 2000. HIV: Challenging the Health Care Delivery System. *American Journal of Public Health* 90:1033–1036.

Lillie-Blanton, M., T. LaVeist. 1996. Race/Ethnicity, the Social Environment, and Health. *Social Science and Medicine* 43:83–91.

Lima, R.M., L.G. Tunala, B. Leme, V. Paiva, N.J. Santos, N. Hearst, C.M. Buchalla. 1998. Motivations to Continue Fighting and Plans for Children After Death Among HIV Positive Women in Sao Paulo, Brazil. *International Conference on AIDS* 12:483 (Abstract No. 24217).

Lin, Y.G., M.W. Melchiono, G.J. Huba, E.R. Woods. 1998. Evaluation of a Linked Service Model of Care for HIV-Positive, Homeless, and At-Risk Youths. *AIDS Patient Care and STDS* 12:787–796.

Lishner, D.M., M. Richardson, P. Levine, D. Patrick. 1996. Access to Primary Health Care among Persons with Disabilities in Rural Areas: A Summary of the Literature. *Journal of Rural Health* 12:45–53.

Lochner, K., E. Pamuk, D. Makuc, B.P. Kennedy, I. Kawachi. 2001. State-Level Income Inequality and Individual Mortality Risk: A Prospective, Multilevel Study. *American Journal of Public Health* 91:351–353.

London, A.S., A.J. LeBlanc, C.S. Aneshensel. 1998. The Integration of Informal Care, Case Management, and Community-Based Seryices for Persons with HIV/AIDS. *AIDS Care* 10:481–503.

Lucas, G.M., R.E. Chaisson, R.D. Moore. 1999. Highly Active Antiretroviral Therapy in a Large Urban Clinic's Risk Factors for Virologic Failure and Adverse Drug Reactions. *Annals of Internal Medicine* 131(2):81–82.

Luginaah, I.N., K.S. Lee, T.J. Abernathy, D. Sheehan, G. Webster. 1999. Trends and Variations in Perinatal Mortality and Low Birthweight: The Contribution of Socio-Economic Factors. *Canadian Journal of Public Health* 90:377–381.

Lundberg, George D. 1998. Rural Communities Struggle with AIDS. *Journal of the American Medical Association* 279:5–6.

Lurie, P., E. Drucker. 1997. An Opportunity Lost: HIV Infections Associated with Lack of a National Needle-Exchange Programme in the USA. *Lancet* 349: 604–608.

Lurie, P., R. Gorsky, T.S. Jones, L. Shomphe. 1998. An Economic Analysis of Needle Exchange and Pharmacy-Based Programs to Increase Sterile Syringe Availability for Injection Drug Users. *Journal of Acquired Immune Deficiency Syndromes* 18 Suppl 1:S126–132.

Lutgendorf, S.K., M.H. Antoni, G. Ironson, N. Klimas, M. Kumar, K. Starr, P. McCabe, K. Cleven, M.A. Fletcher, N. Schneiderman. 1997. Cognitive Behavioral Stress Management Decreases Dysphoric Mood and Herpes Simplex Virus-Type 2 Antibody Titers in Symptomatic HIV Seropositive Gay Men. *Journal of Consulting and Clinical Psychology* 65:31–43.

Lutgendorf, S.K., M.H. Antoni, G. Ironson, K. Starr, N. Costello, M. Zuckerman, N. Klimas, M.A. Fletcher, N. Schneiderman. 1998. Changes in Cognitive Coping Skills and Social Support during Cognitive Behavioral Stress Management Intervention and Distress Outcomes in Symptomatic Human Immunodeficiency Virus (HIV)-Seropositive Gay Men. *Psychosomatic Medicine* 60:204–214.

Lyketsos, C.G., M. Fishman, H. Hutton, T. Cox, S. Hobbs, C. Spoler, W. Hunt, J. Driscoll, G. Treisman. 1997. The Effectiveness of Psychiatric Treatment for HIV-Infected Patients. *Psychosomatics* 38:423–432.

Magnus, S.A., S.S. Mick. 2000. Medical Schools, Affirmative Action, and the Neglected Role of Social Class. *American Journal of Public Health* 90:1197–1201.

Mainous, A.G., S.C. Matheny. 1996. Rural Human Immunodeficiency Virus Health Service Provision. *Archives of Family Medicine* 5:469–473.

Mandelblatt, J.S., K.R. Yabroff, J.F. Kerner. 1999. Equitable Access to Cancer Services: A Review of Barriers to Quality Care. *Cancer* 86:2378–2390.

Marcus, B.H., V.C. Selby, R.S. Niaura, J.S. Rossi. 1992. Self-Efficacy and the Stages of Exercise Behavior Change. *Research Quarterly for Exercise and Sports* 63:60–66.

Marwick, C. 1998. HIV/AIDS Care Calls for Reallocation of Resources. *Journal of the American Medical Association* 279:491–493.

Marx, R., M.H. Katz, M.S. Park, and R.J. Gurley. 1997. Meeting the Service Needs of

HIV-Infected Persons: Is the Ryan White Act Succeeding? *Journal of Acquired Immune Deficiency Syndromes* 14:44–55.

Master, R., T. Dreyfus, S. Connors, C. Tobias, Z. Zhou, R. Kronick. 1996. The Community Medical Alliance: An Integrated System of Care in Greater Boston for People with Severe Disability and AIDS. *Managed Care Quarterly* 4:26–37.

Maslow, A.H. 1987. *Motivation and Personality.* 3d ed. New York: Harper & Row Publishers.

Matsushita, S. 2000. Current Status and Future Issues in the Treatment of HIV-1 Infection. *International Journal of Hematology* 72:20–27.

Mays, V.M., S.D. Cochran. 1996. Is There a Legacy of Tuskegee?: AIDS Misbeliefs among Inner-City African Americans and Hispanics. *International Conference on AIDS* 11:190 (Abstract No.We.D.3789).

McCann, B.S., V.E. Bovjberg, S.J. Curry, B.M. Retzlaff, C.E. Walden, R.H. Knopp. 1996. Predicting Participation in a Dietary Intervention to Lower Cholesterol among Individuals with Hyperlipidemia. *Health Psychology* 15:61–64.

McCoy, C.B., L.R. Metsch, H.V. McCoy, N.L. Weatherby. 1999. HIV Seroprevalence across the Rural/Urban Continuum. *Substance Use and Misuse* 34:595–615.

McCoy, H.V., C.B. McCoy, S. Lai, N.L. Weatherby, S. Messiah. 1999. Behavior Changes among Crack-Using Rural and Urban Women. *Substance Use and Misuse* 34:667–684.

McCracken, L.M., P.A. Klock, D.J. Mingay, J.K. Asbury, D.M. Sinclair. 1997. Assessment of Satisfaction with Treatment for Chronic Pain. *Journal of Pain and Symptom Management* 14:292–299.

McElnay, J.C., C.R. McCallion. 1998. Adherence and the Elderly. In *Adherence to Treatment in Medical Conditions,* eds. L.B. Myers, K. Midence. Amsterdam: Harwood Academic Publishers.

McEwen, B.S., E.A. Gould, R.R. Sakai. 1992. The Vulnerability of the Hippocampus to Protective and Destructive Effects of Glucocorticoids in Relation to Stress. *British Journal of Psychiatry* 160:18–24.

McGinnis, J.M., W.H. Foege. 1993. Actual Causes of Death in the United States. *Journal of the American Medical Association* 270:2207–2212.

McKinney, M.M. 1998. Service Needs and Networks of Rural Women with HIV/AIDS. *AIDS Patient Care and STDS* 12:471–480.

McLeroy, K.R., D. Bibeau, A. Steckler, K. Glanz. 1998. An Ecological Perspective on Health Promotion Programs. *Health Education Quarterly* 15:351–377.

McLoyd, V.C. 1990. The Impact of Economic Hardship on Black Families and Children: Psychological Distress, Parenting, and Socioemotional Development. *Child Development* 61:311–346.

McManus, M.A., P.W. Newacheck, A.M. Greaney. 1990. Young Adults with Special Health Care Needs: Prevalence, Severity, and Access to Health Services. *Pediatrics* 86:674–682.

McVea, K.L. 1997. Lay Injection Practices among Migrant Farmworkers in the Age of AIDS: Evolution of a Biomedical Folk Practice. *Social Science and Medicine* 45:91–98.

Measurement Group, The and HRSA/HAB's SPNS Cooperative Steering Committee. Module 9: Agency Cohesiveness Rating Form, 1997. Available at *http://www. TheMeasurementGroup.com.* Last viewed: October 23, 2001.

Mellins, C.A., E. McCaskill, J. Havens, N. Braine, M. Chesney. 1999. Factors Mediating Medical Adherence in HIV-Infected Mothers. Paper presented at the Annual Conference of the NIMH on "The Role of Families in Preventing and Adapting to HIV-Infection and AIDS." Philadelphia, Pa.

Merwin E.I., H.F. Goldsmith, R.W. Manderscheid. 1995. Human Resource Issue in Rural Mental Health. *Community Mental Health Journal* 31:525–537.

Midgette T., S.S. Meggert. 1991. Multicultural Counseling Instruction: A Challenge for Faculties in the 21st Century. *Journal of Counseling and Development* 70: 136–141.

Miller, P., R. Wikoff, A. Hiatt. 1992. Fishbein's Model of Reasoned Action and Compliance Behaviour of Hypertensive Patients. *Nursing Research* 41:104–109.

Moeller, T.P., G.A. Bachmann, J.R. Moeller. 1993. The Combined Effects of Physical, Sexual, and Emotional Abuse During Childhood: Long-Term Health Consequences for Women. *Child Abuse and Neglect* 17:623–640.

Moneyham, L., B. Seals, A. Demi, R. Sowell, L. Cohen, J. Guillory. 1996. Experiences of Disclosure in Women Infected with HIV. *Health Care for Women International* 17:209–221.

Montoya, I.D. 1998. Social Network Ties, Self-Efficacy, and Condom Use Among Women Who Use Crack Cocaine: A Pilot Study. *Substance Use and Misuse* 33: 2049-2073.

Moon, D.G., M.L. Hecht, K.M. Jackson, R.E. Spellers. 1999. Ethnic and Gender Differences and Similarities in Adolescent Drug Use and Refusals of Drug Offers. *Substance Use and Misuse* 34:1059–1083.

Moon, R.Y., T.L. Cheng, K.M. Patel, K. Baumhaft, P.C. Scheidt. 1998. Parental Literacy Level and Understanding of Medical Information. *Pediatrics* 102:e25.

Moore, R.D., D. Stanton, R. Gopalan, R.E. Chaisson. 1994. Racial Differences in the Use of Drug Therapy for HIV Disease in an Urban Community. *New England Journal of Medicine* 330:763–768.

Mor, V., J.A. Fleishman, S.M. Allen, J.D. Piette. 1994. *Networking AIDS Services.* Ann Arbor, Mich.: Health Administration Press.

Mor, V., J. Piette, J. Fleishman. 1989. Community-Based Case Management for Persons with AIDS. *Health Affairs* 8:139–153.

Mulder, C.L., M.H. Antoni, H.J. Duivenvoorden, R.H. Kauffmann, K. Goodkin 1995. Active Confrontational Coping Predicts Decreased Clinical Progression over a One-Year Period in HIV-Infected Homosexual Men. *Journal of Psychosomatic Research* 39:957–965.

Mulder, C.L., P.M.G. Emmelkamp, M.H. Antoni, J.W. Mulder, T.G.M. Sandfort, M.J. De Vries. 1994. Cognitive-Behavioral and Experiential Group Psychotherapy for HIV-Infected Homosexual Men: A Comparative Study. *Psychosomatic Medicine* 56:423–431.

Murrain, M. 1996. Differential Survival of Blacks and Hispanics with AIDS. *Ethnicity and Health* 1:373–382.

Myers, L.B., K. Midence, ed. 1998. *Adherence to Treatment in Medical Conditions.* London: Harwood Academic Publishers.

Nansel, T.R., M. Overpeck, R.S. Pilla, W.J. Ruan, B. Simons-Morton, P. Scheidt. 2001. Bullying Behaviors among U.S. Youth: Prevalence and Association with Psychosocial Adjustment. *Journal of the American Medical Association* 285:2094–2100.

National Center for Health Statistics. 1994. Health, United States, 1993. Hyattsville, Md.: U.S. Public Health Service.

Nguyen, T.Q., K. Whetten-Goldstein. 2001. Is Anybody Out There?: Integrating HIV Services in Rural Regions. Under review.

Nickens, H.W. 1995. The Role of Race/Ethnicity and Social Class in Minority Health Status. *Health Services Research* 30:151–162.

Norman, P., L. Smith. 1995. The Theory of Planned Behaviour and Exercise: An Investigation into the Role of Prior Behaviour, Behavioral Intentions, and Attitude Variability. *European Journal of Social Psychology* 25:403–501.

North Carolina Department of Health and Human Services. Division of Public Health. 1999. *North Carolina 1998 HIV/AIDS Surveillance Report.* HIV/STD Prevention and Care Branch, Epidemiology, and Special Studies Program. Raleigh, N.C.

North Carolina Division of Medical Assistance, Recipient Services, and Provider Relations. 2000. North Carolina Medicaid: Information about the Medicaid Deductible. Raleigh, N.C.

North Carolina Division of Medical Assistance. 2001. Medicaid Mental Health Survey. Raleigh, N.C.

O'Brien, K., C.B. Wortman, R.C. Kessler, J.G. Joseph. 1993. Social Relationships of Men at Risk for AIDS. *Social Science Medicine* 36: 1161–1167.

Office of the Chief Actuary. 2000. 2000 SSI Annual Report. Washington, D.C.: Social Security Administration.

Office of Disease Prevention and Health Promotion. 2000. *Healthy People 2010: Second Edition Volume 1 and 2.* (November) Washington, D.C.: U.S. Department of Health and Human Services.

Office of Technology Assessment, U.S. Congress. 1993. *Pharmaceutical R and D: Cost, Risks and Rewards.* OTA-H-552. Washington, D.C.: U.S. Government Printing Office.

O'Malley, A.S., C.B. Forrest, P.G. O'Malley. 2000. Low-Income Women's Priorities for Primary Care: A Qualitative Study. *Journal of Family Practice* 49:141–146.

Optenberg, S.A., I.M. Thompson, P. Friedrichs, B. Wojcik, C.R. Stein, B. Kramer. 1995. Race, Treatment, and Long-Term Survival From Prostate Cancer in an Equal-Access Medical Care Delivery System. *Journal of the American Medical Association* 274:1599–1605.

Osher, F.C. 1996. A Vision for the Future: Toward a Service System Responsive to Those with Co-Occuring Addictive and Mental Disorders. *American Journal of Orthopsychiatry* 66:71–76.

Pakenham, K.I., M.R. Dadds, D.J. Terry. 1994. Relationships Between Adjustment to HIV and Both Social Support and Coping. *Journal of Consulting and Clinical Psychology* 62:1194–1203.

Palella, F.J. Jr., K.M. Delaney, A.C. Moorman, M.O. Loveless, J. Fuhrer, G.A. Satten, D.J. Aschman, S.D. Holmberg. 1998. Declining Morbidity and Mortality among Patients with Advanced Human Immunodeficiency Virus Infection. *New England Journal of Medicine* 338:853–860.

Paringer, L., K. Phillips, T. Hu. 1991. Who Seeks HIV Testing? The Impact of Risk, Knowledge, and State Regulatory Policy on the Testing Decision. *Inquiry* 28:226–235.

Parker, J., S. Asher. 1987. Peer Relations and Later Personal Adjustment: Are Low-Accepted Children at Risk? *Psychological Bulletin* 102:357–389.

Patrick, D., P. Erickson. 1993. *Health Status and Health Policy: Quality of Life in Evaluation and Resource Allocation.* New York: Oxford University Press.

Patrick, D., T.M. Wickizer. 1995. Community and Health. In *Society and Health*, eds. B.C. Amick, S. Levine, A.R. Tarlov, D.C. Walsh. New York: Oxford University Press.

Patterson, G.R., B.D. DeBaryshe, E. Ramsey. 1989. A Developmental Perspective on Antisocial Behavior. *American Psychologist* 44:329–335.

Patterson, R.E., A. Kristal, E. White. 1996. Do Beliefs, Knowledge, and Perceived Norms about Diet and Cancer Predict Dietary Change? *American Journal of Public Health* 86:1394–1400.

Pearlin, L.I., C. Schooler. 1978. The Structure of Coping. *Journal of Health Social Behavior* 19:2–21.

Penning, M.J. 1995. Health, Social Support, and the Utilization of Health Services Among Older Adults. *Journals of Gerontology. Series B, Psychological Sciences and Social Sciences* 50:S330–339.

Pharmaceutical Research and Manufacturers of America (PhRMA). 1999. Directory of Prescription Drug Patient Assistance Programs, 1999–2000.

Phillips, L.G., M.H. Nichols, W.D. King. 1995. Herbs and HIV: The Health Food Industry's Answer. *Southern Medical Journal* 88:911–913.

Piette, J.D., J.A. Fleishman, M.D. Stein, V. Mor, K. Mayer. 1993. Perceived Needs and Unmet Needs for Formal Services Among People with HIV Disease. *Journal of Community Health* 18:11–23.

Pillard, R.C., J.M. Bailey. 1998. Human Sexual Orientation Has a Heritable Component. *Human Biology* 70:347–365.

Pinkerton, S.D., D.R. Holtgrave, R.O. Valdiserri. 1997. Cost-Effectivenss of HIV-Prevention Skills Training for Men Who Have Sex with Men. *AIDS* 11:347–357.

Piro, L., J. Doctor. 1998. Managed Oncology Care: The Disease Management Model. *Cancer* 82 Suppl. 10:2068–2075.

Porter, A.L., B.L. Van Cleave, L.A. Milobowski, P.F. Conlon, R.D. Mambourg.1996. Clinical Integration: An Interdisciplinary Approach to a System Priority. *Nursing Administration Quarterly* 20:65–73.

Potvin, L., L. Richard, A.C. Edwards. 2000. Knowledge of Cardiovascular Disease Risk Factors among the Canadian Population: Relationships with Indicators of Socioeconomic Status. *Canadian Medication Association Journal* 162 Suppl 9:S5–11.

Powell, E.C., R.R. Tanz, A. Uyeda, M.B. Gaffney, K.M. Sheehan. 2000. Injury Prevention Education Using Pictorial Information. *Pediatrics* 105:e16.

Powell-Griner, E., J. Bolen, S. Bland. 1999. Health Care Coverage and Use of Preventive Services among the Near Elderly in the United States. *American Journal of Public Health* 89:882–886.

Priest, R. 1991. Racism and Prejudice as Negative Impacts on African American Clients in Therapy. *Journal of Counseling and Development* 70:213–215.

Prochaska, J.O., C.C. DiClemente. 1982. Transtheoretical Therapy: Toward a More Integrative Model of Change. *Psychotherapy: Theory, Research and Practice* 19:276–288.

———. 1983. Stages and Processes of Self-Change of Smoking: Toward an Integrative Model of Change. *Journal of Consulting and Clinical Psychology* 51:390–395.

Public Health Service. 1990. *Healthy People 2000 National Health Promotion and Disease Prevention Objectives* Washington, D.C.: US. Dept. of Health and Human Services, Public Health Service. Government Printing Office.

Qualitative Solutions and Research Pty Ltd. 1997. QSR NUD*IST. Scolari, Sage Publications Software.

Racine, A.D., R.E. Stein, P.F. Belamarich, E. Levine, A. Okun, K. Porder, J.L. Rosenfeld, M. Schechter. 1998. Upstairs Downstairs: Vertical Integration of a Pediatric Service. *Pediatrics.* 102:91–97.

Rask, K.J., M.V. Williams, R.M. Parker, S.E. McNagny. 1994. Predicting Lack of a Regular Provider and Delays in Seeking Care for Patients at an Urban Public Hospital. *Journal of the American Medical Association* 271:1931–1933.

Rathore, S.S., A.K. Berger, K.P. Weinfurt, M. Feinleib, W.J. Oetgen, B.J. Gersh, K.A. Schulman. 2000. Race, Sex, Poverty, and the Medical Treatment of Acute Myocardial Infarction in the Elderly. *Circulation* 102:642–648.

Reif, S., S. Smith, C. Golin. 2001. Adherence Counseling Practices of HIV Case Managers. American Public Health Association Meeting, Atlanta, Ga.

Ren, X.S., B.C. Amick, D.R. Williams. 1999. Racial/Ethnic Disparities in Health: The Interplay between Discrimination and Socioeconomic Sstatus. *Ethnicity and Disease* 9:151–165.

Ricketts, T.C., L.A. Savitz, W.M. Gesler, D.N. Osborne, eds. 1994. *Geographic Methods for Health Services Research: A Focus on the Rural—Urban Continuum*. New York: University Press of America.

Ried, L.D., D.B. Christensen. 1988. A Psychosocial Perspective in the Explanation of Patients' Drug-Taking Behavior. *Social Science and Medicine* 27:277–285.

Ried, L.D., M.A. Oleen, O.B. Martinson, R. Pluhar. 1985. Explaining Intention to Comply with Antihypertensive Regimens: The Utility of Health Beliefs and the Theory of Reasoned Action. *Journal of Social and Administrative Pharmacy* 3:42–52.

Riley, T.A. 1992. HIV-Infected Client Care: Case Management and the HIV Team. *Clinical Nurse Specialist* 6:136–141.

Roberto, K.A., K.R. Allen, R. Blieszner. 1999. Older Women, Their Children, and Grandchildren: A Feminist Perspective on Family Relationships. *Journal of Women and Aging* 11:67–84.

Roberts, K.J., P. Volberding. 1999. Adherence Communication: A Qualitative Analysis of Physician-Patient Dialogue. *AIDS* 13:1771–1778.

Roberts, R.O., T. Rhodes, C.J. Girman, H.A. Guess, J.E. Oesterling, M.M. Lieber, S.J. Jacobsen. 1997. The Decision to Seek Care: Factors Associated with the Propensity to Seek Care in a Community-Based Cohort of Men. *Archives of Family Medicine* 6:218–222.

Rosenberg, M. 1965. *Society and the Adolescent Self-Image*. Princeton, N.J.: Princeton University Press.

Rosenstock, I. 1974. The Health Beliefs Model and Preventative Behavior. *Health Education Monographs* 2:354–386.

Roth, R.H., S.Y. Tam, Y. Ida, J.X. Yang, A.Y. Deutch. 1988. Stress and the Mesocorticolimbic Dopamine Systems. *Annals of the New York Academy of Science* 537: 138–147.

Rothbart, M.K., J.E. Bates. 1997. 5th ed. Temperament. In *Handbook of Child Psychology: Vol 3. Social, Emotional, and Personality Development*, ed. N. Eisenberg. New York: Wiley.

Rotter, J.B. 1966. Generalised Expectancies for Internal Versus External Control of Reinforcement. *Psychological Monographs* 80:1–28.

Rubin, K.H., R.J. Coplan, N.A. Fox, S.D. Calkins. 1995. Emotionality, Emotion Regulation, and Pre-Schoolers' Social Adaptation. *Development and Psychopathology* 7:49–62.

Rumley, R.L., J.D. Esinhart. 1993. AIDS in Rural North Carolina. *North Carolina Journal of Medicine* 54:517–522.

Sallis, J.F., R.M. Grossman, R.B. Pinski, T.L. Patterson, P.R. Nader. 1987. The Development of Scales to Measure Social Support for Diet and Exercise Behaviors. *Preventive Medicine* 16:825–836.

Salmon, P., S. Calderbank. 1996. The Relationship of Childhood Physical and Sexual Abuse to Adult Illness Behavior. *Journal of Psychosomatic Research* 40:329–336.

Samet, J.H., H. Libman, K.A. Steger, R.K. Dhawan, J. Chen, A.H. Shevitz, R. Dewees-Dunk, S. Levenson, D. Kufe, D.E. Craven. 1992. Compliance with Zidovudine Therapy in Patients Infected with Human Immunodeficiency Virus, Type 1: A Cross-Sectional Study in a Municipal Hospital Clinic. *American Journal of Medicine* 92:495–502.

Samuelson, M.C. July 3, 2000. Paying for a Bad Policy: Insurer Settles Charges. *U.S. News and World Report*.

Sansone, R.A., M.W. Wiederman, L.A. Sansone. 1998. Borderline Personality Symptomatology, Experience Multiple Types of Trauma, and Health Care Utilization Among Women in a Primary Care Setting. *Journal of Clinical Psychiatry* 59: 108–111.

Sapolsky, R.M. 1996. Why Stress is Bad for Your Brain. *Science* 273:749–750.

Satcher, D. 1995. Emerging Infections: Getting Ahead of the Curve. *Emerging Infectious Diseases* 1:1–6.

Saunders, E.A., J.A. Edelson. 1999. Attachment Style, Traumatic Bonding, and Developing Relational Capacities in a Long-Term Trauma Group for Women. *International Journal of Group Psychotherapy* 49:465–485.

Saunders, J.M. 1999. Health Problems of Lesbian Women. *Nursing Clinics of North America* 34:381–391.

Scarinci, I.C., J.M. Haile, L.A. Bradley, J.E. Richter. 1994. Altered Pain Perception and Psychosocial Features Among Women with Gastrointestinal Disorders and History of Abuse: A Preliminary Model. *American Journal of Medicine* 97:108–118.

Schiltz, M.A., T.G. Sandfort. 2000. HIV-Positive People, Risk, and Sexual Behaviour. *Social Science and Medicine* 50:1571–1588.

Scholer, S.J., G.B. Hickson, W.A. Ray. 1999. Sociodemographic Factors Identify U.S. Infants at High Risk for Injury Mortality. *Pediatrics* 103:1183–1188.

Schor, E.L., E.G. Menaghan. 1995. Family Pathways to Child Health. In *Society and Health*, eds. B.C. Amick, S. Levine, A.R. Tarlov, D.C. Walsh. New York: Oxford University Press.

Schulman, K.A., E. Rubenstein, F.D. Chesley, J.M. Eisenberg. 1995. The Roles of Race and Socioeconomic Factors in Health Services Research. *Health Services Research* 30:179–195.

Schulz, A., B. Israel, D. Williams, E. Parker, A. Becker, S. James. 2000. Social Inequalities, Stressors, and Self-Reported Health Status among African American and White Women in the Detroit Metropolitan Area. *Social Science and Medicine* 51:1639–1653.

Schur, C.L., S.J. Franco. 1999. Access to Health Care. In *Rural Health in the United States*, ed. T.C. Ricketts, III. New York: Oxford University Press.

Schuster, M.A., R.M. Bell, S.H. Berry, D.E. Kanouse. 1998. Impact of a High School Condom Availability Program on Sexual Attitudes and Behaviors. *Family Planning Perspectives* 30:67–72, 88.

Schuster, M.A., D.E. Kanouse, S.C. Morton, S.A. Bozzette, A. Miu, G.B. Scott, M.F. Shapiro. 2000. HIV-Infected Parents and Their Children in the United States. *American Journal of Public Health* 90:1074–1081.

Schwarzer, R., R. Fuchs. 1996. Self-Efficacy and Health Behaviors. In *Predicting Health Behaviour*, eds. M. Conner, P. Norman. Buckingham, U.K.: Open University Press.

Schwartz, P. 1996. Medical Ethics Under Managed Care. *International Journal of Fertility and Menopausal Studies* 41:124–128.

Shapiro, M.F., S.C. Morton, D.F. McCaffrey, J.W. Senterfitt, J.A. Fleishman, J.F. Perlman, L.A. Athey, J.W. Keesey, D.P. Goldman, S.H. Berry, S.A. Bozzette. 1999. Variations in the Care of HIV-Infected Adults in the United States. *Journal of the American Medical Association* 281:2305–2315.

Shi, L., B. Starfield, B. Kennedy, I. Kawachi. 1999. Income Inequality, Primary Care, and Health Indicators. *Journal of Family Practice* 48:275–284.

Siegel, K., B.J. Krauss. 1991. Living with HIV Infection: Adaptive Tasks of Seropositve Gay Men. *Journal of Health and Social Behavior* 32:17–32.

Siegel, K., I.H. Meyer. 1999. Hope and Resilience in Suicide Ideation and Behavior of Gay and Bisexual Men Following Notification of HIV Infection. *AIDS Education and Prevention* 11:53–64.

Siegel, K., V.H. Raveis, E. Gorey. 1997. Barriers and Motivating Factors Impacting Delaying Seeking Medical Care Among HIV-Infected Women. *National Conference on Women with HIV*, May 4–7 (Abstract No. 108.1).

Siegel, M., L. Biener. 2000. The Impact of an Antismoking Media Campaign on Progression to Established Smoking: Results of a Longitudinal Youth Study. *American Journal of Public Health* 90:380–386.

Siegler, M. 1982. Confidentiality in Medicine—A Decrepit Concept. *New England Journal of Medicine* 307(24):1518–1521.

Singh, N., S.M. Berman, S. Swindells, J.C. Justis, J.A. Mohr, C. Squier, M.M. Wagener. 1999. Adherence of Human Immunodeficiency Virus-Infected Patients to Antiretroviral Therapy. *Clinical Infectious Diseases* 29:824–830.

Sloan, F.A., E. Stout, K. Whetten-Goldstein. 2000. *Drinkers, Drivers, and Bartenders: Balancing Private Choices and Public Accountability*. Chicago: University of Chicago Press.

Smith, C.A., M. Pratt. 1993. Cardiovascular Disease. In *Chronic Disease Epidemiology and Control*, eds. R.C. Brownson, P.I. Remington, J.R. Davis. Washington, D.C.: American Public Health Association.

Smith, V.K., D.H. Taylor, F.A. Sloan. 2001. Longevity Expectations and Death: Can People Predict their Own Demise? *American Economic Review* (29):1–29.

Social Security Administration. 1995. Social Security Benefits For People Living With HIV/AIDS. SSA Publication No. 05-10019. Washington, D.C.

———. 1997(a). Social Security Handbook, 13th ed. SSA Publication No. 65-008. Washington, D.C.

———. 1997(b). Social Security: A Guide to Social Security and SSI Disability Benefits for People with HIV Infection. Publication No. 05-10020. Washington, D.C.

———. 1999. Social Security Disability Benefits. SSA Publication No. 05-10029. Washington, D.C.

Solano, L., M. Costa, S. Salvati, R. Coda, F. Aiuti, I. Mezzaroma, M. Bertini. 1993. Psychological Factors and Clinical Evolution in HIV-1 Infection: A Longitudinal Study. *Journal of Psychosomatic Research* 37:39–51.

Song, J. 1999. HIV/AIDS and Homelessness: Recommendations for Clinical Practice and Public Policy. Washington, D.C.: National Health Care for Homelessness Council.

Sonsel, G.E. 1989. Case Management in a Community-Based AIDS Agency. *Quality Review Bulletin* 15:31–36.

Sorensen, G., A. Stoddard, E. Macario. 1998. Social Support and Readiness to Make Dietary Changes. *Health Education and Behavior* 25:586–598.

Sowell, R.L., P. Christensen. 1996. HIV Infection in Rural Communities. *Nursing Clinics of North America* 31:107–123.

Sowell, R.L., T.R. Misener. 1997. Decisions to Have a Baby by HIV-Infected Women. *Western Journal of Nursing Research* 19:56–70.

Sowell, R.L., K.D. Phillips, J. Grier. 1998. Restructuring Life to Face the Future: The Perspective of Men After a Positive Response to Protease Inhibitor Therapy. *AIDS Patient Care* 12:33–42.

Spasoff, R.A. 1999. *Epidemiologic Methods for Health Policy*. New York: Oxford University Press.

Springs, F.E., W.N. Friedrich. 1992. Health Risk Behaviors and Medical Sequelae of Childhood Sexual Abuse. *Mayo Clinic Proceedings* 67:527–532.

Stansfeld, S.A. 1999. Social Support and Social Cohesion. In *Social Determinants of Health*, eds. M. Marmot, R.G. Wilkinson. Oxford: Oxford University Press.

Stanton, A.L., P.R. Snider. 1993. Coping with Breast Cancer Diagnosis: A Prospective Study. *Health Psychology* 12:16–23.

Stefanski, W., H. Engler. 1998. Effects of Acute and Chronic Social Distress on Blood Cellular Immunity in Rats. *Physiology and Behavior* 64:733–741.

Stein, J.A., M. Riedel, M.J. Rotheram-Borus. 1999. Parentification and Its Impact on Adolescent Children of Parents with AIDS. *Family Process* 38:193–208.

Stein, M.D., S. Crystal, W.E. Cunningham, A. Ananthanarayanan, R.M. Andersen, B.J. Turner, S. Zierler, S. Morton, M.H. Katz, S.A. Bozzette, M.F. Shapiro, M.A. Schuster. 2000. Delays in Seeking HIV Care Due to Competing Caregiver Responsibilities. *American Journal of Public Health* 90:1138–1140.

Stephenson, J. 1998. Studies Reveal Early Impact of HIV Infection, Effects of Treatment. *Journal of the American Medical Association* 279:641–642.

Strathdee, S.A., A. Palepu, P.G.A. Cornelisse, B. Yip, M.V. O'Shaughnessy, J.S.G. Montaner, M.T. Schechter, R.S. Hogg. 1998. Barriers to Use of Free Antiretroviral Therapy in Injection Drug Users. *Journal of the American Medical Association* 280:547–549.

Strathdee, S.A., D.M. Patrick, C.P. Archibald, M. Ofner, P.G. Cornelisse, M. Rekart, M.T. Schechter, M.V. O'Shaughnessy. 1997. Social Determinants Predict Needle-Sharing Behaviour Among Injection Drug Users in Vancouver, Canada. *Addiction* 92:1339–1347.

Strauss, A.L., J.M. Corbin. 1998. *Basics of Qualitative Research: Techniques and Procedures for Developing Grounded Theory*. Thousand Oaks, Calif.: Sage Publications.

Stokols, D. 2000. Social Ecology and Behavioral Medicine: Implications for Training, Practice, and Policy. *Behavioral Medicine* 26:129–138.

Susser, M., E. Susser. 1996. Choosing a Future for Epidemiology: I. Eras and Paradigms. *American Journal of Public Health* 86:668–673.

Swindells, S., J. Mohr, J.C. Justis, S. Berman, C. Squier, M.M. Wagener, N. Singh. 1999. Quality of Life in Patients with Human Immunodeficiency Virus Infection: Impact of Social Support, Coping Style, and Hopelessness. *International Journal of STD and AIDS* 10:383–391.

Switzer, G.E., M.A. Dew, K. Thompson, J.M. Goycoolea, T. Derricott, S.D. Mullins. 1999. Posttraumatic Stress Disorder and Service Utilization among Urban Mental Health Center Clients. *Journal of Traumatic Stress* 12:25–39.

Tardiff, K., P.M. Marzuk, A.C. Leon, C.S. Hirsch, L. Portera, N. Hartwell. 1998. Human Immunodeficiency Virus among Trauma Patients in New York City. *Annals of Emergency Medicine* 32:151–154.

Teicher, M.H., C.A. Glod, J. Surry, C. Swett, Jr. 1993. Early Childhood Abuse and Limbic System Ratings in Adult Psychiatric Outpatients. *Journal of Neuropsychiatry and Clinical Neurosciences* 5:301–306.

Tesh, S. N. 1988. *Hidden Arguments: Political Ideology and Disease Prevention Policy*. New Brunswick, N.J.: Rutgers University Press.

Theorell, T., V. Blomkvist, H. Jonsson, S. Schulman, E. Berntorp, L. Stigendal. 1995. Social Support and the Development of Immune Function in Human Immunodeficiency Virus Infection. *Psychosomatic Medicine* 57:32–35.

Thomas, J.C., M. Clark, J. Robinson, M. Monnett, P.H. Kilmarx, T.A. Peterman. 1999. The Social Ecology of Syphilis. *Social Science and Medicine* 48:1081–1094.

Thomas, P. Associated Press. June 9, 2000. Justice Department: King Assassination Was Not a Conspiracy: Report Follows 18-Month Investigation.

Thomas, S.B., S.C. Quinn. 1991. The Tuskegee Syphilis Study, 1932 to 1972: Implications for HIV Education and AIDS Risk Education Programs in the Black Community. *American Journal of Public Health* 81:1498–1505.

Thomas, S.B., S.C. Quinn, A. Billingsley, C. Caldwell. 1994. The Characteristics of Northern Black Churches with Community Health Outreach Programs. *American Journal of Public Health* 84:575–579.

Thompson, N.J., J.S. Potter, C.A. Sanderson, E.W. Maibach. 1997. The Relationship of Sexual Abuse and HIV Risk Behaviors among Heterosexual Adult Female STD Patients. *Child Abuse and Neglect* 21:149–156.

Tortu, S., M. Goldstein, S. Deren, M. Beardsley, R. Hamid, K. Ziek. 1998. Urban

Crack Users: Gender Differences in Drug Use, HIV Risk, and Health Status. *Women and Health* 27:177–189.

Tramarin, A., S. Campostrini, K. Tolley, F. De Lalla. 1997. The Influence of Socioeconomic Status on Health Service Utilisation by Patients with AIDS in North Italy. The North-East Italian Group for Planning of AIDS Health Care. *Social Science and Medicine* 45:859–866.

Tramarin, A., F. Milocchi, K. Tolley, A. Vaglia, F. Marcolini, V. Manfrin, F. deLalla. 1992. An Economic Evaluation of Home-Care Assistance for AIDS Patients: A Pilot Study in a Town in Northern Italy. *AIDS* 6:1377–1383.

Turner, B.J., L.E. Markson, L.J. McKee. 1994. Health Care Delivery, Zidovudine Use, and Survival of Women and Men with AIDS. *Journal of Acquired Immune Deficiency Syndrome* 7:1250–1262.

Turner, M.A., F. Skidmore. 1999. *Mortgage Lending Discrimination: A Review of Existing Evidence.* Urban Institute.

Turner, P. 1993. *I Heard it Through the Grapevine: Rumor in African American Culture.* Berkeley: University of California Press.

Ubel, P.A., M.M. Zell, D.J. Miller, G.S. Fischer, D. Peters-Stefani, R.M. Arnold. 1995. Elevator Talk: Observational Study of Inappropriate Comments in a Public Space. *American Journal of Medicine* 99:190–194.

Ulmer, C., D. Lewis-Idema, M. Falik, T.P. Raggio, P. Stoessel, T. Coughlin, D. Butterworth, J. Tillman. 1997. Categorical Funding to Seamless Systems of Care: The Challenge of Community-Based Primary Care Providers. *Journal of Case Management* 6:97–103.

Ungvarski, P.J., H. Grossman. 1999. Health Problems of Gay and Bisexual Men. *Nursing Clinics of North America* 34:313–331.

U.S. Census Bureau. 1995 Urban and Rural Population: 1900 to 1990. 1990 Census of Population and Housing, "Population and Housing Unit Counts," CPH-2-1.

———. 1997. 1990 Census of Population and Housing Unit Counts (CPH-2); and ST-97-1 Estimates of the Population of States: Annual Time Series, 1 July 1990 to 1 July 1997. Washington, D.C.

———. 1998. Estimates of the Population of States by Race and Hispanic Origin; 1July 1997; published 4 September. Washington, D.C.

———. March 1999, 1998, and 1997. Current Population Surveys. Washington, D.C.

U.S. Department of Housing and Urban Development. 2000. Housing Opportunities for People with AIDS B HOPWA. Washington, D.C.

U.S. Department of Health and Human Services, Public Health Service. Substance Abuse and Mental Health Services Administration, Center for Substance Abuse Treatment. 1999. *Enhancing Motivation for Change in Substance Abuse Treatment: Treatment Improvement Protocol (TIP) Series 35.* Rockville, Md.: D.H.H.S. Publication No. (SMA) 99-3354.

van Ryn, M., J. Burke. 2000. The Effect of Patient Race and Socio-Economic Status on Physicians' Perceptions of Patients. *Social Science and Medicine* 50:813–828.

van Servellen, G., G. Padilla, M. Brecht, L. Knoll. 1993. The Relationship of Stressful Life Events, Health Status, and Stress-Resistance Resources in Persons with AIDS. *Journal of the Association of Nurses in AIDS Care* 4:11–22.

Veatch, R. M. 1997. Consent, Confidentiality, and Research. *New England Journal of Medicine,* 336: 869–870.

Velicer, W.F., J.O. Prochaska, J.S. Rossi, M.G. Snow. 1992. Assessing Outcome in Smoking Cessation Studies. *Psychological Bulletin* 111:23–41.

Voelker, R. 1998. Rural Communities Struggle with AIDS. *Journal of the American Medical Association* 279:5–6.

Vogt, B.A., D.M. Finch, C.R. Olson. 1992. Functional Heterogeneity in Cingulate

Cortex. The Anterior Executive and Posterior Evaluative Regions. *Cerebral Cortex* 2:435–443.

Von Bargen, J. 1998. How Many Pills Do Patients with HIV Infection Take? *Journal of the American Medical Association* 280:29.

Wainberg, M., G. Friedland. 1998. Public Health Implications of Antiretroviral Therapy and HIV Drug Resistance. *Journal of the American Medical Association* 279:1977–1983.

Walker, E.A., A.N. Gelfand, M.D. Gelfand, M.P. Koss, W.J. Katon. 1995. Medical and Psychiatric Symptoms in Female Gastroenterology Clinic Patients with Histories of Sexual Victimization. *General Hospital Psychiatry* 17:85–92.

Walker, E.A., A.N. Gelfand, W.J. Katon, M.P. Koss, M. Von Korff, D. Berstein, J. Russo. 1999(a). Adult Health Status of Women with Histories of Childhood Abuse and Neglect. *American Journal of Medicine* 107:332–339.

Walker, E.A., J. Unutzer, C. Rutter, A. Gelfand, K. Saunders, M. VonKorff, M.P. Koss, W. Katon. 1999(b). Costs of Health Care Use by Women HMO Members with a History of Childhood Abuse and Neglect. *Archives of General Psychiatry* 56:609–613.

Walling, M.K., M.W. O'hara, R.C. Reiter, A.K. Milburn, G. Lilly, S.D. Vincent. 1994. Abuse History and Chronic Pain in Women: II. A Multivariate Analysis of Abuse and Psychological Morbidity. *Obstetrics and Gynecology* 84:200–206.

Ward, J.W., J.S. Duchin. 1997–1998. The Epidemiology of HIV and AIDS in the United States. *AIDS Clinical Review* 1–45.

Ware, J.E., K.K. Snow, M. Kosinski, B. Gandek. 1993. SF-36 Health Survey: Manual and Interpretation Guide. Boston: Health Institute, New England Medical Center.

Washington Post. 26 February 1999. An Angry Judge. A26.

Wehrwein, T.C., M.E. Eddy. 1993. Breast Health Promotion: Behaviors of Midlife Women. *Journal of Holistic Nursing* 11:223–236.

Weidle, P.J., C.E. Ganera, K.L. Irwin, J.P. McGowan, J.A. Ernst, N. Olivo, S.D. Holmberg. 1999. Adherence to Antiretroviral Medications in an Inner-City Population. *Journal of Acquired Immune Deficiency Syndromes* 22:498–502.

Whetten-Goldstein K., J. Driscoll, K. Scott. 2001(a). Mental Health Integration Project. Report to the Kate B. Reynolds Charitable Trust.

Whetten-Goldstein, K., E. Kulas, F. Sloan, G. Hickson, S. Entman. 1999. Compensation for Birth Related Injury: No-Fault Compared to Tort Systems. *Archives of Pediatric and Adolescent Medicine* 153:41–48.

Whetten-Goldstein, K., T.Q. Nguyen, A.E. Heald. 2001(b). Characteristics of Individuals Infected with the Human Immunodeficiency Virus and Provider Interaction in the Predominantly Rural Southeast. *Southern Medical Journal.* 94: 212–222.

Whetten-Goldstein, K., T. Nguyen, S. Kim. 2000(a). Lessons Learned: Creating an Integrated Service Delivery System for Underserved, Rural-Living Men and Women with HIV/AIDS. In *Lessons Learned.* Washington, D.C.: HRSA HIV/AIDS Bureau, SPNS Program and Department of Housing and Urban Development, HOPWA Program.

Whetten-Goldstein, K., T.Q. Nguyen, J. Sugarman. 2001(c). So Much for Keeping Secrets: Patients' Perspectives on Confidentiality and the Use of Computers in Medicine. *AIDS Care* 13.

Whetten-Goldstein, K., F.A. Sloan, E. Kulas, M. Schenkman, T. Cutson. 1997. The Burden of Parkinson's Disease on Society, Family and Individual. *Journal of the American Geriatrics Society* 45(7):844–847.

Whetten-Goldstein, K., F.A. Sloan, E. Stout, L. Liang. 2000(b). Civil Liability, Criminal Law, and Other Policies and the Reduction of Alcohol-Related Motor Vehicle Fatalities in the United States: 1984–1995. *Accident Analysis and Prevention* 32:723–733.

Whitmire, L.E., L.L. Harlow, K. Quina, P.J. Morokoff. 1999. *Childhood Trauma and HIV: Women at Risk.* Ann Arbor, Mich. Brunner/Mazel Taylor and Francis Group.

Widom, C.S. 1999. Posttraumatic Stress Disorder in Abused and Neglected Children Grown Up. *American Journal of Psychiatry* 156:1223–1229.

Wight, R.G., A.J. LeBlanc, C.S. Aneshensel. 1995. Support Service Use by Persons with AIDS and Their Caregivers. *AIDS Care* 7:509–520.

Wilfert, C., J.E. Aronson, D.T. Beck, A.R. Fleischman, M.W. Kline, L.M. Mofenson, G.B. Scott, D.W. Wara, P.N. Whitley-Williams. 1999. Planning for Children Whose Parents are Dying of HIV/AIDS. American Academy of Pediatrics. Committee on Pediatric AIDS, 1998–1999. *Pediatrics* 103:509–511.

Wilkinson, D.Y., G. King. 1987. Conceptual and Methodological Issues in the Use of Race as a Variable: Policy Implications. *The Milbank Quarterly.* Milbank Memorial Fund. 65 Suppl 1:56–71.

Wilkinson, R.G. 1992. Income Distribution and Life Expectancy. *British Medical Journal* 304:165–168.

Willard, C.L., P. Liljestrand, R.H. Goldschmidt, K. Grumbach. 1999. Is Experience with Human Immunodeficiency Virus Disease Related to Clinical Practice? *Archives of Family Medicine* 8:502–509.

Williams, D.R. 1997. Race and Health: Basic Questions, Emerging Directions. *Annals of Epidemiology* 7:322–333.

———. 1999. Race, Socioeconomic Status, and Health. The Added Effects of Racism and Discrimination. *Annals of the New York Academy of Science* 896:173–188.

Williams, D.R., R. Lavizzo-Mourey, R.C. Warren. 1994. The Concept of Race and Health Status in America. *Public Health Reports* 109:26–41.

Wingood, G.M., R.J. DiClemente. 1997. Child Sexual Abuse, HIV Sexual Risk, and Gender Relations of African-American Women. *American Journal of Preventive Medicine* 13:380–384.

———. 1998. Rape among African American Women: Sexual, Psychological, and Social Correlates Predisposing Survivors to Risk of STD/HIV. *Journal of Women's Health* 7:77–84.

Wolk, L.I., R. Rosenbaum. 1995. The Benefits of School-Based Condom Availability: Cross-Sectional Analysis of a Comprehensive High School-Based Program. *Journal of Adolescent Health* 17:184–188.

Woodward, B. 1995. The Computer-Based Patient Record and Confidentiality. *New England Journal of Medicine* 333:1419–1422.

———. 1997. Medical Record Confidentiality and Data Collection: Current Dilemmas. *Journal of Law, Medicine and Ethics* 25:88–97.

Wu, A.W., H.R. Rubin, W.C. Mathews, J.E. Ware, Jr., L.T. Brysk, W.D. Hardy, S.A. Bozzette, S.A. Spector, D.D. Richman. 1991. A Health Status Questionnaire Using 30 Items From the Medical Outcomes Study: Preliminary Validation in Person with Early HIV Infection. *Medical Care* 29:786–798.

Zheng, D., J.E. Ferguson, C.A. Macera, Y. Boateng, S.P. Temple, F.C. Wheeler. 1997. Self-Reported Prevalence of Diabetes and Preventive Health Care Practices among People with Diabetes in South Carolina. *South Carolina Medical Association* 93:93–98.

Zierler, S., W.E. Cunningham, R. Andersen, M.F. Shapiro, T. Nakazono, S. Morton, S. Crystal, M. Stein, B. Turner, P. St Clair, S.A. Bozzette. 2000. Violence Victimization after HIV Infection in a U.S. Probability Sample of Adult Patients in Primary Care. *American Journal of Public Health* 90(2):208–215.

Zimmerman, R.S., D. Verhberg.1994. Models of Preventive Health Behaviour: Comparison, Critique and Meta-Analysis. *Advances in Medical Sociology* 4:45–67.

Index

abortion, 35–36

abstinence, promotion of, 228

abuse: emotional, 55; stopping cycle of, 146–148, 149; symptoms of, 80. *See also* sexual abuse

acquired immunodeficiency syndrome (AIDS): change in rates of, 15, 17g; early research on, 176. *See also* human immunodeficiency virus (HIV)

action, in health behavior, 205f, 207

activities of living, in SHIPS, 238

activity patterns, mortality associated with, 212

addiction, hospitalizations and, 90

adherence, 7, 9; and barriers to care, 193; and confidentiality policy, 179; counseling for, 9, 190, 197; dangers of non-adherence, 191; determinants of, 203f, 204f, 205f; environmental factors affecting, 217–218; gender differences in, 213; health policy affecting, 219–221; health service utilization and, 202; and health status, 208; and internal decision making, 203–208; and locus of control, 162; and medication regimen, 220; and personal characteristics, 213–214; physician involvement in, 191; SHIPS study of, 192–193, 193t; and young children, 149. *See also* nonadherence

adoption, among study participants, 33

African Americans, 232; AIDS conspiracy theory believed by, 174–175; and discrimination, 75; effective treatment of, 222; health care utilization of, 214; HIV seen as genocide by, 176; and physician communication, 192; prevalence of HIV infection among, 15; survival expectancies of, 213

aggressive behavior, predicting, 72

aggressive therapy, problems associated with, 8–9

Agriculture, U.S. Dept. of: discrimination against black farmers of, 175; Food Stamp Program of, 27

AIDS Drug Assistance Programs (ADAPs), 181; eligibility guidelines for, 25, 26t; funding for, 25; funding of, 219–221

AIDS Education and Training Networks, Health Resources and Services Administration-funded, 225. *See also* education

AIDS service organizations, in NC HIV Provider Survey, 240

Alabama: case managers in, 197, 225; HIV characteristics of, 14–15; mental health services in, 222; poverty in, 19t; SHIPS in, 237; urban vs. rural residents in, 18t

Alabama, University at Birmingham, 237

alcohol consumption, and health policy, 219

Alcoholics Anonymous group, 168

alcoholism, 42–43; and childhood physical abuse, 79; among study participants, 33, 36, 37, 48, 52, 53, 56, 60, 65, 68, 69

American General Life and Accidental Insurance Co., 176

About the Authors

Kathryn Whetten-Goldstein is an assistant professor of public policy and community and family medicine in the Terry Sanford Institute of Public Policy, the Center for Health Policy, Law and Management, and Duke University Medical Center. She is the director of Duke's Health Inequalities Program and a health services researcher focused on the health of poor and disenfranchised individuals.

Trang Quyen Nguyen received a Master of Public Health from the Johns Hopkins University School of Public Health and is currently a doctoral student at the University of North Carolina–Chapel Hill School of Public Health. She plans to continue work identifying personal and structural characteristics and behaviors that determine health care access and utilization, particularly among disenfranchised communities both nationally and internationally.